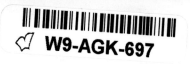

Perinatal Substance Abuse

*The Johns Hopkins Series in
Environmental Toxicology*

Zoltan Annau, Series Editor

Also in This Series:

Neurobehavioral Toxicology, edited by Zoltan Annau

*Monitoring the Worker for Exposure and Disease: Scientific, Legal,
and Ethical Considerations in the Use of Biomarkers*,
Nicholas A. Ashford, Christine J. Spadafor, Dale B. Hattis, and
Charles C. Caldart

*Variations in Susceptibility to Inhaled Pollutants: Identification,
Mechanisms, and Policy Implications*, edited by Joseph D. Brain,
Barbara D. Beck, A. Jane Warren, and Rashid A. Shaikh

*Aging and Environmental Toxicology: Biological and Behavioral
Perspectives*, edited by Ralph L. Cooper, Jerome M. Goldman,
and Thomas J. Harbin

The Toxicity of Methyl Mercury, edited by Christine U. Eccles
and Zoltan Annau

Lead Toxicity: History and Environmental Impact, edited by
Richard Lansdown and William Yule

Toxic Chemicals, Health, and the Environment, edited by
Lester B. Lave and Arthur C. Upton

Indoor Air Pollution: A Health Perspective, edited by
Jonathan M. Samet and John D. Spengler

Perinatal Substance Abuse

Research Findings and Clinical Implications

Edited by

Theo B. Sonderegger

Professor, Department of Psychology

University of Nebraska, Lincoln

The Johns Hopkins University Press

Baltimore and London

The Johns Hopkins University Press
701 West 40th Street
Baltimore, Maryland 21211-2190
The Johns Hopkins Press Ltd., London

The paper used in this book meets the minimum
requirements of American National Standard for
Information Sciences—Permanence of Paper
for Printed Library Materials, ANSI Z39.48-1984.

Library of Congress Cataloging-in-Publication Data

Perinatal substance abuse : research findings and
    clinical implications / edited by Theo B. Sonderegger.
        p.   cm.—(The Johns Hopkins series in
    environmental toxicology)
    Includes index.
    ISBN 0-8018-4275-1 (alk. paper)
    1. Fetus—Effect of drugs on.   I. Sonderegger,
Theo.   II. Series.
    [DNLM: 1. Infant, Newborn, Diseases—
chemically induced.   2. Prenatal Exposure Delayed
Effects.   3. Substance Abuse—complications.
4. Substance Abuse—in pregnancy.   WM 270 P445]
RC627.6.D79P443   1992
618.3′268—dc20
DNLM/DLC
for Library of Congress   91-20861

Contents

Preface   *ix*

Introduction, *Theo B. Sonderegger*   *1*

1. Methodological Issues: Laboratory Animal Studies of   *13*
Perinatal Exposure to Alcohol or Drugs and Human Studies
of Drug Use during Pregnancy, *Joanne Weinberg,*
Theo B. Sonderegger, and Ira J. Chasnoff

2. Gender-specific Effects of Perinatal Exposure to Alcohol   *51*
and Other Drugs, *Joanne Weinberg, Betty Zimmerberg,*
and Theo B. Sonderegger

3. Risk Factors for Alcohol-related Birth Defects: Threshold,   *90*
Susceptibility, and Prevention, *Robert J. Sokol*
and Ernest L. Abel

4. Clinical Considerations Pertaining to Adolescents and   *104*
Adults with Fetal Alcohol Syndrome, *Robin A. LaDue,*
Ann P. Streissguth, and Sandra P. Randels

5. Paternal Exposure to Alcohol, *Ernest L. Abel*   *132*

6. The Effects of Marijuana Use on Offspring,   *161*
Susan L. Dalterio and Peter A. Fried

7. Cocaine Use during Pregnancy: Neurobehavioral Changes in the Offspring, *Diana Dow-Edwards, Ira J. Chasnoff, and Dan R. Griffith*   *184*

8. The Perinatal Opioid Syndrome: Laboratory Findings and Clinical Implications, *Ian S. Zagon and Patricia J. McLaughlin*   *207*

9. Heroin Use during Pregnancy: Clinical Studies of Long-term Effects, *Geraldine S. Wilson*   *224*

10. Methadone Maintenance during Pregnancy: Implications for Perinatal and Developmental Outcome, *Karol Kaltenbach and Loretta P. Finnegan*   *239*

11. Phencyclidine: Experimental Studies in Animals and Long-term Developmental Effects on Humans, *Gaylia Jean Harry and Judy Howard*   *254*

12. The Effects of Maternal Use of Tobacco Products or Amphetamines on Offspring, *Joan C. Martin*   *279*

13. Policy Responses When Women Use Drugs during Pregnancy: Using Child Abuse Laws to Combat Substance Abuse, *Alan J. Tomkins and Sam S. Kepfield*   *306*

Index   *347*

Contributors

Ernest L. Abel, Ph.D., professor, Department of Obstetrics-Gynecology, Wayne State University School of Medicine, and director, C. S. Mott Center for Human Development, Hutzel Hospital, Detroit

Ira J. Chasnoff, M.D., director, National Association for Perinatal Addiction Research and Education, and associate professor, Departments of Pediatrics and of Psychiatry, Northwestern University Medical School, Chicago

Susan L. Dalterio, Ph.D., lecturer and consultant, University of Texas at San Antonio

Diana Dow-Edwards, Ph.D., associate professor, Department of Pharmacology, State University of New York, Brooklyn

Loretta P. Finnegan, M.D., professor, Department of Pediatrics Psychiatry and Human Behavior, Jefferson Medical College, and executive director, Family Center, Thomas Jefferson University, Philadelphia

Peter A. Fried, Ph.D., professor, Department of Psychology, Carleton University, Ottawa

Dan R. Griffith, Ph.D., clinical associate, National Association for Perinatal Addiction Research and Education, Chicago

Gaylia Jean Harry, Ph.D., research associate toxicologist, Biological Sciences Research Center, University of North Carolina, Chapel Hill

Judy Howard, M.D., professor of clinical pediatrics, Intervention Program for Handicapped Children, Division of Child Development, Department of Pediatrics, School of Medicine, University of California, Los Angeles

Karol Kaltenbach, Ph.D., assistant professor, Department of Pediatrics Psychiatry and Human Behavior, Jefferson Medical College, and acting director and research director, Family Center, Thomas Jefferson University, Philadelphia

Sam S. Kepfield, J.D., attorney, private practice, Lincoln, Nebraska

Robin A. LaDue, Ph.D., clinical psychologist, Department of Psychiatry and Behavioral Sciences, Child Development and Mental Retardation Center, Alcoholism and Drug Abuse Institute, University of Washington, Seattle

Patricia J. McLaughlin, D.Ed., senior research associate, Department of Neuroscience and Anatomy, M. S. Hershey Medical Center, Pennsylvania State University, Hershey

Joan C. Martin, Ph.D., professor, Department of Psychiatry and Behavioral Sciences, University of Washington, Seattle

Sandra P. Randels, M.S.N., public health nurse, Department of Psychiatry and Behavioral Sciences, Child Development and Mental Retardation Center, Alcoholism and Drug Abuse Institute, University of Washington, Seattle

Robert J. Sokol, M.D., dean, Wayne State University School of Medicine, Detroit

Ann P. Streissguth, Ph.D., professor of psychology, Department of Psychiatry and Behavioral Sciences, Child Development and Mental Retardation Center, Alcoholism and Drug Abuse Institute, University of Washington, Seattle

Alan J. Tomkins, J.D., Ph.D., assistant professor of psychology and law, Department of Psychology, and associate director for policy studies, Center on Children, Families, and the Law, University of Nebraska, Lincoln

Joanne Weinberg, Ph.D., associate professor, Department of Anatomy, Faculty of Medicine, University of British Columbia, Vancouver

Geraldine S. Wilson, M.D., associate professor, Department of Pediatrics, and associate director, Meyer Center for Developmental Pediatrics, Baylor College of Medicine, Houston

Ian S. Zagon, Ph.D., professor of anatomy, neuroscience, and cell and molecular biology, Department of Neuroscience and Anatomy, M. S. Hershey Medical Center, Pennsylvania State University, Hershey

Betty Zimmerberg, Ph.D., assistant professor, Department of Psychology, Williams College, Williamstown, Massachusetts

Preface

SINCE 1973, when Kenneth Jones and David Smith described the effects that alcohol may produce in the developing organism as the "fetal alcohol syndrome" (*Lancet* 1:1267–71), extensive research with other licit and illicit drugs by both clinicians and laboratory researchers has revealed a multiplicity of problems in infants of drug-using mothers and fathers. Data concerning the effects of perinatal drug exposure appear widely in the journals of many different disciplines and, hence, often go unnoticed by those who could most benefit from the knowledge. The unusual observations made in the laboratory, too few sometimes to reach statistical levels of significance, and the anomalies seen by the clinician are frequently not reported except anecdotally in informal conversations among participants at meetings.

In 1979, Emery Zimmermann, an endocrinologist and psychiatrist at UCLA, and I decided to address the communication problems by organizing a satellite session of the Committee on Problems of Drug Dependence to provide a forum for the presentation of research findings and to facilitate communication between clinicians and animal researchers on perinatal drug research. The success of this meeting led to other satellite sessions in 1982, 1984, 1986, and 1987, the last with Loretta Finnegan as co-organizer. In 1985 I organized a symposium on this topic for the meetings of the American Psychological Association.

The enthusiastic cooperation of and stimulating interchange of information by the participants in these conferences led to the development of this book. Many of the contributors to this volume presented papers at the earlier meetings; all have a commitment to furthering our knowledge in this area. I express my heartfelt thanks to them for cooperating in this endeavor.

Emery Zimmermann introduced me to some of the problems of perinatal drug research when I was on a sabbatical leave at UCLA in 1974. His continued interest and support are much valued and appreciated. I also express special appreciation to another colleague, Patricia

Rand, for her encouragement and valuable editorial suggestions. Thanks, too, to Wendy Harris of the Johns Hopkins University Press for her initial recognition that this material might make a book and for her patience and guidance in reaching this goal.

This book was conceived to serve as a resource for individuals working in the broad arena of health care, child protective services, and other agencies concerned with issues that arise from working with drug-exposed infants. Individuals who work in any capacity with these infants and their parents should know the nature and extent of the problem and the procedures used to investigate the consequences of drug exposure during the perinatal period. They should maintain an awareness of developments in the field and have available "state of the art" information about the consequences, including policy issues, that may result for the child, the caregivers, and society as a whole. It is also essential that informed individuals not limit their understanding to only a phase or two of the work, but that they recognize the importance of the information emerging from both the research laboratories and the clinics. All types of information are necessary to understand the difficult and far-reaching problems created by parental drug abuse.

Perinatal Substance Abuse

Introduction

Theo B. Sonderegger, Ph.D.

THE UNITED STATES is currently experiencing a drug epidemic whose ramifications permeate all facets of society. Daily reports attest to the extent and the costs of our struggle, now called a "war," against the use of illegal drugs. The real victims of this war are neither the drug dealers nor the drug users, unfortunate though their circumstances may be, but the children of drug-abusing parents. Concern for such children increases as we learn more about the immediate and long-term effects of drugs on development and behavior.

Irrevocably enmeshed with the drug epidemic is the spread of AIDS (acquired immunodeficiency syndrome) through the population. We now know that the majority of the perinatal AIDS victims are children of women who use drugs intravenously or who have had an intravenous drug user as a sexual partner. Blood transfusions, the other major source of perinatal AIDS, add another avenue of transmission.

The complex problems experienced by these "youngest victims" and their caregivers, both immediate and at the professional level, as well as the problems generated for all of society will be with us through the life-span of these children and may be compounded in future generations as well. The potential costs to society are incalculable and beyond ordinary comprehension.

Although the 1989 U.S. Department of Health and Human Services *National Household Survey on Drug Abuse* showed significant declines in the "current use" (i.e., 1988) of illicit drugs in the United States, drug abuse remains a serious problem (U.S. Department of Health and Human Services 1989). The survey also indicated a continued problem with heavy drug users, especially those who use cocaine. Even though there was a decrease of 37% in the use of illicit drugs in 1988 when compared with a similar survey conducted in 1985, the survey found continued intense use of cocaine in some segments of the population.

Some 862,000 people used cocaine once a week or more in 1988, compared with 647,000 in 1985; 292,000 in 1988 used the drug daily or almost daily, compared with 246,000 such users in 1985. Of relevance to the topic of substance abuse during the perinatal period is the survey finding that more than 5 million (9%) of the nearly 60 million women 15–44 years of age, the childbearing years, used an illicit drug during a one-month period in 1988. How many of these already were pregnant or conceived a child during this time?

The popularity of specific drugs of abuse changes over the years. Cocaine, for example, and its freebase derivative, crack, have been the most popular of the abused drugs until quite recently. Now the use of "speed," "crank," or "zip" (or whatever street name currently is popular for the methamphetamines) is said to be rising (U.S. Department of Health and Human Services 1988/1989, 15). The Drug Abuse Warning Network, or DAWN (1988), reported a fivefold increase in medical emergencies due to cocaine since 1984—from 8,831 to more than 46,000 in 1988; the number of cocaine-related deaths more than doubled during the same period even though the number of cocaine users was reduced from almost 6 million to less than 3 million in the population as a whole.

As a drug increases in popularity, its use rises among pregnant women. In Chicago, for instance, the use of illicit drugs during pregnancy was reported to be between 0.4 and 27% and that of cocaine alone was between 0.2 and 17%, depending upon the hospital studied; data from these studies suggest that 11% of the infants born each year—about 375,000 nationwide—are suffering from the effects of in utero drug exposure (Chasnoff 1989). Statistics from other cities throughout the country verify the popularity of cocaine use among pregnant women (Jones and Lopez 1988). These authors reported a prevalence rate of perinatal cocaine exposure in Miami of 12%. In Philadelphia, data from an eight-week survey of eight city hospitals showed that more than 16% of the women who delivered there used cocaine. In Boston, as reported in one study of 579 women receiving prenatal care, prevalence rates were 17% for the use of cocaine and 28% for the use of marijuana.

The epidemic of drug use during pregnancy, although widely publicized as a problem in the large cities of the east and west coasts of the United States, clearly is not confined to these areas. In Kansas City, for example, 40% of the infants in the intensive care units in inner city hospitals that care for indigent cases reportedly either have a positive urine screen test for cocaine or else have a mother who does (David Mundy, M.D., and Howard Kilbride, M.D., telephone interviews, January 1990).

The consequences of exposing the immature organism to drugs are far reaching. Among other outcomes, drug addiction in pregnant women has increased the infant mortality rate in the United States at a time when the rate is already one of the highest among the industrialized nations (*Newsweek* 1989). Moreover, alcohol use during pregnancy is now recognized as the leading known cause of mental retardation in the Western world (Abel and Sokol 1987).

In addition to costs in human suffering, the economic costs associated with perinatal drug exposure are tremendous. Abel and Sokol (1987) estimated that 7,000 infants with fetal alcohol syndrome are born yearly in the United States. Treatment costs for infants with fetal alcohol syndrome were $321 million in 1987. This sum does not include treatment of infants damaged by perinatal exposure to other drugs. One example of the treatment costs is provided by data from Kansas City hospitals on intensive-care treatment for cocaine-exposed infants. The average stay for a cocaine-exposed baby with minor problems is four to five extra days of intensive care. This adds around $3,000 to infant delivery costs (Howard Kilbride, M.D., telephone interview, January 1990). For infants who are very sick, costs run from $40,000 to $300,000. At the time of the interview, one sick infant in a Kansas City facility had already run up charges of $700,000. These costs, large as they are, do not approach the costs to society as perinatal damage becomes apparent during development and growth of the child (e.g., the cost of educating children who manifest attention-span difficulties, low achievement, or other problems in the school situation).

THE PLAN OF THE BOOK

All drugs—therapeutic, legal, or illegal—affect a developing organism in many ways. Some of these effects may have long-term consequences. For human infants as well as the young of other species, drug exposure early in life may produce a broad spectrum of changes that range from short-term physiological and behavioral effects to long-term morphological, physiological, and behavioral alterations. Changes may not manifest themselves until later in childhood or young adulthood. Some may persist throughout life or, in some instances, into the second generation. The combined efforts of clinicians and researchers, using all available research models, are needed to understand the complexity of drug-exposure effects in order to plan interventions for and possible ameliorations of the detrimental effects of perinatal drug exposure.

The following chapters present state-of-the-art data on several common drugs of abuse—alcohol, marijuana, cocaine, phencyclidine (PCP), amphetamines, and tobacco. Data from laboratories where animal models are used are presented together with observations from clinical populations. Both animal and clinical findings are necessary to understand the array of consequences to the developing organism of exposure to substances of abuse. Each of the chapter contributors is a well-respected researcher and/or clinician who has worked with specific drugs and has published widely concerning the effects of the drug on humans and other animals.

The book begins with an introduction to general methodological issues in chapter 1. The authors here emphasize the value of animal research to the clinician and of the insights the clinician can contribute to the animal researcher. For example, some data from work with animals suggest that certain consequences of drug exposure early in life do not manifest themselves until adulthood. Since experimental animal lifespans are measured in months, it is possible to collect data from all life stages during a relatively short period, a feat impossible with human subjects. Although caution must be exercised when one generalizes from animal models to humans, well-planned and well-controlled studies using animals are one of the most feasible ways to obtain the data necessary to plan intervention strategies and ways to ameliorate effects that may occur in human infants exposed early in life to drugs. The need to deal with the large numbers of drug-exposed infants is urgent; we cannot afford to wait 20 years for results from long-term studies with these infants before beginning treatment. Furthermore, the ethics of using the present generation of drug-exposed infants as experimental models, watching as they mature and waiting to prescribe treatments until abnormal conditions develop, is highly questionable. Data from longitudinal studies with short-generation-span animals, on the other hand, may provide clues to ways to treat the thousands of drug-exposed infants now being born. It is apparent, therefore, that information is needed at once from both the laboratory and the clinic to elucidate and treat the problems associated with perinatal drug exposure. To reiterate, the clinician and the researcher each must be aware of developments in the other's area to deal adequately with the far-reaching problems of perinatal substance abuse. This book is designed to facilitate such an exchange of information.

When data from both the clinic and the laboratory were examined during the preparation of this book, some unexpected results emerged. For one thing, data from a variety of studies suggest that exposure to drugs early in life produces gender-specific effects; that is, exposure to drugs early in life appears to affect males and females differently. Many of these effects are described in the second chapter. Gender-specific effects of early drug exposure have been demonstrated as differences in morphology (e.g., in the structure of the corpus callosum), sexual development and differentiation, neuroendocrine functioning, and an assortment of behaviors. In some studies males and in others females seem more vulnerable to drug exposure and are affected to a greater extent. Although the underlying mechanisms are not yet understood, the authors of this chapter join other researchers in the contention that both male and female members of a species must be studied to delineate accurately the effects on the organism of drug or alcohol exposure early in life.

Consequences of perinatal exposure to specific drugs of abuse currently in vogue are discussed in separate chapters because many of the drugs are pharmacologically different and, hence, can be expected to produce different effects. For the most part, information about one kind of drug obtained from both laboratory researchers and clinicians is combined in a single chapter. Three chapters, however, are devoted to alcohol, the substance of abuse which has been studied for the longest period. Chapter 3 discusses threshold effects, defining, for example, the amount of alcohol ingested by a pregnant woman that likely will affect her fetus. Other factors that increase the risk for alcohol-related birth defects are also described here. Chapter 4 contains information gained from longitudinal studies already conducted; such studies have shown the consequences of exposure to alcohol early in life in children who have now reached adolescence or early adulthood. The findings reported from these longitudinal studies with alcohol-exposed human infants lend credence to data from animal studies which suggest that drug exposure early in life may lead to effects still present in adulthood. In chapter 5, relatively new information about paternal alcohol abuse, which can be detrimental to offspring, is described. Information presented in these three chapters should be of immense value to individuals

planning and implementing educational treatment programs that deal
with children who suffer from the fetal alcohol syndrome (FAS) or fetal
alcohol effects (FAE).

Marijuana is discussed next. The use of marijuana, or "pot," has
declined; nevertheless, 6% or 3.8 million of the women of childbearing
age were reported by the National Household Survey to have used
marijuana during a one-month period (U.S. Department of Health and
Human Services 1989). Effects of this drug upon the developing organism range from abnormalities in the size of the eyes, also seen in some
babies exposed to alcohol or cocaine, to a wide variety of neuroendocrine or behavioral changes. Compared to alcohol, however, much less
is known about the long-term effects of exposure to this drug early in
life and the conditions under which these effects may become apparent.
One suggestion made by the authors of chapter 6 is that the effects may
manifest themselves only in some cases as the child becomes older or
has more demands placed upon the nervous system.

Cocaine use during the perinatal period is discussed in chapter 7.
As stated earlier, the use of cocaine by women who are delivering
babies in hospitals in our major cities has reached epidemic proportions.
Although reports on the teratology of cocaine appeared as early as 1980,
almost 1 million (2%) of women of childbearing age used cocaine during
a one-month period in 1988 (U.S. Department of Health and Human
Services 1989). Only now are we beginning to get data from the clinic
and from a rapidly growing number of laboratory studies using animal
models and cocaine. Data from the latter studies indicate that low birth
weight, abruptio placentae, cephalic hemorrhage, and other effects reported in some clinical studies are the effects of cocaine per se and not
the result of other factors such as polydrug interactions. Although there
are many similarities between cocaine-exposed infants and those exposed to alcohol or marijuana, an important difference is discussed in
this chapter. The majority of the infants subjected to early contact with
cocaine do not seem able to protect themselves from overstimulation
and still exhibit these characteristics at the age of one month. Consequently, these infants cannot be held or cuddled in the same way as non-
drug-exposed infants. Many of these babies still displayed abnormal
reflexes and hypertonicity even at four months of age. Little is known
about the long-term effects of exposure of the immature organism to
cocaine. The chapter authors believe that there are enough similarities
between the findings of human and animal studies to suggest that the

latter may serve well to warn of the long-term risks to human growth and development of cocaine exposure early in life.

Opioid use during pregnancy and its consequences have been of concern to researchers and clinicians for a much longer time than has the use of many other currently available street drugs. Changes in the behavior of the fetus/neonate exposed to opium were reported as early as the 1870s. Opioid use is still widespread; current estimates suggest that 1 in every 1,000 of the population in the United States was exposed to opioids early in life (chapter 8), and a broad spectrum of information from both the laboratory and the clinic exists. For these reasons, three chapters are devoted to information about opioid exposure in the developing organism. Chapter 8 presents some of the extensive laboratory data, including new information about the receptor sites where opioids act on the central nervous system. Ways by which exogenous opioids such as heroin and methadone interact with endogenous opioids to control growth are only now beginning to be explored.

Chapter 9 includes findings from longitudinal studies of heroin-exposed infants. Among the concerns of clinicians who work with heroin-addicted infants are the lack of long-term commitment on the part of the drug-dependent personality, the absence or poor quality of prenatal care, and the difficulties in obtaining an accurate drug history. Long-term detrimental effects seem to be related to factors associated with the life-style of the drug-dependent woman. Consequently, it is suggested that intervention efforts should be directed toward improving the environment of the infant and child as well as improving the in utero environment.

Cessation from opioid use may produce a withdrawal process with severe consequences. The withdrawal process, therefore, must be recognized and treated in both addicted mothers and infants. Methadone, a synthetic opioid, is used in maintenance therapy for pregnant women to stabilize addictive behavior and to prevent erratic periods of drug withdrawal; some of the effects of methadone treatment with pregnant women are described in chapter 10. Perinatal outcome is much improved in women on supervised methadone maintenance compared to those addicted women who do not seek treatment for chemical dependence. Another factor of paramount importance to be considered with drugs that are injected intravenously, as is often the case with the opioids, is the possibility of getting infections, particularly AIDS, if intravenous drug use is continued during pregnancy.

Phencyclidine (PCP or "angel dust") is another drug used by pregnant women, and chapter 11 is devoted to joint findings from the laboratory and the clinic. PCP was introduced as an anesthetic in 1957, and evidence of the abuse of this drug, as "angel dust," began to be reported in emergency rooms across the country soon after. After a decline in its use, PCP again emerged as a major drug of abuse in 1982; by 1988, 120,000 women of childbearing age were reported to be using PCP (U.S. Department of Health and Human Services 1989). Findings reported in this chapter again underscore the concerns of researchers reporting on other abused substances—there are subtle but long-term effects of early exposure that may not manifest themselves until later in the development of the exposed young. Moreover, as reported for other drugs, these effects may be exhibited simply as delays in the appearances of various developmental indices (e.g., onset of puberty), or they may not become apparent until the child is expected to use some cognitive skill in a school or other situation.

Because licit as well as illicit drugs are abused by pregnant women and their partners to the detriment of their offspring, a chapter has been devoted to tobacco and amphetamine, both central nervous system stimulants. Tobacco reportedly is the most widely abused stimulant drug of this class and one that pregnant women have more difficulty giving up than alcohol. Like many of the drugs previously discussed, the effects of in utero nicotine exposure for human infants include an increased risk for stillbirths, low-birth-weight infants, and the sudden infant death syndrome (SIDS). Animal study data indicate deficits in whole brain and cerebellar weights in addition to other specific metabolic changes in the brains of the nicotine-exposed offspring. A broad array of changes in activity and learning tasks is also noted.

Amphetamine dropped out of popularity with drug users in the 1970s, but there now is a rise in the street use of the drug, particularly in the form of methamphetamine with the street names of "crank" or "ice." Growth deficits, increased motor activity, perceptual changes (e.g., altered taste preferences), and changes in performance in learning tasks are reported in one or more studies as a consequence of methamphetamine use. As was the case with nicotine, exposure in utero to methamphetamine produces lower sex ratios of males to females, indicating that males seem to be more adversely affected than females by the exposure to nicotine or methamphetamine.

Chapter 12 presents provocative data suggesting that exposure to either nicotine or methamphetamine in utero may increase the risk for tumor development later in life. Similar findings have been observed in our laboratories in older female rats exposed early in life to morphine or alcohol (T. B. Sonderegger, unpublished data) and in the laboratory of Susan Dalterio with older female mice exposed at an earlier age to marijuana (personal communication, June 1986).

The final chapter of the book covers a topic of concern to all citizens, i.e., the law and the human fetus. The issue of perinatal substance abuse has entered the judicial system in the form of "protecting the fetus" or "punishment of the pregnant woman who takes drugs." Efforts to protect the fetus may run counter to the right of the mother to be protected from an invasion of her privacy. Parents who take drugs may be prone to abuse and/or neglect their children. Such infants (e.g., cocaine-exposed babies) are difficult to nurture and may require specialized care.

Although definitive answers are yet to come from the U.S. Supreme Court, lower courts have made relevant decisions on several types of cases (e.g., abortion and forced medical care or employment restriction cases where fetal rights have outweighed maternal rights). Child welfare laws also have been used to protect the fetus against harm from substances ingested by the mother during the perinatal period. The chapter authors point out that, although there are laws in all states that bear directly or indirectly on maternal substance abuse during pregnancy, there is no consistency in the way in which these statutes are applied.

CONCERNS FOR THE FUTURE

Where have our investigations led us and what direction should they take in the future? Several conclusions emerge from the studies and discussions of this book: specific drugs have specific effects, but all drugs produce both immediate and potentially long-term effects on the developing organism. Although we know something of the outward manifestations of perinatal drug abuse (i.e., morphological and behavioral changes), much remains to be learned in the laboratory and in investigations in vitro to determine the mechanisms underlying drug effects.

What is lacking also in the information on all drugs discussed here, with the possible exception of alcohol, are adequate data on the long-term effects on the human organism of drugs administered perinatally.

As Gaylia Jean Harry and Judy Howard write in chapter 11, "Is it possible that some children will improve once higher centers of learning have matured? Or will we continue to see dysfunction in the growing child similar to that observed in some adults who have abused PCP?" Data from animal studies are clear: effects often are not apparent until the organism reaches a critical developmental stage. In organisms with long lifespans, such as humans, years may pass before an effect is noted. Well-controlled prospective longitudinal studies in both the clinic and the laboratory should be initiated at once to identify such long-term effects. The data are critical for the programs now being undertaken to treat the large numbers of drug-affected infants entering society today.

It is difficult to monitor and collect drug use data from human subjects over long periods. The parents in perinatal drug use studies usually are polydrug users, and drug intake often is not accurately reported by them. Because of their drug intake, they often are careless or inadequate parents, and their children suffer from neglect. Clinicians and researchers are adamant: intervention efforts, therefore, must be directed toward improving the environment of the growing child as well as the in utero environment of the fetus. No matter what drug has been studied, clinicians stress the need for good prenatal care and a supportive environment to help ameliorate the effects of early drug exposure. Appropriate educational procedures to recognize and handle these drug-exposed children as they reach school age and classes in parenting to help those at home who work with the children have also been suggested in many of these chapters.

Regardless of the state of the scientific data, the law and the courts have moved into the arena of perinatal drug effects. Decisions are being made now which are antithetical to our understanding of the needs of mothers and their children. A deplorable solution currently is being advanced to deal with the consequences of drug-taking during pregnancy: punishment of the chemically dependent woman who most likely is a victim of abuse herself. Seventy-four percent of alcohol- and drug-dependent women are the victims of sexual abuse including rape and incest (Wilsnack 1984, 215). Moreover, many agencies deny treatment to the chemically dependent pregnant woman because of fear of subsequent liability charges. According to a survey of 78 drug treatment programs in New York City, for instance, 54% of the programs refused treatment to pregnant addicts; 67% denied treatment to pregnant addicts on Medicaid and 87% denied treatment to Medicaid patients addicted specifically to crack-cocaine (Chavkin 1989).

The consequences of treatment denial are disastrous for both mother and child. Not only is the parenting frequently inadequate, but the drug-exposed infants often are placed in foster homes [e.g., in California, up to 60% of drug-exposed babies are placed in foster care (Halfon 1989)]. Compounding the problem is the widespread prevalence of the AIDS virus in the drug-taking population. Nearly 1 infant in 50 born in inner-city New York, for example, is now HIV-infected (Landsman et al. 1987). New York is not alone in this problem; data from other cities confirm the presence of the virus in the drug-abusing population.

It is imperative that correct information about the extent and consequences of exposure to drugs during the perinatal period reach the public, particularly those individuals who make and administer our laws. Scientists must make clear the limitations of their findings, not only to their scientific colleagues but also to the public at large, for "science," the "scientific method," and "scientific data" are now being invoked, rightly or wrongly, to justify all manner of societal actions. If scientists do not contribute to the process by which scientific information is assimilated into the public domain, essential interpretations and understandings may be lost as legislators address issues that are connected to exposure of the developing organism to drugs. Informed individuals can provide legislators and judges with accurate insights by testifying formally before legislatures or courts or by submitting amicus curia ("friend of the court") briefs (Morris and Sonderegger 1986). Informal contacts with lawmakers and their staffs are also effective. No matter which procedures are used to provide assistance, it is critical that those who generate the data take an active role in assuring that the information is correctly understood and interpreted when it is applied to the needs of society. The littlest victims of the war on drugs deserve all the help we can give them.

REFERENCES

Abel, E. L., and Sokol, R. J. 1987. Incidence of fetal alcohol syndrome and economic impact of FAS-related anomalies. *Drug Alcohol Depend* 19:51–70.

Chasnoff, I. 1989. Drug use and women: Establishing a standard of care. *Ann NY Acad Sci* 562:208–10.

Chavkin, W. 1989. Born hooked: Confronting the impact of perinatal substance abuse. Hearing, Select Committee on Children, Youth and Families, U.S. House of Representatives, April 27, 1989.

DAWN. 1988. *Drug Abuse Warning Network*. Rockville, Md.: National Institute on Drug Abuse.

Halfon, N. 1989. Born hooked: Confronting the impact of perinatal substance abuse. Hearing, Select Committee on Children, Youth and Families, U.S. House of Representatives, April 27, 1989.

Jones, C. L., and Lopez, R. E. 1988. Direct and indirect effects on the infant of maternal drug abuse, 1–33. Report of the Expert Panel on Prenatal Care, U.S. Department of Health and Human Services/ National Institutes of Health.

Landsman, S., Minkoff, H., Holman, S., McCalla, S., and Suin, O. 1987. Serosurvey of human immunodeficiency virus in parturients. *JAMA* 258:2701–3.

Morris, R., and Sonderegger, T. 1986. Perinatal toxicology and the law. *Neurobehav Toxicol Teratol* 8:325–419.

Newsweek. 1989. Vital statistics. October 16, p. 10.

U.S. Department of Health and Human Services. 1988/1989. *NIDA Notes*, Winter, p. 15.

U.S. Department of Health and Human Services. 1989. National household survey on drug abuse: Population estimates 1988. National Institute of Drug Abuse. DHHS Publication (ADM) 89-1636.

Wilsnack, S. 1984. Drinking and sexuality and sexual dysfunction in women. In *Alcohol Problems in Women*, p. 215. New York: Guilford Press.

1

Methodological Issues: Laboratory Animal Studies of Perinatal Exposure to Alcohol or Drugs and Human Studies of Drug Use during Pregnancy

Joanne Weinberg, Ph.D., Theo B. Sonderegger, Ph.D., and Ira J. Chasnoff, M.D.

ANIMAL MODELS

INFORMATION about the effects of perinatal exposure to drugs can be obtained effectively through the use of animal studies. Chemical dependency clinics in every major city have a large number of patients who continue to take one or more drugs throughout pregnancy, and one might think that adequate information about the consequences of perinatal alcohol and/or drug abuse could be obtained from the unfortunate infants of these women. However, the information gained from these patients is often limited in value for several reasons, including (1) polydrug use by the mother; (2) inaccurate reports of the quantity of the drugs taken or the frequency of use; (3) other detrimental factors affecting the infant's development, such as malnutrition, inadequate maternal care, and poor medical care (prenatal and postnatal); (4) little knowledge about the father; and (5) the presence of uncontrolled or unknown factors, since it is, of course, unethical as well as impossible to put the mother and infant in controlled conditions with the measured drug manipulations necessary to make cause-and-effect statements. These issues are discussed in more detail later in this chapter.

Animal studies permit the use of genetic and environmental controls as well as the use of regulated drug treatment protocols. Exposure of the developing organism to drugs/alcohol may produce short-term and perhaps transitory as well as long-term and relatively persistent effects. Much work has been done on the recognition and treatment of the short-term effects (e.g., the withdrawal effects seen in an infant born addicted), but it is often much more difficult to recognize some of the long-term effects (e.g., behavioral hyperactivity). There are a few human longitudinal studies, but data from animal studies provide the most substantial clues as to what happens to the adolescent/adult exposed prenatally or neonatally to alcohol and other drugs. The use of animal models is also essential if we are to ascertain the biological mechanisms underlying such long-term effects. Moreover, animal models may provide useful information about possible methods of ameliorating the effects of alcohol/drug exposure early in development. It goes without saying, however, that caution and judgment must be used in applying findings from research obtained from one mammalian species to another. On the other hand, information gained from the animal work may not only guide research in the study of human infants born to addicted mothers but also provide insights useful to the clinician planning intervention strategies.

The nature of the effects produced by perinatal exposure of the immature animal to substances of abuse will depend upon many factors. These include (1) the chemical structure of the drug; (2) the mode of administration; (3) the dose of the drug; (4) the duration of drug administration; (5) the developmental stage of the organism at the time of drug administration; and (6) the susceptibility of the species, as well as the individual, to the particular drug (Coyle, Wayner, and Singer 1976).

Of these factors, the developmental stage at the time of drug exposure has been of considerable interest to researchers because this knowledge can be useful in predicting and understanding the nature of the drug-induced damage. The rate of development of the central nervous system in mammals differs according to the species being investigated. Wilson (1973) conceptualized teratogenic susceptibility to various developmental insults by means of a hypothetical curve that spans the embryonic and fetal periods.

Drug effects will depend upon the animal subject being studied. In general, the highest sensitivity to structural malformations is found if an insult occurs during the period of organogenesis (embryonic period). Minor structural changes and functional changes, however, are more likely to occur with insult during the period of histogenesis (the fetal period). These changes are also likely to be reflected in behavior alterations. Another important developmental stage is the brain growth spurt, a period when the brain is particularly vulnerable to drugs (Dobbing and Sands 1979). This period of rapid growth occurs at different times for different species and is a time when there is axonal growth, dendritic arborization, maximal synaptogenesis, gliogenesis, myelination, and maturation of synaptic neurotransmission. Both structural and functional or behavioral alterations may result from an insult during this period. In the human, the brain growth spurt period is perinatal, beginning about the middle of pregnancy and extending to the third or fourth postnatal year, when myelination is still taking place. In the rat, the period is postnatal and extends from birth until about 24 days postnatal (Dobbing 1974, 1976).

Animal models of perinatal alcohol/drug exposure may be characterized by the developmental stage during which the alcohol/drug exposure occurred: (1) period before conception; (2) prenatal period; (3) prenatal and lactation periods; (4) lactation period only (postnatal). When administered before conception, the drug is administered to the adult animal that will then be used in breeding. When given prenatally or both prenatally and during lactation, the substance is typically administered to the pregnant female. If the postnatal period is of interest, the substance may be administered to the lactating animal or given directly to the offspring. Administration of alcohol/drugs during each of these periods can present a number of methodological problems. In this chapter, some of the issues involved in perinatal drug exposure are reviewed. Much of the discussion is based upon previously published work.

Although this chapter focuses primarily on perinatal alcohol administration, examples of other drugs will be used where appropriate. The reader should be aware that the researcher takes into account the characteristics of the drug to be studied (i.e., whether it is stimulant, depressant, psychoactive, etc.) before designing an experiment. For example, to achieve levels of morphine that are tolerable to the animal, one must increase the doses gradually at daily intervals to reach the desired dose level. In turn, it is necessary to taper the doses after the treatment period to minimize withdrawal effects, as demonstrated in a study in which adult behavior and adrenocortical functions were examined after postnatal treatment with morphine (Sonderegger and Zimmermann 1978). It is also typically necessary to do preliminary studies to determine the range of doses of each drug necessary to produce a minimal effect up to the LD_{50} (i.e., the dose that is lethal 50% of the time). To determine the amount of alcohol that rat pups could tolerate when fed the drug intragastrically, for example, a preliminary study was conducted where rat pups were fed doses of ethanol ranging from 0.8 to 7.0 g/kg (Sonderegger et al. 1982).

Models of Drug Administration

Drugs may be administered to affect the developing organism over a broad time period, ranging from the period before conception through adolescence. Development is a continuous process. Although birth is an important event, it does not necessarily divide development into distinct phases as birth occurs at different developmental stages for various species (Vorhees 1986). For example, rats are relatively less developed at birth, compared to humans, whereas guinea pigs are relatively more developed. The rat is the animal most frequently used in behavioral teratology studies, and it is the laboratory animal most widely discussed in this chapter.

Preconception

Administration of drugs before conception is one of the less frequently used treatment procedures but has received more attention recently with the increased interest in the effects of paternal drug exposure. Typically, the prospective sire is treated with the drug for a period and then bred with a non-drug-treated female. Effects on the offspring have been found with methadone (Joffee et al. 1976), marijuana (Fried 1976), and alcohol (Abel 1984; Abel and Tan 1988; Meadows, Schmidt, and Friedler 1987). The methodological issues of paternal drug exposure are discussed in detail in chapter 5. As an example of such a study, male mice were given alcohol (ethanol is typically used in experiments) by gavage (3.5 g/kg) twice daily for 8½ days (Friedler et al. 1987). This was followed by ad libitum access to food and water for 7 days, and animals were then bred. Paternal exposure to ethanol resulted in offspring with an increase in pivoting locomotion at 10 days of age and an altered activity profile at 12 weeks of age.

The Prenatal Period

ADMINISTRATION PROCEDURES

The five main methods that have been used to expose animals to alcohol (ethanol) during the prenatal period are injection, intubation, administration in the drinking water, addition to a liquid diet, and administration through an implanted osmotic pump.

Placing ethanol in the drinking water and providing this as the only source of fluid is technically the simplest method of administering alcohol and was used in many early animal studies. However, most rodents find the taste of ethanol aversive and will not voluntarily consume very concentrated solutions. Therefore, if ethanol is placed unadulterated in the drinking water, fluid intake will typically decrease. With water intake suppressed, the amount of ethanol ingested and therefore the blood alcohol levels are also reduced (Abel 1980; Wiener 1980). Furthermore, food intake often decreases concomitantly with the decrease in drinking. This probably occurs partly because eating and drinking are very closely related in the typical laboratory setting (Marwine and Collier 1979). More important, however, is the fact that ethanol-derived calories replace the calories that would normally be supplied by food. Although this problem occurs regardless of method of alcohol administration, it is particularly severe when high concentrations of ethanol are presented in the drinking water. Thus, this method of alcohol administration is often unsatisfactory because it produces neither adequate nutrition nor substantially elevated blood alcohol levels.

Both injection and intubation have the technical advantage that ethanol can be administered in uniformly controlled and timed doses, resulting in high blood alcohol levels. However, both of these methods involve handling and restraint, which can be stressful to the pregnant animal. Because prenatal stress in itself can affect hormonal, physiological, and behavioral responsiveness of rodent offspring (Archer and Blackman 1971; Barlow, Knight, and Sullivan 1978; Herrenkohl 1979; Sproul 1974), these may not be the methods of choice for many investigations.

Adding ethanol to a liquid diet and providing this as the only source of nutrition seems to be an effective method of administering alcohol to pregnant females (Lieber and DeCarli 1982). The liquid diet method has been shown to result in consistent intake of high doses of ethanol and consistently elevated blood alcohol levels (Lieber and DeCarli 1982). In addition, the stress associated with alcohol administration is minimized in the liquid diet model because pregnant animals need not be handled or restrained, as during injection or intubation procedures. Finally, nutrient composition of liquid diets can easily be adjusted and controlled according to the requirements of each experimental situation. (For further discussion of these methodological issues, see Lieber and DeCarli 1982; Riley and Meyer 1984; Weinberg 1984; Wiener 1980). Several concerns about this method have been raised (Abel 1980; Wiener 1980). One is that animals consume greater amounts of water with liquid diet than they would with pelleted diet (approximately 60–80 ml of liquid diet daily). It is possible that increased fluid intake could affect water balance and/or kidney function and thus contribute to fetal distress. Although neither diarrhea nor excessive urination have been observed in our own studies with liquid diet (Gallo and Weinberg 1982; Weinberg 1985), this is an issue to keep in mind. In addition, many of the liquid diets used are based on commercial food products such as Slender or Nutrament. Because these products have not been formulated for rodents, their nutritional adequacy is sometimes questionable. Further, diet composition may vary over several months, and flavorings or preservatives are generally present. Use of a semipurified diet formulated specifically for rodents and tailored to meet the needs of the particular experimental situation overcomes some of these problems and allows the investigator more control over nutrient composition and intake (Lieber and DeCarli 1982).

Osmotic minipumps are typically used to administer drugs other than alcohol. They usually are implanted subcutaneously and have been used to reduce the amount of handling involved in drug administration as well as to deliver the drug at a steady rate. For example, in a recent study on the effects of prenatal nicotine exposure, Fung and Lau (1989) were concerned that administration of nicotine to pregnant animals through parenteral injections or through drinking water could expose both mother and fetus to spike concentrations of nicotine which could result in maternal vasculature constriction and subsequent fetal hypoxia (Murrin et al. 1987). Consequently, they elected to implant osmotic minipumps (model 2ML4; Alza Corp., Palo Alto, California) containing either physiological saline or nicotine (released at the rate of 1.5 mg/kg/day) into pregnant female rats. They found that the number of pups in the drug-treated litters was significantly reduced compared to that in the saline-treated litters. Interestingly, this effect was due to a significant reduction in the number of male pups but not female pups. Nicotine-treated pups also had reduced body lengths and, by day 9, reduced body weights compared to saline-treated controls. In addition, a decrease in the number of striatal dopaminergic receptor binding sites was found in male pups but not female pups.

NUTRITIONAL ISSUES

Once a method of drug administration has been chosen, the investigator is faced with the problem that drug intake may alter nutritional status. This is particularly critical for studies involving alcohol because of the complex interactions of alcohol and nutrition.

Nutrient Intake. Addition of ethanol to an animal's diet may directly affect nutrient intake. Because of its high energy value (providing 7.1 kcal/g), ethanol may readily displace other food in the diet. Animals exposed to ethanol thus typically consume less food than animals given ad libitum access to nonethanol diets (Gallo and Weinberg 1981, 1982; Wiener et al. 1981). Because calories in ethanol are not associated with vitamins, minerals, protein, or other essential nutrients, intake of these "empty" calories can result in nutrient deficiencies. This situation is especially critical for pregnant and/or lactating females whose nutritional requirements are known to be greater than those of nonpregnant/ nonlactating adults (National Academy of Sciences 1978). For example, the energy requirement for gestation appears to be 10–30% greater than that for a nonpregnant adult fed ad libitum, and it has been shown that food intake can increase by as much as 140% by the end of gestation. Similarly, the protein requirement for maintenance of adult rats is 4.2% net protein, whereas that for maintenance during gestation and lactation is at least three times greater (National Academy of Sciences 1978). In addition to displacing nutrient-rich foods in the diet, ethanol has an anorexigenic effect (Smith 1979; Sorette et al. 1980), further compromising nutrient intake. This effect is compounded in animal models of fetal alcohol syndrome because, as noted, most experimental animals find the taste of ethanol aversive and will not voluntarily consume very concentrated solutions (Abel 1980). [Miniature swine (Dexter et al. 1980) and certain specially bred strains of rats and mice (Church, Fuller, and Dann 1979; Duckett, Schneider, and Hartline 1981) are exceptions.] Thus, for a variety of reasons and across a variety of species, alcoholism is associated with decreased nutrient intake, and nutritional deficiencies ranging from undernutrition to severe malnutrition can occur (Lieber 1979; Smith 1979).

Secondary Malnutrition. Dietary deficiencies are only one cause of the undernutrition or malnutrition that typically accompanies alcohol intake in both humans and laboratory animals. Alcohol also has deleterious effects at almost every level of the gastrointestinal tract, as well as direct toxic effects on many organs, including the liver, pancreas, and placenta. Thus, alcohol consumption may alter metabolism, transport, utilization, activation, and storage of almost every essential nutrient, including vitamins and minerals (folate, thiamin, vitamin A, vitamin B_6, and zinc deficiencies are among the most commonly reported), proteins, and amino acids (Lieber 1979; Lieber 1982).

Nutrient Requirements.   It has been suggested that alcohol ingestion may cause a "wastage" of specific nutrients, including energy. Chronic alcohol intake may increase the body's energy requirements, possibly through energy wastage secondary to induction of the hepatic microsomal ethanol-oxidizing system (MEOS) (Lieber 1979). Although the primary metabolic pathway for alcohol involving alcohol dehydrogenase is economical, yielding high-energy phosphate bonds, oxidation via the hepatic MEOS is inefficient. This latter pathway could normally account for as much as 20–25% of the oxidation of alcohol and for much more after chronic consumption of high doses of alcohol. The MEOS pathway seems to result in a loss of chemical energy as heat without any effective coupling to adenosine triphosphate (ATP) synthesis. Similar considerations apply to the oxidation of other drugs by liver microsomal pathways. Thus, with repeated intake of alcohol or other drugs, the energy balance of the body may be seriously compromised.

Alcohol consumption might also increase the need for certain vitamins and minerals. Simple supplementation, however, cannot always solve the problem because toxicity may increase with alcohol intake. For pregnant animals, the effects of alcohol on nutrient availability is even more critical, since nutrient requirements are so much greater. Therefore, during pregnancy and/or lactation, it might be necessary to supply nutrients at levels above the minimum daily requirements (but with monitoring for toxicity) if animals are consuming high doses of ethanol.

Alcohol-Nutrition Interactions.   As noted above, food intake and therefore nutrient intake are invariably reduced in both animals and humans consuming alcohol. Most investigators working with animal models of fetal alcohol syndrome include a control group that is "yoked" or "pair-fed" to the alcohol group to control for this reduced intake. Each animal in the pair-fed group receives control diet (with carbohydrate isocalorically substituted for alcohol) in the amount consumed by its alcohol-fed partner each day. Animals in pair-fed and alcohol-fed groups should be matched for body weight; alternatively, feeding can be equated in terms of grams per gram of body weight. In a pregnancy study, animals should also be matched for day of gestation. Inclusion of a pair-fed group enables one to begin to separate effects due to direct pharmacological actions of alcohol from those that are secondary to alcohol-induced undernutrition.

Recently, several investigators have presented data suggesting that, even with the inclusion of appropriate pair-fed control groups, undernutrition or malnutrition may still be a confounding variable in studies of maternal alcoholism. Furthermore, some of the adverse effects of alcohol, particularly on fetal growth and development, may be nutritionally mediated or may occur primarily under conditions of inadequate nutrition. For example, Sorette et al. (1980) reported that maternal consumption of moderate levels of ethanol [a diet with 15% ethanol-derived calories (EDC)] produced significant adverse effects on fetal body weight, organ weights, and organ deoxyribonucleic acid (DNA) and protein content. Adverse effects of higher levels of ethanol intake (25% EDC), however, were due primarily to an ethanol-induced suppression of maternal food intake rather than to direct effects of ethanol per se. Gallo and Weinberg (1986) similarly reported adverse effects of the maternal consumption of moderate doses of ethanol on offspring body weight as well as weights of brain, heart, liver, and kidney. Effects on brain, heart, and kidney were attributed to a direct effect of maternal ethanol intake, whereas effects on the liver were attributed primarily to an ethanol-induced nutritional deficit. Interactive effects of moderate ethanol consumption and maternal nutritional status on fetal body weight and brain development in the BALB/c mouse have also been demonstrated (Wainwright, Ward, and Blom 1985). It was shown that ethanol intake resulted in higher blood alcohol levels in protein-malnourished than in well-nourished dams and that these higher blood alcohol levels correlated with greater effects on fetal body and brain growth. Wiener et al. (1981) also reported interactive effects of ethanol and nutrition during gestation using a rat model. Offspring of ethanol-exposed dams that were undernourished weighed even less than the growth-stunted offspring of undernourished pair-fed dams. Protein-supplementation of the maternal diets eliminated these deficits in pup body weight. Moreover, despite equivalent alcohol intake, blood alcohol levels of well-nourished females were lower than those of undernourished females. It should be noted, however, that protein supplementation of the experimental diets in that study reduced the percentage of ethanol-derived calories from 36% to 30%, and this may have influenced the outcome obtained.

To examine possible alcohol-nutrition interactions in pregnant rats consuming consistently high doses of ethanol (36% EDC), a recent study compared three diet regimens (Weinberg 1985). A marginal protein diet (18% of kilocalories as protein) provided a model of the fetal alcohol syndrome in which maternal females were mildly undernourished. Two additional diet regimens provided optimal (25% of kilocalories as protein) or supraoptimal (32% of kilocalories as protein) nutrition to pregnant females regardless of ethanol intake and allowed an assessment of the effects of ethanol in well-nourished animals. The data indicated that, although a marginal protein diet increased the adverse effects of alcohol on some measures, consumption of adequate or even protein-enriched diets did not attenuate the deleterious effects of high doses of ethanol on fetal growth and development. Such high ethanol doses resulted in the high blood alcohol levels (140–190 mg/dl) that seem to be necessary for the increased mortality and morbidity associated with maternal alcoholism.

Two more recent studies have shown that outcome measures chosen for study may influence the results obtained, as certain outcome measures may be more sensitive than others in reflecting alcohol-nutrition interactions. For example, an optimal maternal diet was shown to attenuate deficits in certain aspects of skeletal development in fetuses exposed to high doses of ethanol (Weinberg, D'Alquen and Bezio 1990). Pregnant, ethanol-consuming females were fed marginal (18% protein) or optimal (25% protein) diets, and the degree of skeletal ossification was determined on gestation day 21. Ethanol-exposed fetuses showed retarded ossification of the tibia and radius, regardless of maternal nutritional status. In contrast, the optimal maternal diet enhanced the degree of skeletal ossification of the ulna, the sternum, the humerus, and the ilium-ischium. For the ulna, ethanol-exposed fetuses from dams fed a 25% protein diet showed greater ossification than ethanol-exposed fetuses from dams fed an 18% protein diet, but their ulnar ossification was still retarded compared to pair-fed and control fetuses. For the sternum, humerus, and ilium-ischium, however, ossification in the fetuses from dams fed a 25% protein diet was increased to the levels observed in pair-fed and control groups. Vavrousek-Jakuba, Baker, and Shoemaker (1991) also investigated alcohol-nutrition interactions by comparing females given one of three liquid diet formulations that all provided 36% EDC but that differed in protein and carbohydrate content. Maternal weight gain (adjusted for diet intake), blood alcohol levels (particularly at 2:00 P.M.), parturition delay, stillbirths, and neonatal mortality were all more adversely affected in alcohol-consuming females fed a low protein diet than in those fed an optimal or enriched protein diet.

Taken together, these studies clearly indicate that diet composition (protein content and percentage of ethanol-derived calories) is a critical factor in prenatal/perinatal alcohol effects. In addition to diet composition, method of alcohol administration and timing and duration of alcohol exposure are important variables in determining blood alcohol levels achieved, the effects of alcohol on both the dam and the fetus/neonate, and the possible interactive effects of alcohol and nutritional variables. Finally, sensitivity of the outcome measures selected may influence the effects that can be observed.

PAIR-FEEDING AS A TREATMENT AS WELL AS A CONTROL

Although inclusion of a pair-fed group allows one to control for the reduced food intake typically observed in alcohol-fed animals, pair-feeding is not a simple procedure.

First, although alcohol and pair-fed subjects may be matched for body weight, there is still a possibility that metabolic rates of the paired subjects may differ. Thus, animals in the pair-fed group may actually be underfed or overfed relative to animals in the alcohol group (Abel 1980). In addition, pair-feeding can never completely control for alcohol's effects on the digestion, absorption, and utilization of nutrients. One must acknowledge that part of what are called "alcohol effects," particularly with high doses of alcohol, may occur through a complex interaction with at least certain aspects of nutrition.

Second, pair-feeding in itself is a type of experimental treatment. Because pair-fed animals are fed a reduced ration (i.e., equivalent to that consumed by their alcohol-exposed partners), they are getting less food than they want and are constantly hungry. Therefore, these animals frequently consume their limited portion almost immediately (or within the first few hours after presentation) and are effectively on a meal-feeding schedule, being fed once daily and then deprived until the next day's feeding. Restricted meal-feeding can override the influence of the light-dark cycle and serve as the *zeitgeber* or synchronizer for the circadian rhythms of numerous variables including enzymes, biogenic amines, hormones, body temperature, and running activity (Gallo and Weinberg 1981). Gallo and Weinberg (1981) examined the effects of restricted feeding on the circadian rhythm of plasma corticosterone in the adult rat. To simulate the typical pair-feeding regimen, they matched experimental animals to ad libitum-fed controls and fed 80% of control food intake, an amount that was consumed within one or two hours of presentation. Three experimental schedules were examined: (1) animals were fed in the early morning, at 9:00; (2) animals were fed in the late afternoon, at 5:00; (3) animals were fed by automated feeder gradually throughout the 24-hour day. The first two procedures provided a single daily meal in a manner similar to most pair-feeding regimens. The third procedure was an attempt to provide food continuously so that animals could eat in a more typical manner throughout the day and night. It was found that control animals fed ad libitum exhibited a typical corticosterone circadian rhythm, with corticoids lowest at 8:00 A.M. and a peak at 8:00 P.M. Animals fed at 9:00 A.M. exhibited a 12-hour shift in peak corticoids (i.e., a peak at 8:00 A.M. and a nadir at 12:00 M.), with no significant peak at 8:00 P.M. For animals fed by automated feeder, the circadian rhythm was virtually abolished. Offering the restricted ration at 5:00 P.M., however, resulted in a diurnal rhythm similar to that of controls (i.e., lowest values at 8:00 A.M. and a peak in the late afternoon). These results clearly indicated that, although pair-feeding provides an important nutritional control, it is also an experimental treatment in itself. This interrelationship between feeding schedule and diurnal rhythm should not be ignored in the design of studies using pair-fed control groups.

Further evidence for this point comes from an experiment that examined the effects of ethanol consumption on pituitary-adrenal activity in pregnant females (Weinberg and Gallo 1982). Compared to pair-fed animals, ethanol-consuming females exhibited elevated basal levels of corticosterone and a greater initial response to stress. In contrast, pair-fed females showed no change in absolute levels of corticosterone but did show prolonged corticoid activation after stress compared to controls. Thus, both ethanol and pair-feeding regimens altered pituitary-adrenal responsiveness in pregnant females; ethanol treatment produced a greater stress response, whereas pair-feeding altered the pattern of the stress response.

Other studies have shown that pair-feeding may alter maternal weight gain, adrenal weights, and adrenocortical response to stress, as well as offspring organ weights and behavioral and physiological responsiveness (Weinberg and Gallo 1982; Weinberg 1984; Weinberg 1985). Taylor and co-workers (1986) also noted significant effects of pair-feeding during pregnancy on the ontogeny of pituitary-adrenal responses to ethanol and morphine challenges. Typically, pair-feeding has significantly less effect on both the dam and the offspring than does prenatal ethanol exposure. Nevertheless, these data indicate that alcohol-induced nutritional effects may occur, particularly with high doses of alcohol (Weinberg 1984).

Because of the problems inherent in pair-feeding, it may be important to include a control group fed ad libitum in studies where aspects of behavioral or physiological responsiveness could be affected. However, it is not clear what type of diet should be fed to this control group. Laboratory chow is a standard reference for many experimental situations. Unfortunately, nutrient composition often varies slightly between batches of chow, and it is difficult to determine its exact nutrient composition because only "minimum" amounts of each nutrient are listed. Even more important is the fact that the nutrient composition of chow may differ from that of both the commercial and the experimental liquid diets typically used to feed alcohol and pair-fed groups.

Ad libitum access to liquid control diet has occasionally been provided to control animals (e.g., Weinberg 1985). This procedure has the advantage of providing controls with an isocaloric diet that is matched for all nutrients to the diets consumed by ethanol-fed and pair-fed animals. The disadvantage of this procedure is that animals may tend to overeat liquid diets that are provided ad libitum (Wiener et al. 1981; J. Weinberg, unpublished data) and may actually be "overnourished" and gain weight at a faster rate than animals consuming a pelleted control diet. This could result in skewed values for comparison with ethanol and pair-fed groups. One option is to limit access to the control diet to the extent that caloric intake is equivalent to that of animals consuming either laboratory chow or a semipurified pelleted control diet. The obvious problem is that it is difficult to restrict intake to just the right extent and still maintain the animals as an "ad libitum" control group.

One solution (Weinberg 1985) is to formulate a pelleted diet with nutrient density adjusted so that daily intake of nutrients and calories is equivalent to that of animals consuming the liquid diets. This procedure seems to resolve most of the problems described above because nutrient intakes are equated and controlled. However, because the physical state of the diet can affect digestion and the absorption of nutrients, this procedure is still not completely unconfounded.

In summary, although pair-feeding is not a simple procedure and cannot perfectly control for all of the interactions of alcohol and nutrition, it does allow one to begin to differentiate the effects of alcohol from nutritional effects. Depending upon the question under investigation, the effects of alcohol might be assessed adequately in a comparison of ethanol-fed and pair-fed groups alone. However, because pair-feeding can constitute an experimental treatment, it is often important to include a control group fed ad libitum as well.

The Prenatal and Postnatal Periods

In some studies, the object has been to continue the administration of alcohol to the pregnant dam after the prenatal period and through the lactation (preweaning) period. It is possible, of course, to administer the alcohol (1) during the gestation period only; (2) during both the gestation and the lactation periods; and (3) during the lactation period only. Aberrant maternal behavior may result from all of these treatment procedures (Hill and Means 1982; Mathews and Jameson 1982). In the first instance, where drug treatment stops after parturition, aberrant maternal behavior may be eliminated by the use of cross-fostering procedures. When alcohol administration is continued through the gestation and lactation periods or is given just during the lactation period, one may encounter both atypical maternal behavior and the effects produced by the interaction of nutrition with alcohol.

THE INTERACTION OF ETHANOL AND NUTRITION DURING LACTATION

It is known that alcohol passes freely from the maternal circulation into the breast milk (Kesaniemi 1974; Vorherr 1974) and therefore to the nursing infant. Relatively few studies have examined the effects of exposure to alcohol during lactation. In those that have, however, marked effects on growth, development, and behavior have been observed in offspring of lactating females consuming ethanol (Abel 1974, 1975; Martin et al. 1977; Rawat 1975, 1976).

Unfortunately, when extending the period of ethanol exposure through lactation, it is difficult to evaluate the influence of ethanol per se. First, females consuming ethanol during lactation frequently show suppressed weight gains (e.g., Abel 1974; Martin et al. 1977). Maternal undernutrition can decrease the amount of milk available to offspring and thus compromise offspring nutritional status. In addition, alcohol can directly affect milk secretion by depressing the milk-ejection reflex through an inhibitory effect on oxytocin release (Fuchs 1969). This would also have a deleterious effect on offspring weight gain and nutritional status. Finally, alcohol might affect offspring development indirectly through effects on the mother-infant relationship. Bond (1979) demonstrated that females consuming ethanol in a liquid diet through postpartum days 1–17 spent more time in the nest nursing the young on days 7–15. Because motor development and development of the exploratory drive occur during this period, Bond suggested that this change in maternal behavior could have long-term effects on the development of pup behavior. In contrast, DaSilva, Ribeiro, and Masur (1980) found a persistent deficit in retrieving and nest-building activities of ethanol-consuming females. Once again, it was suggested that an altered mother-infant relationship could have long-term effects on offspring development. Clearly, it is difficult to develop appropriate control procedures for postnatal alcohol exposure, regardless of the method of alcohol administration. Although alcohol undoubtedly can have direct effects on the neonate [e.g., enough alcohol can be consumed via breast milk for the development of tolerance (Abel 1974)], one must be careful to differentiate the effects of alcohol from effects that are secondary to undernutrition.

CROSS-FOSTERING

Cross-fostering or surrogate-fostering is a procedure that minimizes the confounding of pre- and postnatal factors and thus enables the investigator to begin to separate direct effects of alcohol on the offspring from indirect effects that may occur through persistent alterations in maternal behavior or responsiveness.

There has been some controversy over the need to cross-foster offspring at birth. Several studies have argued strongly that cross-fostering is essential to avoid the confounding of alcohol effects with the aftereffects of drug treatment on maternal behavior (e.g., Abel 1978; Abel and Dintcheff 1978), whereas others have demonstrated that cross-fostering does not significantly affect the results. For example, using a complete fostering/cross-fostering design, Osborne, Caul, and Fernandez (1980) showed that neither the fostering procedure nor postweaning rearing conditions had any influence on the effects of prenatal ethanol on offspring growth, viability, or behavior. Similarly, Martin et al. (1978) showed that hyperactivity resulting from prenatal ethanol exposure was not attenuated by cross-fostering. In both of these studies, ethanol was administered to females by intubation. In a recent review of data using the liquid diet model, Abel (1982) also concluded that the pup and not the mother was primarily responsible for the residual effects of ethanol on mother-offspring interactions and therefore suggested that surrogate-fostering is not an important procedure for minimizing residual effects of ethanol exposure during pregnancy.

Nevertheless, Weinberg, Nelson, and Taylor (1986) suggested that one cannot dismiss the issue of cross-fostering. The mother-pup interaction is complex. Subtle changes in the mother-pup interaction that might not be detected in standard tests could still influence offspring development. Similarly, residual effects of alcohol on the dam might influence only certain aspects of development, and it might not be possible to predict those aspects that would be most affected. If an investigator is following a procedure in which cross-fostering has already been shown to have no effect on outcome, then this procedure can be eliminated from the experimental design. If, however, there is any doubt as to whether the prenatal manipulation might produce long-lasting effects on the dam, cross-fostering should be considered as an additional control procedure in the experimental design.

The Lactation Postnatal Period

Treatment of the rat mother during the lactation period is one way to treat the rat pup postnatally. Although this approach is sometimes used, results may be confounded because of the interaction of alcohol and nutrition, as discussed previously. An alternative is to administer the study substance to the preweaning animal directly by injection or intubation.

METHODOLOGICAL ISSUES

As noted, the early postnatal period in the rat is equivalent to the third trimester of pregnancy in the human in that it is the period when the brain is particularly vulnerable to drugs (i.e., the brain growth spurt period). Thus, direct treatment of the rat pup can be used to examine "third-trimester-equivalent" effects of drugs. As with administration models in the prenatal rat, however, there are advantages as well as disadvantages to the use of the postnatal approach.

Known Drug Dose.   One advantage of postnatal treatment of the animal is that it permits known doses of drugs to be administered directly to the developing organism. Amounts in the bloodstream can be verified through appropriate measurement techniques.

Nutritional Control.   One of the confounding factors in animal models of drug abuse, in both prenatal and postnatal exposure paradigms, may be malnutrition or undernutrition, as discussed earlier. In postnatal administration procedures, however, this problem can be overcome by giving the drug to the rat pup in a nutriment solution. This tactic allows the body weight of the drug-treated animal to be maintained so as to be comparable to that of its littermates.

Aberrant Maternal Behavior.   Administration of drugs to the pregnant female during the prenatal period may produce aberrant maternal behavior; this difficulty can be eliminated or evaluated by cross-fostering the rat pups at birth, as discussed previously. Administration of drugs directly to the offspring after birth, however, may also alter maternal behavior and/or the mother-pup interaction. In some forms of postnatal administration models, the pup remains with its mother except during the treatment period. In others the pup is kept in an isolated, environmentally regulated condition. Unfortunately, there are problems of methodological confounding with either of these approaches, as discussed below.

Handling.   Direct treatment of the rat pup requires that it be removed from the mother and handled briefly during treatment; the number of times that it is handled depends upon the procedure used. Handling/disturbance effects may be minimized in the treatment protocols by keeping the treatment periods as brief as possible and by keeping the pups in a warm huddle. The consequences of handling may be partially evaluated in postnatal administration studies through the use of handled but not treated same-sex controls and unhandled controls from same-sized litters not disturbed during the preweaning period.

In one study, for example, it was shown that preweaning handling not only influenced development, but also interacted differentially with prenatal drug exposure (Weinberg and Gallo 1982). In that study, one-half of the litters from each prenatally ethanol-fed, pair-fed, and control group were part of a study on neuromotor development (Gallo and Weinberg 1982) and were therefore handled and tested daily from day 2 of age until weaning. Pups in the remaining litters were completely undisturbed until weaning at 21 days of age. At 39 days of age, all animals showed a significant corticoid elevation in response to ether stress, although handled animals exhibited higher corticosterone levels overall than did nonhandled animals. In addition, however, fetal ethanol-exposed animals subjected to preweaning handling showed a significant sex difference in their corticoid response to stress; females had higher corticosterone levels than had males. Thus, preweaning handling differentially affected the corticoid response of ethanol-exposed males and females but not of animals in pair-fed and control groups.

Other studies have also shown interactive effects of early handling and early dietary treatment on both the behavioral and physiological development of offspring. For example, malnourished pups handled during the preweaning period exhibit higher basal levels of corticosterone than do nonhandled malnourished pups (Wiener and Levine 1978). Similarly, handling can attenuate or eliminate behavioral deficits produced both by early malnutrition (Cines and Winick 1979; Levitsky and Barnes 1972) and prenatal ethanol exposure (Gallo and Weinberg 1982). Preweaning handling is often inadvertently introduced into developmental studies during routine procedures such as weighing or cage cleaning. The data reviewed here clearly indicate that the investigator should take this variable into account in the design of any study on development.

Isolation.   In some postnatal administration models, pups remain with their mothers except during brief treatment periods; in others to be discussed subsequently, however, the pup is maintained in a regulated environment away from its mother. Studies conducted on rats reared in isolation from the mother have shown profound effects on adult behavior [e.g., males exhibited impaired copulatory behavior (Gruendel and Arnold 1969)]. Effects on adult behavior have also been demonstrated in litters where the mother was disturbed, as by removal of the pups (Levine and Thoman 1968). Again, such effects should be evaluated through the use of same-sex, unhandled controls from litters not disturbed before weaning.

ADMINISTRATION PROCEDURES

Several types of postnatal administration models have been reported in the literature. The major differences among them are the type of alcohol/drug administration procedure used and the system used to maintain the animal.

Injection. One widely used method is to inject a drug solution once or twice daily for a designated period. Typically, pups are kept with the mother except during the short time when they are weighed and receive injections. The injection procedure permits littermate controls to receive injections of the vehicle or to be handled. It is also possible to use a treatment protocol that allows the animal to develop tolerance to higher doses of drugs. Graduated doses can also be used to minimize withdrawal effects. In addition, doses can be varied from the minimal dose necessary to produce effects to those just below toxicity. Treatment periods can be adjusted to maximize effects on the development of a particular physiological system. With some drugs, if the doses are high enough, the animals will lose weight as there are periods when they do not suckle because of the drug treatment. In some instances these effects may be counteracted by intubating the animal with a nutriment solution. In other instances, the undernutrition effects may be evaluated by using a pair-underfed control. In this procedure, a same-sex littermate is placed with a nonlactating female for a period sufficient to match its body weight with that of the same-sex, drug-treated littermate (Sonderegger et al. 1984).

Morphine is one of the drugs with which this procedure has been used. In one study, Sonderegger and Zimmermann (1978) injected morphine subcutaneously into female rat pups either on days 3–12 (maximum dose, 8 mg/kg) or on days 12–21 (maximum dose, 16 mg/kg). All animals showed a diminished analgesic response (hot-plate test) on day 156. In addition, animals treated during days 3–12 but not those treated during days 12–21 showed impaired learning of a conditioned emotional response on days 90–95. In another study (Zimmermann, Sonderegger, and Bromley 1977), female rat pups were given morphine injections during postnatal weeks 1, 2, or 3. Animals that received injections during week 3 showed impaired activity in the open field and an impaired corticosterone rise in response to a morphine challenge on day 62.

Other laboratories have used the postnatal injection technique to study naltrexone (Paul, Diaz, and Bailey 1978), phenobarbital (Diaz and

Schain 1978; Diaz 1983), and, more recently, cocaine (Dow-Edwards, Freed, and Milhorat 1988). The work on phenobarbital is of particular interest as barbiturates have been prescribed in pregnancy as an antiseizure medication. Diaz and Schain (1978) gave two doses of phenobarbital daily for two weeks to infant rats. They found increased responses to novel stimuli and dose-dependent reductions in brain growth. Diaz (1983) found that phenobarbital (either 15 or 60 mg/kg) injected as late as postnatal days 25–39 affected brain growth. This latter finding suggests that brain growth may be vulnerable to disruption even in late stages and that barbiturates may constitute a threat to normal brain growth.

Animal studies with cocaine are also of great importance. Infants damaged by cocaine have appeared in clinics in many large cities (see chapter 7), but relatively little is known about the long-term effects of this insult. Dow-Edwards, Freed, and Milhorat (1988) injected doses of cocaine of up to 50 mg/kg into pregnant female rats on prenatal days 6–20 or pups on postnatal days 1–10 and reported changes in glucose utilization in the limbic system of the females. The authors felt that these findings could reflect an imbalance of the dopaminergic pathways.

From these studies, it can be concluded that postnatal administration of drugs such as morphine, naltrexone, phenobarbital, and cocaine can produce immediate as well as persistent effects ranging from impaired neuroendocrine and behavioral responses to altered brain growth or neurochemical changes as adults.

Pellet Implantation.   To reduce handling, one can implant slow-release drug pellets or placebos subcutaneously on the flank of a lightly anesthetized rat pup. Except for the brief implantation procedure, the pup remains with its littermates, some of which will serve as untreated controls. This method has proven effective in studying the effects of morphine (pellets implanted on postnatal days 5 or 11) on adult behaviors in female rats (Sonderegger, O'Shea, and Zimmermann 1979). Activity measures (open-field test) did not differentiate among the treatment groups, but morphine-treated females showed impaired learning as adults on the Lashley III maze. Although resting plasma corticosterone levels were comparable, morphine-treated animals showed altered neuroendocrine functioning as evidenced by impaired ether stress-induced elevations of corticosterone on day 239 and a diminished steroid response to a challenge dose of morphine (30 mg/kg) on day 301. Similar results were obtained in a later study using male rats (Sonderegger, Bromley, and Zimmermann 1977; Sonderegger, O'Shea, and Zimmermann 1980).

In a third study, groups of females that had received implants of morphine pellets on day 5 or 11 of age were bred with non-drug-treated males (Zimmermann and Sonderegger 1980). The reproductive capacity of these animals did not seem to be affected; neither litter sizes, sex ratios, nor birth weights differed among the groups except for six pups, to be described later. By day 28, however, untreated offspring of morphine-treated mothers weighed less than littermate controls. On day 67, offspring of day 5- but not day 11-implanted animals seemed more sensitive to the effects of morphine in the hot plate test for analgesia. Untreated offspring of the day 11 morphine-treated animals showed protracted tolerance to the pituitary-adrenal stimulating effects of a challenge dose of morphine (30 mg/kg). The other six pups showed a striking syndrome of growth, sensory, and motor defects. They lacked pain sensation and fine motor control.

In general, findings from the postnatal pellet administration models show that exposure of the developing organism to morphine during the brain growth spurt period produces differential long-term effects upon behavior and pituitary-adrenal responses. They also serve to illustrate the complexity of the data obtained in many studies of postnatal drug exposure.

Artificial Rearing-Intragastric Feeding.   The problems encountered in exposing neonates to ethanol by feeding the ethanol to lactating dams have been discussed above. To avoid these confounding factors and to gain control over the alcohol dose that gets into the pup, as well as the pup's caloric intake, one team of researchers (Diaz and Samson 1980) developed a postnatal administration procedure in which pups receive implants of intragastric cannulae. After the gastrostomy feeding tubes are implanted, the pups are reared individually in plastic cups containing bedding. The cups are floated in an aquarium filled with aerated heated water (40°C), and the area above the aquarium is enclosed with a vented cover to maintain constant levels of temperature and humidity. Pups are fed a milk formula containing ethanol or an isocaloric amount of maltose-dextrin via timer-controlled infusion pumps. Pups are typically handled at least twice daily and gently stroked to stimulate urination and defecation. In addition, both gastrostomy and suckle control groups are reared simultaneously for comparison purposes. Artificial rearing allows good control over the alcohol dose, the timing of administration, and nutrition. One possible drawback of this procedure, however, is that pups are reared for a significant part of the preweaning period without the presence of littermates and normal maternal care. Work by Gruendel and Arnold (1969), for example, has shown that male pups reared in isolation from their mother exhibit atypical sexual behavior as adults. Furthermore, one must be aware that, like the interaction of alcohol and nutrition, there may be an interaction of alcohol and isolation rearing which cannot be fully controlled, even with the inclusion of appropriate control groups.

A few examples of the utility of the artificial rearing procedure follow. Grant, Choi, and Samson (1983) used the artificial rearing technique developed by Diaz and Sampson (1980) to give ethanol to animals on postnatal days 4–18; pups were then given ad libitum access to food. Body weights of these animals were comparable to those of littermates left with their mothers. At 30 days of age, no differences between drug-exposed animals and controls were found on a battery of behavioral tasks except that ethanol-exposed female rats showed increased activity compared to controls in the open field. Examination of brain growth parameters indicated that ethanol-treated males did not differ from controls on any measure of growth. Brains of ethanol-treated females, however, continued to show microcephaly, with the most severe effects on the cerebellum. In a second study, these same investigators found that an ethanol dose of at least 6 g/kg was required to produce reduced brain weights in animals exposed on postnatal days 5, 6, 7, and 8; blood alcohol concentrations (BACs) below 100 mg/100 ml failed to result in significant brain weight reductions (Samson and Grant 1984).

Pierce and West (1987) used this artificial rearing technique to administer ethanol (9.8 g/kg/day) or isocaloric maltose/dextrin to rat pups on postnatal days 4–10. BACs reached 345.8 mg/dl on postnatal day 10. At that time, body weights of treated animals and controls did not differ significantly, but a 30% reduction in brain growth was found in the ethanol-exposed animals. Researchers also found growth deficits in specific brain regions, including the sublaminae within the hippocampus, the midsagittal (vermal) cerebellum, and the dentate gyrus (West, Hamre, and Cassell 1985). These data suggested that most regions of the brain are not affected equally by alcohol exposure during the brain growth spurt period. Phillips and Harper (1987) used the Sampson and

Diaz model and fed ethanol to rat pups on postnatal days 5–9. They found that the overall cortex was decreased to 80% of that of controls.

One very important finding that has emerged from the work of Dr. James West and co-workers using this artificial rearing procedure concerns the effects of bingeing or concentrated alcohol exposure on brain growth (Bonthius and West 1990; Bonthius, Goodlett, and West 1988; Pierce and West 1986). Studies from this laboratory have demonstrated that the peak BAC is a reliable predictor of the severity of alcohol-induced microencephaly and behavioral dysfunction; that is, the severity of microencephaly increased in a dose-dependent manner with increasing BACs. Importantly, peak BACs seem to be a function not only of the dose of ethanol infused into the pup but also of the rate of infusion. Thus, exposure to a given volume of ethanol over a short period can produce higher maximum BACs than exposure to an equal or even larger dose over a longer period. Using the artificial rearing procedure, Bonthius and West (1990) exposed two groups of pups (postnatal days 4–10) to an ethanol dose of 4.5 g/kg/day, administered either as a 10.2% ethanol solution in 2 of the 12 daily feedings or as a 5.1% ethanol solution in 4 of the 12 daily feedings. A third group received a higher dose of ethanol (6.6 g/kg/day), administered as a 2.5% ethanol solution in each of the 12 daily feedings. The smaller ethanol dose (4.5 g/kg/day) concentrated into 2 or 4 consecutive daily feedings induced more severe microencephaly and greater cell loss than the larger (6.6 g/kg/day) dose administered in equal fractions throughout the day. The more concentrated the dose, the more severe the damage. The authors emphasized the important clinical implications of these data: binge alcohol consumption is particularly injurious to the offspring because it lowers the minimum dose of alcohol necessary to induce alcohol teratogenicity.

Results from studies using the artificial rearing procedure clearly allow the effects of the drug administered during the postnatal period to be separated from those of underfeeding and have demonstrated marked changes in brain growth and in various brain structures that are specific to ethanol. This procedure has also enabled investigators to examine dose-dependent effects of alcohol during the "third-trimester-equivalent" period of brain development (postnatal days 1–10 in the rat, which is equivalent to the third trimester of human pregnancy) and to begin to understand the relationship between blood alcohol level and alcohol teratogenicity.

Intragastric Intubation. Another way to administer drugs, particularly alcohol, has been through intubation. In this procedure, rat pups have been given known quantities of ethanol in a nutriment vehicle (Sustagen, Mead Johnson). Gastric intubation is accomplished through a piece of Silastic tubing attached to a hypodermic syringe. In an initial study of animals intubated intragastrically with ethanol (0.8, 1.2, or 2.0 g/kg of ethanol [20% w/v] on days 2–8), body weights of the drug-treated animals were comparable to those of vehicle-treated animals (Sonderegger et al. 1982). Pups were kept in a warm huddle except during the minute or so taken to weigh and intubate them; they were then returned immediately to the mother. On day 8, BACs were determined 30 minutes or 4 hours after intubation of a challenge dose of 2 g/kg ethanol. After 30 minutes, BACs of both control and ethanol-treated animals were elevated; after 4 hours only the BACs of the control group had fallen significantly. This procedure thus provides a technique whereby one can separate the effects of a drug from the confounding effects of underfeeding.

These findings were substantially verified by data collected in another laboratory (Serbus, Young, and Light 1986). Animals given single or multiple intubations of 3.0 or 3.6 g/kg of ethanol in a 20% Sustacal (Mead Johnson) vehicle were found to have high BACs for up to four hours after intubations. The BACs were dose dependent and reduced by repeated ethanol exposure, and body weights were not compromised, supporting the viability of the procedure for postnatal administration studies.

Doses of ethanol as high as 5 g/kg on days 2–6 can be tolerated by rat pups; at these doses, however, body weight impairment occurs and mortality rate increases (40%). A higher dose of 7 g/kg produces a 100% mortality (Sonderegger et al. 1982). These findings are compatible with those of Abel and Dintcheff (1978), who found that ethanol doses of 4 to 6 g/kg/day to pregnant rats (producing peak BACs of 150 and 270 mg/100 ml, respectively, which are equivalent to those produced by 5–10 drinks consumed by a 64-kg woman in one hour) significantly reduced pup body weight at birth and increased postnatal mortality.

Postnatal ethanol exposure via intragastric intubation has also been shown to have long-term effects on behavior. In male pups ethanol was intubated on postnatal days 1–8, reaching a peak dose of 4 g/kg on days 4–5 (Sonderegger et al. 1984). Vehicle-intubated (isocaloric Sustagen), handled and nonhandled controls were included. Body weights did not differ at weaning (day 21) nor on day 150 when activity was tested in an open field. Ethanol-treated animals exhibited less activity (total squares entered) and longer start latencies than other groups.

As discussed earlier, handling rat pups during the preweaning period affects adult behaviors, including open-field activity. Dennenberg and Zarrow (1971) found that adult male rats handled during the preweaning period had lower open-field activity on test day 1 and higher activity on test days 2–4; the reverse pattern was found for the nonhandled animals (i.e., they were more active on test day 1 and less active on days 2–4). The nonhandled animals in the ethanol intubation study discussed above behaved as did the nonhandled animals in the Dennenberg and Zarrow study, showing decreasing activity from day 1 to days 2–4. Ethanol-treated animals showed lower activity on day 1, which would be characteristic of handled animals, but their activity scores declined on the succeeding test days rather than increasing, as happened with the handled (non-drug-exposed) animals in the Dennenberg and Zarrow study. Thus, the behavior of the ethanol-treated animals was similar to that of the nonhandled animals but at a lower level. Although handling may have masked some of the drug effects, the ethanol group clearly displayed a lower activity level. Findings of lowered activity in adult animals as a consequence of ethanol treatment have also been reported in other laboratories (Abel 1989).

Meaney et al. (1987) found that postnatal handling attenuated age-related changes in the adrenocortical stress response and spatial memory in the rat. One implication of these findings is that handling reduces any obtained adrenocortical responses so that the actual effects are possibly much greater than the measured changes.

Burns and co-workers (1986) used a slightly different gavage procedure to treat four groups of animals: (1) ethanol (4 g/kg), with two doses three hours apart on days 6–16; (2) ethanol (4 g/kg) on day 6 only; (3) isocaloric milk; (4) handled only. Significant differences in whole brain weights, a disproportionately decreased cerebellar weight, altered balancing ability, and a decreased number of cerebellar cells were observed on days 17 and 70 in both ethanol-treated groups compared to controls. The researchers concluded that episodic exposure to ethanol during the brain growth spurt period could be as devastating to brain development as chronic exposure during that period.

Inhalation.   When it is feasible, the postnatal pup may also be treated through inhalation procedures. Bauer-Moffett and Altman (1977) treated rats on postnatal days 3–20 with ethanol vapor to produce BACs of 268 mg/100 ml. Cerebellar weights and number of Purkinje cells were reduced up to 90 days of age. Body weights did not differ from those of controls.

In general, these studies show that exposure of rat neonates to alcohol during the brain growth spurt period, when undernutrition is controlled, produces dose-dependent changes in activity and possible changes in brain weights and numbers of cerebellar cells. Breeding capabilities of the females do not seem to be unequivocally affected. Differences in behavior and growth, however, have been found in some instances in the untreated progeny.

Behavior-dependent Variables

A broad array of dependent variables may be used to monitor behavioral changes that occur as a consequence of exposure to drugs early in life. Some of these have already been described in the studies discussed in this chapter.

Careful consideration must be given to the selection of tests for assessment of behavioral or developmental changes that are appropriate for the age of the animal at the time of testing. Further, one should recognize that an effect may change over time (e.g., drug-exposed animals may be hyperactive compared to controls before early adulthood but not thereafter). It must also be recognized that a single behavioral test may not be sensitive to all drug-induced effects, so a battery of tests may be required. For the young rodent, developmental indices such as pinna unfolding, incisor tooth eruption, or time of eye opening may be affected by drug exposure early in life. Altman and Sudarshan (1975) provided one battery of tests that are sensitive to drug exposure effects in the young rodent. These tests include such measures as rivoting behavior, negative geotaxis or movement on an inclined plane, ability to ascend a wire mesh ladder, ability to support body weight by hindlimbs when suspended by forepaws on a wire rod, and ability to balance and/or walk on a slowly revolving rod. For older animals, the time of onset of puberty as well as reproductive behaviors have been studied. Other measures used for older animals include learning ability using either appetitive or aversive stimuli and performance in tasks involving classical conditioning, operant conditioning, active avoidance learning, passive avoidance learning, and a variety of discrimination tasks. Measurement of conditioned emotional responses may also provide a useful indicator of drug effects. Changes in the ability to habituate to repetitive stimulation, particularly auditory startle responses, have also been used. In addition, a variety of activity measures have been employed, ranging from a study of behaviors that result from placing an animal in an open arena (open-field testing) to exploratory activity observed when an animal is placed in a wooden box with holes in the floor and the animal dips its head to explore the holes.

For a discussion of additional measures and other methodological issues, the reader is referred to an excellent chapter on the subject by Jane Adams (1986). She pointed out that, when little information is available about the compound to be tested, there are test batteries to satisfy both scientific and regulatory needs. These batteries include assessments of growth and development, sensory functions, learning abilities, and activity levels. One attempt to develop a screening battery of tests which produce comparable results although administered in different laboratories was developed as a consequence of a National Center for Toxicology Research collaborative study involving several laboratories. For the interested reader, a complete discussion of the project may be found in a special issue of *Neurobehavioral Toxicology and Teratology* edited by Buelke-Sam, Kimmel, and Adams (1985).

The Differential Effects of Perinatal Alcohol/Drug Exposure on Males and Females

Data from many recent studies suggest that perinatal insults may affect male and female offspring differently. An increased vulnerability to perinatal drug effects or, conversely, an increased protection from perinatal drug effects in one sex versus the other is potentially important in terms of understanding the mechanism of action of teratogenic drugs. The following chapter provides a detailed review of data demonstrating differential effects of drugs on male and female offspring body weight, brain growth and development, sexual differentiation, hormonal responsiveness, sexual behavior, and a number of nonreproductive behaviors.

IN VITRO RESEARCH

The material in this chapter thus far has dealt primarily with procedural considerations for animal research. This direction has been followed primarily because of the authors' familiarity with these issues through their own research.

It should be emphasized, however, that procedures other than research with live animals can also be used effectively to obtain information about the effects of drugs and alcohol on the developing organism. Clearly, in vitro techniques such as cell culture or computer simulation cannot provide the same information as that obtained in the whole animal; for example, they cannot provide data on behavioral changes reflecting damage to one or more developing physiological systems in drug-exposed animals. However, these methodological approaches can provide insights into mechanism(s) of toxicity as well as other valuable information that cannot be obtained through work with live animals. A complete picture of the broad array of drug-exposure effects would best be obtained by a combination of information from in vivo, ex vivo, and in vitro approaches. In practice, however, many scientists have only the facilities to focus on work either in vivo or in vitro.

It is beyond the scope of this book to review all of the methodological issues associated with in vitro research, but the reader should be alerted to the fact that some of the most exciting and valuable information on drug-induced changes is coming from cell culture work. Ornoy and Zusman (1984) pointed out that in vitro whole embryo cultures are free of metabolic changes caused by maternal metabolism or placental modification and in many ways are superior for studies of teratogenic action. These same authors, however, also cautioned that embryonic cell investigations are limited to the time periods when the embryos can be kept in a cultured state, which may preclude the study of drug effects on later developmental periods of the brain. Such cell culture work on early developmental stages, however, may provide clues to effects on the brain at later developmental stages. Shuster (1989), for example, observed that the addition of morphine to cultured embryonic chick brain cells increased the activity of two enzymes, acetyltransferase and acetylcholinesterase. These observations, along with other information of this type, led him to conclude that morphine could affect the developing neuronal cells and led to subsequent experiments with young rodents.

HUMAN STUDIES

Studies of human pregnancy and teratogens are hampered by numerous methodological issues that make the results vulnerable to criticism. This is especially true when one attempts to evaluate the effect of maternal use of licit or illicit drugs on pregnancy and neonatal outcome. Examination of several studies of cocaine use in pregnancy gives examples of the problems that arise.

The first difficulty arises when researchers attempt simply to identify the drug they wish to study. Polydrug use is the most common form of drug use in the United States. Numerous studies focus on only cocaine, for example, and do not allow for the effects of tobacco, alcohol, marijuana, or multiple other drugs the woman may be combining with her cocaine. A study may purport to focus on the influence of cocaine on pregnancy outcome, but the women under study may actually be heroin-addicted, methadone-maintained women who also used cocaine.

The purity and concentration of cocaine is a factor that cannot be included in the analysis of outcome measures. These characteristics of cocaine vary from city to city and can change within a particular geographic area over the course of a woman's pregnancy. Thus, the dose/response relationship of cocaine to pregnancy outcome cannot be accurately assessed. In addition, the effect of biologically active contaminants that may be present in cocaine bought on the street has never been assessed.

Patterns of cocaine use, including dosage, route of use, and timing, are another aspect difficult to assess in the human population. Few users of cocaine can reliably estimate the amount of cocaine they have used. The route of administration of the drug can alter the biological effect on both the mother and the fetus. Cocaine can be used by inhalation, intravenously, or intranasally; however, no studies have specifically addressed this issue. Timing of use is more easily assessed but is accurate only if this assessment is ongoing throughout the pregnancy. Reliance on maternal recall at the time of delivery impedes any real estimate of drug use patterns. This becomes especially important when investigators have used a single urine toxicological analysis at the time of delivery or maternal recall history to separate cocaine-using women from non-drug-using women (Bingol et al. 1987; Oro and Dixon 1987; Chouteau, Namerow, and Leppert 1988; Cherukuri et al. 1988; Little et al. 1989). It is most probable that cocaine-using women were included in the drug-free comparison group because of the women's inaccurate denial of drug use and/or a negative urine toxicological analysis at the time of delivery, which accounts for drug use only during the 48 to 72 hours before testing. This major flaw hampers multiple studies.

The environment in which a woman is living before and during her pregnancy will also have an important influence on pregnancy outcome. Although some groups (Chasnoff, Burns, and Burns 1987; Chasnoff et al. 1985, 1989; MacGregor et al. 1987; Bingol et al. 1987; Ryan, Ehrlich, and Finnegan 1987; Little et al. 1989; Zuckerman et al. 1989) utilized as controls women from the same obstetric population as their study group to reflect a similar socioeconomic background, these investigators could not control for factors related to living in a drug-seeking environment: violence, poor nutrition, inadequate prenatal care, impaired health, homelessness, and a host of other issues.

Finally, the genetic makeup of the woman and of the fetus and the efficiency at which each may metabolize and excrete cocaine is another area that could have a profound influence on pregnancy and neonatal outcome. However, researchers are not even close to understanding these issues. Thus, current debates regarding "threshold" amounts of cocaine which can affect outcome are futile, since individual fetal susceptibility is an important yet unpredictable factor in the outcome of the fetus exposed in utero to cocaine.

Although studies of human pregnancy are fraught with many of the methodological issues discussed, consistent patterns of outcome have begun to emerge. These patterns can guide researchers and clinicians in the development of further studies that can address some of the important issues remaining in the understanding of the effect of cocaine and other drugs on pregnancy and neonatal outcome.

SUMMARY AND CONCLUSIONS

In this chapter we have reviewed the methodological issues critical in animal experimentation as well as many of the experimental strategies used to investigate the consequences of exposing the immature organism to alcohol/drugs. The advantages and disadvantages of a variety of drug administration strategies used during the prenatal, perinatal, or postnatal periods were discussed. Nutritional issues that frequently confound interpretation of the results of research with both animals and humans were reviewed in detail, and the limitations inherent in the development of appropriate nutritional control groups were described. Finally, some of the critical methodological issues in drug research with human subjects were discussed. This latter discussion described the many complex and confounding variables that may influence the interpretation of results from human studies and further highlight the need for animal models in which variables can be more tightly controlled.

This review of methodological issues and experimental findings makes it clear that, although most adverse effects of drugs on offspring seem to be due to the drugs themselves and not to other factors, these other factors may interact with and/or modify drug effects. This review also makes clear the complex nature both of the data collected and the data-collecting procedures. It is apparent that the information is far from complete and that many major scientific questions remain to be answered.

REFERENCES

Abel, E. L. 1974. Alcohol ingestion in lactating rats: Effects on mothers and offspring. *Arch Int Pharmacodyn* 210:121–27.

———. 1975. Emotionality in offspring of rats fed alcohol while nursing. *J Stud Alcohol* 36:654–58.

———. 1978. Effects of ethanol on pregnant rats and their offspring. *Psychopharmacology (Berlin)* 57:5–11.

———. 1980. Procedural considerations in evaluating prenatal effects of alcohol in animals. *Neurobehav Toxicol* 2:167–74.

———. 1982. In utero alcohol exposure and development delay of response inhibition. *Alcohol Clin Exp Res* 6:369–76.

———. 1984. *Fetal Alcohol Syndrome and Fetal Alcohol Effects*. New York: Plenum Press.

———. 1989. Paternal and maternal alcohol consumption: Effects on offspring in two strains of rats. *Alcohol Clin Exp Res* 13:533–41.

Abel, E. L., and Dintcheff, B. A. 1978. Effects of prenatal alcohol exposure on growth and development in rats. *J Pharmacol Exp Ther* 207:916–21.

Abel, E. L., and Tan, S. E. 1988. Effects of paternal alcohol consumption on pregnancy outcome in rats. *Neurotoxicol Teratol* 10:187–93.

Adams, J. 1986. Methods in behavioral teratology. In *Handbook of Behavioral Teratology*, ed. E. Riley and C. Vorhees, 49–67. New York: Plenum Press.

Altman, J., and Sudarshan, K. 1975. Postnatal development of locomotion in the developing rat. *Anim Behav* 23: 896–920.

Archer, J. E., and Blackman, D. E. 1971. Prenatal psychological stress and offspring behavior in rats and mice. *Dev Psychobiol* 4:193–248.

Barlow, S. M., Knight, A. F., and Sullivan, F. M. 1978. Delay in postnatal growth and development of offspring produced by maternal restraint stress during pregnancy in the rat. *Teratology* 18:211–18.

Bauer-Moffett, C., and Altman, J. 1977. The effect of ethanol chronically administered to preweanling rats on cerebellar development: A morphological study. *Brain Res* 119:249–68.

Bingol, N., Fuchs, M., Diaz, V., Stone, R. K., and Gromisch, D. S. 1987. Teratogenicity of cocaine in humans. *J Pediatr* 110:93–96.

Bond, N. W. 1979. Effects of postnatal alcohol exposure on maternal nesting behavior in the rat. *Physiol Psychol* 7:396–98.

Bonthius, D. J., Goodlett, C. R., and West, J. R. 1988. Blood alcohol concentration and severity of microencephaly in neonatal rats depend on the pattern of alcohol administration. *Alcohol* 5:209–14.

Bonthius, D. J., and West, J. R. 1990. Alcohol-induced neuronal loss in developing rats: Increased brain damage with binge exposure. *Alcohol Clin Exp Res* 14:107–18.

Buelke-Sam, J., Kimmel, A. C., and Adams, J. 1985. Design considerations in screening for behavioral teratogens: Results of the collaborative behavior teratology study. *Neurobehav Toxicol Teratol* 7:537–793.

Burns, E. M., Kruckeberg, M., Kanak, F., and Stibler, H. 1986. Ethanol exposure during brain ontogeny: Some long-term effects. *Neurobehav Toxicol Teratol* 8:383–91.

Chasnoff, I. J., Burns, K. A., and Burns, W. J. 1987. Cocaine use in pregnancy: Perinatal morbidity and mortality. *Neurotoxicol Teratol* 9:291–93.

Chasnoff, I. J., Burns, W. J., Schnoll, S. H., and Burns, K. A. 1985. Cocaine use in pregnancy. *N Engl J Med* 313:666–69.

Chasnoff, I. J., Griffiths, D. R., MacGregor, S., Dirkes, K., and Burns, K. 1989. Temporal patterns of cocaine use in pregnancy. *JAMA* 261:1741–44.

Cherukuri, R., Minkoff, H., Feldman, J., Parekh, A., and Glass, L. 1988. A cohort study of alkaloidal cocaine ("crack") in pregnancy. *Obstet Gynecol* 72:147–51.

Chouteau, M., Nemerow, P. B., and Leppert, P. 1988. The effect of cocaine abuse on birth weight and gestational age. *Obstet Gynecol* 72:351–54.

Church, A. C., Fuller, J. L., and Dann, L. 1979. Alcohol intake in selected lines of mice: Importance of sex and genotype. *J Comp Physiol Psychol* 93:242–46.

Cines, B. M., and Winick, M. 1979. Behavioral and physiological effects of early handling and early malnutrition in rats. *Dev Psychobiol* 12:381–89.

Coyle, I., Wayner, M. J., and Singer, G. 1976. Behavioral teratogenesis: A critical evaluation. *Pharmacol Biochem Behav* 4:191–200.

DaSilva, V. A., Ribeiro, M. J., and Masur, J. 1980. Developmental, behavioral and pharmacological characteristics of rat offspring from mothers receiving ethanol during gestation or lactation. *Dev Psychobiol* 13:653–60.

Dennenberg, V. H., and Zarrow, M. X. 1971. Effects of handling in infancy upon adult behavior and adrenocortical activity: Suggestions for a neuroendocrine mechanism. In *The Development of Self-Regulatory Mechanisms*, ed. D. Walcher and D. Peters, 39–71. New York: Academic Press.

Dexter, J. D., Tumbleson, M. E., Decker, J. C., and Middleton, C. C. 1980. Fetal alcohol syndrome in Sinclair (S-1) miniature swine. *Alcohol Clin Exp Res* 4:146–51.

Diaz, J. 1983. Disruption of the brain growth spurt in adolescent rats by chronic phenobarbital administration. *Exp Neurol* 79:559–63.

Diaz, J., and Samson, H. H. 1980. Impaired brain growth in neonatal rats exposed to ethanol. *Science* 208:751–53.

Diaz, J., and Schain, R. J. 1978. Effects of long-term administration of phenobarbital on behavior and brain of artificially reared rats. *Science* 199:90–91.

Dobbing, J. 1974. The later growth of the brain and its vulnerability. *Pediatrics* 53:2–6.

———. 1976. Vulnerable periods in brain growth and somatic growth. In *The Biology of the Human Fetus*, ed. D. F. Roberts, 137–47. London: Taylor and Francis.

Dobbing, J., and Sands, J. 1979. Comparative aspects of the brain growth spurt. *Early Hum Dev* 3:79–83.

Dow-Edwards, D. L., Freed, L. L., and Milhorat, T. H. 1988. The effects of cocaine on development. *Brain Res* 42:137–41.

Duckett, S., Schneider, C. W., and Harline, R. A. 1981. Liquidation of alcohol in free-moving mice from high and low preference strains. *Pharmacol Biochem Behav* 15:495–99.

Fried, P. A. 1976. Short- and long-term effects of prenatal cannabis inhalation on rat offspring. *Psychopharmacology (Berlin)* 50:285–91.

Friedler, G., Brown, D. R., Wooten, V., and Meadows, M. E. 1987.

Paternal ethanol alters behavior of mouse progeny. *Soc Neurosci Abstr* 13:691.

Fuchs, A. R. 1969. Ethanol and the inhibition of oxytocin released in lactating rats. *Acta Endocrinol (Copenh)* 62:546–54.

Fung, Y. K., and Lau, Y. 1989. Effects of prenatal nicotine exposure on rat striatal dopaminergic and nicotinic systems. *Pharmacol Biochem Behav* 33:1–6.

Gallo, P. V., and Weinberg, J. 1981. Corticosterone rhythmicity in the rat: Interactive effects of dietary restriction and schedule of feeding. *J Nutr* 111:208–18.

———. 1982. Neuromotor development and response inhibition following prenatal ethanol exposure. *Neurobehav Toxicol Teratol* 4:505–13.

———. 1986. Organ growth and cellular development in ethanol-exposed rats. *Alcohol* 3:261–67.

Grant, K. A., Choi, E. Y., and Samson, H. H. 1983. Neonatal ethanol exposure: Effects on adult behavior and brain growth parameters. *Pharmacol Biochem Behav* 18(Suppl 1):331–36.

Gruendel, A. D., and Arnold, W. J. 1969. Effects of early social deprivation on reproductive behavior of male rats. *J Comp Physiol Psychol* 67:123–28.

Herrenkohl, L. R. 1979. Prenatal stress reduces fertility and fecundity in female offspring. *Science* 206:1097–99.

Hill, L. G. J., and Means, L. W. 1982. Effects of alcohol consumption during pregnancy on subsequent maternal behavior in rats. *Pharmacol Biochem Behav* 17:125–29.

Joffee, T. J., Peterson, J. M., Smith, D. J., and Soyka, L. F. 1976. Sublethal effects in offspring of male rats treated with methadone before mating. *Res Commun Chem Pathol Pharmacol* 13:611–21.

Kesaniemi, Y. A. 1974. Ethanol and acetaldehyde in the milk and peripheral blood of lactating women after ethanol administration. *J Obstet Gynaecol Br Commonw* 81:84–86.

Levine, S., and Thoman, E. B. 1968. Role of maternal disturbance and temperature change in early experience studies. *Physiol Behav* 4:142–45.

Levitsky, D. A., and Barnes, R. H. 1972. Nutritional and environmental interactions in the behavioral development of the rat: Long-term effects. *Science* 176:68–71.

Lieber, C. S. 1979. Alcohol-nutrition interactions. In *NIAAA Monograph 2: Alcohol and Nutrition*, ed. T. K. Li, S. Schenker, and L. Lumeng, 47–63. DHEW Publication (ADM) 79–780. Washington, D.C.: U.S. Government Printing Office.

————. 1982. *Medical Disorders of Alcoholism: Pathogenesis and Treatment.* Philadelphia: Saunders.

Lieber, C. S., and DeCarli, L. M. 1982. The feeding of alcohol in liquid diets: Two decades of applications and 1982 update. *Alcohol Clin Exp Res* 6:523–31.

Little, B. B., Snell, L. M., Klein, V., and Gilstrap, L. 1989. Cocaine abuse during pregnancy: Maternal and fetal implications. *Obstet Gynecol* 73:157–60.

MacGregor, S. N., Keith, L. G., Chasnoff, I. J., Rosner, M. A., Chisum, G. M., Shaw, P., and Minogue, J. P. 1987. Cocaine use during pregnancy: Adverse perinatal outcome. *Am J Obstet Gynecol* 157:686–90.

Martin, J. C., Martin, D. C., Sigman, G., and Radow, B. 1977. Offspring survival, development and operant performance following maternal ethanol consumption. *Dev Psychobiol* 10:435–46.

————. 1978. Maternal ethanol consumption and hyperactivity in cross-fostered offspring. *Physiol Psychol* 6:362–65.

Marwine, A., and Collier, G. 1979. The rat at the waterhole. *J Comp Physiol Psychol* 93:391–402.

Mathews, D., and Jameson, S. 1982. Effects of ethanol consumption on maternal behavior in the female rat. *Physiol Behav* 29:595–97.

Meadows, M. E., Schmidt, J., and Friedler, G. 1987. Paternal ethanol alters side preference in mouse offspring. Paper presented at the International Society for Developmental Psychobiology, New Orleans, La., November 1987.

Meaney, M. J., Aitken, D. H., van Berkel, C., Bhatnagar, S., and Sapolsky, R. M. 1987. Effect of neonatal handling on age-related impairments associated with the hippocampus. *Science* 239:766–68.

Murrin, L. C., Ferrer, J. R., Zeng, W., and Haley, N. J. 1987. Nicotine administration to rats: Methodological considerations. *Life Sci* 40:1699–708.

National Academy of Sciences. 1978. *Nutrient Requirements of Laboratory Animals.* Washington, D.C.: Office of Publications.

Ornoy, A., and Zusman, I. 1984. In vitro embryo cultures as a method for the study of central nervous system malformations. In *Neurobehavioral Teratology*, ed. J. Yanai, 93–107. New York: Elsevier Science Publishers BV.

Oro, A. S., and Dixon, S. D. 1987. Perinatal cocaine and methamphetamine exposure: Maternal and neonatal correlates. *J Pediatr* 111:571–78.

Osborne, G. L., Caul, W. F., and Fernandez, K. 1980. Behavioral effects of prenatal ethanol exposure and differential early experience in rats. *Pharmacol Biochem Behav* 12:393–401.

Paul, L., Diaz, J., and Bailey, B. 1978. Behavioral effects of chronic narcotic antagonist administration to infant rats. *Neuropharmacology* 17:655–57.

Phillips, D. E., and Harper, E. A. 1987. Effects of limited postnatal ethanol on the rat cerebral cortex. *Soc Neurosci Abstr* 13:692.

Pierce, D. R., and West, J. R. 1986. Blood alcohol concentration: A critical factor for producing fetal alcohol effects. *Alcohol* 3:269–72.

———. 1987. Differential deficits in regional brain growth induced by postnatal alcohol. *Neurotoxicol Teratol* 9:129–41.

Rawat, A. K. 1975. Ribosomal protein synthesis in the fetal and neonatal brain as influenced by maternal ethanol consumption. *Res Commun Chem Pathol Pharmacol* 12:723–32.

———. 1976. Effect of maternal ethanol consumption on fetal and neonatal rat hepatic protein synthesis. *Biochem J* 160:653–61.

Riley, E. P., and Meyer, L. S. 1984. Considerations for the design, implementation, and interpretation of animal models of fetal alcohol effects. *Neurobehav Toxicol Teratol* 6:97–101.

Ryan, L., Ehrlich, S., and Finnegan, L. 1987. Cocaine abuse in pregnancy: Effects on the fetus and newborn. *Neurotoxicol Teratol* 9:295–99.

Samson, H. H., and Grant, K. A. 1984. Ethanol-induced microcephaly in neonatal rats: Relation to dose. *Alcohol Clin Exp Res* 8:201–3.

Serbus, D. C., Young, D. W., and Light, K. E. 1986. Ethanol exposure during brain ontogeny: Some long-term effects. *Neurobehav Toxicol Teratol* 8:403–7.

Shuster, L. 1989. Pharmacogenetics of drugs of abuse. In *Prenatal Abuse of Licit and Illicit Drugs*, ed. D. E. Hutchings. *Ann NY Acad Sci* 562:56–74.

Smith, J. C., Jr. 1979. Marginal nutritional states and conditioned deficiencies. In *NIAAA Monograph 2: Alcohol and Nutrition*, ed. T. K. Li, S. Schenker, and L. Lumeng, 23–46. DHEW Publication (ADM) 79–780. Washington, D.C.: U.S. Government Printing Office.

Sonderegger, T. B., Bromley, B., and Zimmermann, E. 1977. Tolerance in adult male rats after early morphine pellet implantation. *Proc West Pharmacol Soc* 20:435–38.

Sonderegger, T. B., Calmes, H., Corbitt, S., Colbern, D., and Simmermann, E. G. 1982. Methodological note: Intragastric intubation of ethanol to rat pups. *Neurobehav Toxicol Teratol* 4:477–83.

Sonderegger, T., O'Shea, S., and Zimmermann, E. 1979. Consequences of neonatal morphine pellet implantation in adult female rats. *Neurobehav Toxicol* 1:161–69.

————. 1980. Protracted effects of neonatal morphine pellet implantation in male rats. *Pharmacol Biochem Behav* 11:29–33.

Sonderegger, T. B., Ritchie, A. J., Bernye-Key, S., Flowers, J., and Zimmermann, E. G. 1984. Microcomputer-assisted openfield measures of rats given ethanol on postnatal days 1–8. *Neurobehav Toxicol Teratol* 6:325–31.

Sonderegger, T. B., and Zimmermann, E. G. 1978. Adult behavior and adrenocortical function following postnatal morphine treatment. *Psychopharmacology (Berlin)* 56:103–9.

Sorette, M. P., Maggio, C. S., Starpoli, A., Boissevain, A., and Greenwood, M. R. C. 1980. Maternal ethanol affects rat organ development despite adequate nutrition. *Neurobehav Toxicol* 2:181–88.

Sproul, M. 1974. The role of maternal adrenocortical hormones in the ontogeny of the rat hypothalamo-hypophyseal-adrenal axis. Ph.D. dissertation, Stanford University, Palo Alto, Calif.

Taylor, A. N., Branch, B. J., Nelson, L. R., Love, L. A., and Poland, R. E. 1986. Prenatal ethanol and ontogeny of pituitary-adrenal responses to ethanol and morphine. *Alcohol* 3:255–59.

Vavrousek-Jakuba, E. M., Baker, R. A., and Shoemaker, W. J. 1991. Effect of ethanol on maternal and offspring characteristics: Comparison of three liquid diet formulations fed during gestation. *Alcohol Clin Exp Res* 15:129–35.

Vorhees, C. 1986. Principles of behavioral teratology. In *Handbook of Behavioral Teratology*, ed. E. Riley and C. Vorhees, 23–31. New York: Plenum Press.

Vorherr, H. 1974. Drug excretion in breast milk. *Postgrad Med* 56:97–104.

Wainwright, P., Ward, G. R., and Blom, K. 1985. Combined effects of moderate ethanol consumption and a low protein diet during gestation on brain development in BALB/c mice. *Exp Neurol* 90:422–33.

Weinberg, J. 1984. Nutritional issues in perinatal alcohol exposure. *Neurobehav Toxicol Teratol* 6:261–69.

————. 1985. Effects of ethanol and maternal nutritional status on fetal development. *Alcohol Clin Exp Res* 9:49–55.

Weinberg, J., D'Alquen, G., and Benzio S. 1990. Interactive effects of ethanol intake and maternal nutritional status on skeletal development of fetal rats. *Alcohol* 7:383–388.

Weinberg, J., and Gallo, P. V. 1982. Prenatal ethanol exposure: Pituitary-adrenal activity in pregnant dams and offspring. *Neurobehav Toxicol Teratol* 4:515–20.

Weinberg, J., Nelson, L. R., and Taylor, A. N. 1986. Hormonal effects of fetal alcohol exposure. In *Alcohol and Brain Development*, ed. J. R. West, 310–42. New York: Oxford Press.

West, J. R., Hamre, K. M., and Cassell, M. D. 1985. Effects of ethanol exposure during the third trimester equivalent on neuron number in the rat hippocampus and dentate gyrus. *Alcohol* 10:190–97.

West, J. R., Hamre, K. M., and Pierce, D. R. 1984. Delay in brain growth induced by alcohol in artifically reared rat pups. *Alcohol* 1:213–22.

Wiener, S. G. 1980. Nutritional considerations in the design of animal models of the fetal alcohol syndrome. *Neurobehav Toxicol* 2:175–79.

Wiener, S. G., and Levine, S. 1978. Perinatal malnutrition and early handling: Interactive effects on the development of the pituitary-adrenal system. *Dev Psychobiol* 11:335–52.

Wiener, S. G., Shoemaker, W. J., Koda, L. Y., and Bloom, F. E. 1981. Interaction of ethanol and nutrition during gestation: Influence on maternal and offspring development in the rat. *J Pharmacol Exp Ther* 216:572–79.

Wilson, J. G. 1973. *Environment and Birth Defects*. New York: Academic Press.

Zimmermann, E., and Sonderegger, T. 1980. A syndrome of drug-induced delay of maturation. In *Biogenic Amines and Development*, ed. H. Parvez and S. Parvez, 591–607. New York: Elsevier, North Holland Press.

Zimmermann, E., Sonderegger, T., and Bromley, B. 1977. Development and adult pituitary-adrenal function in female rats injected with morphine during different postnatal periods. *Life Sci* 20:639–44.

Zuckerman, B., Frank, D. A., Hingson, R., Amaro, H., Levenson, S. M., Kayne, H., Parker, S., Vinci, R., Aboagye, K., Fried, L. E., Cabral, H., Timperi, R., and Bauchner, H. 1989. Effects of maternal marijuana and cocaine use on fetal growth. *N Engl J Med* 320:762–68.

2

Gender-specific Effects of Perinatal Exposure to Alcohol and Other Drugs

Joanne Weinberg, Ph.D., Betty Zimmerberg, Ph.D., and Theo B. Sonderegger, Ph.D.

EARLY INSULTS to an organism, such as exposure to alcohol or other drugs during the prenatal and/or early postnatal periods, may significantly alter normal growth and development as well as the organism's ability to cope successfully with its environment later in life. Children born to women who are chronic alcoholics, for example, may exhibit multiple birth defects that together are termed the fetal alcohol syndrome (FAS) (Lemoine et al. 1968; Jones and Smith 1973; Jones et al. 1973). The major features of FAS include prenatal and postnatal growth deficiency, central nervous system dysfunction (e.g., retarded mental and motor development, tremulousness, and hyperactivity), and a characteristic facial dysmorphology. In addition to these features, almost every organ system of the body may be vulnerable to the teratogenic effects of alcohol (Streissguth et al. 1980). However, FAS is just one end—the extreme end—of the spectrum of prenatal effects of alcohol. Lower levels of prenatal alcohol exposure may also have a variety of adverse effects, even on offspring who do not exhibit the pattern of morphological defects characteristic of the FAS. In particular, these lower-dose adverse effects appear as behavioral dysfunctions including learning disabilities, hyperactivity, attentional deficits, increased reaction time, and decrements in performance over time on a task (e.g., Streissguth et al. 1986).

Morphological and functional abnormalities similar to those observed in humans have been observed in laboratory animals after prenatal and/or early postnatal (third trimester equivalent) alcohol exposure. Adverse effects on body weight and brain weight (Samson 1986; Weinberg 1985; West, Hamre, and Pierce 1984), abnormalities in brain growth and development (West, Hodges, and Black 1981; West et al. 1984; West, Hamre, and Cassell 1986), changes in hormonal responsiveness (Weinberg, Nelson, and Taylor 1986), deficits in learning and memory, deficits in active and passive avoidance learning (Abel 1981), and hyperactivity and deficits in response inhibition (Riley, Lochry, and Shapiro 1979; Shaywitz, Griffith, and Warshaw 1979) have been reported.

Prenatal exposure to drugs other than alcohol may also result in deficits in physical and psychological development. Children born to methadone- or morphine-addicted mothers, for example, may exhibit behavioral disturbances including brief attention spans, temper tantrums, mood lability, and impaired fine motor coordination (Zimmermann and Sonderegger 1980). Gestational or neonatal exposure of rats to opiate drugs typically results in a syndrome consisting of impaired growth, altered behavior, and evidence of altered neurochemical development. This pattern of effects has been termed the syndrome of drug-delayed maturation. Similarly, perinatal exposure to barbituates (Middaugh et al. 1981), benzodiazepines (Grimm 1984; Kellogg, Ison, and Miller 1983), haloperidol (Hull et al. 1984), nicotine (Martin and Becker 1971), and cocaine (Hutchings, Fico, and Dow-Edwards 1989; Smith et al. 1989; Spear et al. 1989) may result in long-lasting or permanent changes in exposed offspring. These sequelae include significant developmental delays as well as alterations in activity levels, learning and memory, rate of sexual development, sexual behavior, and insensitivity to later exposure to the same agent.

An interesting finding emerging from many of these studies on perinatal alcohol or drug exposure is that perinatal insults may affect male and female offspring differently. An increased vulnerability to perinatal drug effects or, conversely, an increased protection from perinatal drug effects in one sex versus the other is potentially important in terms of understanding the mechanism of action of teratogenic drugs. In this chapter, we review data indicating differential effects of drugs on male and female offspring body weight, brain growth and development, sexual differentiation, hormonal responsiveness, sexual behavior, and a number of nonreproductive behaviors.

Although the review of studies revealing gender-specific effects of exposure to drugs early in life reported here is extensive, it is not exhaustive. For the most part, published articles neither list sex differences in drug-exposure effects as a key word nor describe them as such in the abstract. Often drug-exposure consequences are reported as occurring in males but not females, or vice versa. In some cases, a study was performed only with animals of one sex, and it is necessary to compare the findings of a second study from the same laboratory using the opposite sex to understand the consequences of early drug treatment for the two sexes. We have chosen representative studies from those found in the literature to illustrate our points. We hope that an increased awareness of gender-specific outcomes may lead to a more systematic reporting of such findings in the future.

SEX-DEPENDENT EFFECTS SHOWN BY ANIMAL STUDIES

The Effects of Ethanol and Other Drugs on Body Weight and Brain Weight

Body Weight

In general, prenatal exposure to ethanol or other drugs reduces body weights and brain weights of fetuses and neonates (e.g., Abel, Dintcheff, and Day 1980; Weinberg 1985, 1989; West et al. 1984). In many studies, body weights of males and females are not reported separately. However, in studies where gender is considered, data suggest that prenatal drug exposure may differentially alter offspring body weight. For example, Abel, Dintcheff, and Day (1980) administered marijuana to pregnant females by intubation from gestation day 3 until parturition. Although litter size and neonatal mortality were not affected, pup birth weight was decreased by 10% in drug-treated pups compared to pair-fed controls. At 11 weeks of age, it was noted that drug-treated males had caught up and were similar in body weight to pair-fed control males. Body weights of drug-treated females, however, were still significantly less than those of pair-fed females. Neonatal naltrexone administration may also differentially affect body weight of males and females. Male rat pups treated with naltrexone on postnatal days 1–21 weighed less than saline controls; female weight gain, however, was unaffected (Caldarone and Kehoe 1988).

Other laboratories reported gender-dependent effects of nicotine upon body weight. Nicotine was given to adult female rats in the drinking water for a period of six weeks before mating and throughout pregnancy (Peters and Tang 1982). Litters were cross-fostered to control dams at birth. Prenatal nicotine treatment reduced both the number of male pups born and the male birth weights; females were not significantly affected.

Sex differences in body weights were also found when inbred Buffalo and Fischer rats were treated daily with nicotine or alcohol; alcohol treatment was both pre- and postnatal, and nicotine treatment was from day 10 of age until six months (Riesenfeld 1985). Body weights of males from both strains treated with nicotine were significantly depressed compared to controls, whereas body weights of females were not consistently depressed or were depressed to a lesser extent than those of males. The author stated that the females tolerated growth depression as a consequence of the nicotine exposure better than did the males. When the skeletons of these animals were examined, it was found that, although lumbar, pelvic, tail, and skull weights were significantly depressed in nicotine-treated males, these depressions were not significant in females.

In the alcohol portion of the experiment, the Buffalo rats were found to show a greater tolerance to alcohol than did Fischer rats, and males tolerated the alcohol better than did females. Buffalo females showed less depression of bone growth length in the cervical area, the humerus, radius, ulna, femur, and tibia than did the males. However, the Buffalo females lost more weight in their long bones than did males, with the exception of the lumbar section. This researcher believed that hypocalcemia may be one of the factors contributing to the growth-depressing reactions reported.

Perinatal exposure of the rat to morphine has also produced gender-specific effects on body weight (Zimmermann et al. 1974). Rat pups were given two daily subcutaneous injections of morphine sulfate; the dose began at 0.5 mg/kg and was doubled each day from day 0 to day 7 and then maintained at 8 g/kg from days 8 to 18. The dose was tapered on days 19–21 and then discontinued. Compared to those of saline-treated controls, the body weights of morphine-treated females were significantly depressed until day 105. In the males, a similar pattern of ponderal depression was observed, but it persisted throughout the observation period of four months. Thus, it seems that males were more adversely affected than females by early exposure to morphine.

In some instances, sex differences in body weights were reported in the second generation (i.e., untreated offspring of drug-treated animals). Gender-specific changes in body weights were found in the untreated progeny of male rats given subcutaneous implants of a slow-release morphine pellet on postnatal day 5 or 11 (Sonderegger, O'Shea, and Zimmermann 1979). When adult, the morphine-treated rats and placebo controls were bred with non-drug-treated females. Mean body weight differences of the untreated progeny did not differ from those of controls on postnatal day one. By day 35, however, both male and female offspring of the day 11 morphine-implanted males had body weights significantly below those of controls. By day 126, the significantly reduced body weights persisted in the female but not the male offspring.

Brain Weight

Only a few studies have examined sex-related differences in effects of perinatal drug exposure on brain weights. A recent study by West, Hamre, and Pierce (1984) used an artificial rearing procedure to expose rat pups to ethanol on postnatal days 4–10, which is during the major brain growth spurt for the rat. When examined at the end of this exposure period (i.e., day 10 of age), females showed greater deficits than males. Alcohol-exposed females had a reduced brain volume compared to their suckle controls and a significantly lower brain weight/body weight ratio compared to both suckle and pair-fed controls. Females also exhibited a trend toward greater deficits in brain weights than males. A similar trend was found in another study designed to correlate microencephaly with alcohol dose and blood alcohol level (Pierce and West 1986). For each dose (ranging from 6.6–9.8 g/kg), females exhibited greater reductions in brain weights and also higher blood alcohol levels than males. However, more males than females died at the highest alcohol dose and, therefore, males may be more vulnerable to the effects of high blood alcohol levels than are females.

Using a similar artificial rearing procedure and ethanol exposure on postnatal days 4–7, Grant and Samson (1982) found no sex differences in ethanol effects on forebrain or hindbrain weight or on brain weight/body weight ratio at 18 days of age; on all measures, ethanol-exposed offspring showed deficits compared to controls. At 60 days of age, ethanol-treated males had forebrain and hindbrain weights as well as brain weight/body weight ratios that were similar to those of their controls, indicating significant catch-up growth. Ethanol-exposed females, however, continued to exhibit microcephaly on all three measures compared to their controls, with growth of the cerebellum most severely impaired.

Cerebellar growth in females was also shown to be deficient at 90 days of age in a study in which artificially reared animals were exposed to alcohol in a condensed pattern (resulting in cyclic blood alcohol levels with high peaks) (Kelly, Pierce, and West 1987). Both males and females showed reduced weights of the whole brain, cerebrum, and cerebellum compared to their suckle and gastrostomy controls. However, when data were calculated to measure recovery or catch-up growth from day 10 to day 90, it was found that males exhibited a catch-up growth of 9.9% for cerebellar weight while females showed no catch-up, but rather a 6.1% decrease in cerebellar weight. Interestingly, males still showed a deficit in brain stem weight at 90 days of age.

The Effects of Ethanol on Neuroanatomy and Neurochemistry

Prenatal exposure to alcohol has also been shown to alter certain brain nuclei or structures. These effects may occur differentially in males and females and in some cases may thus affect sexually dimorphic neuroanatomical features or sexual differentiation of the brain.

The Corpus Callosum

In one study (Zimmerberg and Scalzi 1989), sex differences in the size of the corpus callosum were examined in 3-day-old neonates from fetal alcohol-exposed (FAE), pair-fed, and control groups. It was found that male control pups had significantly larger callosal areas than did females. Prenatal alcohol exposure abolished this sexual dimorphism; FAE male pups had significantly smaller callosal areas than had males from pair-fed and control conditions. This finding of prenatal alcohol effects on male but not female offspring suggested that this alcohol-related birth defect was hormonally mediated.

Neocortical Asymmetry

Prenatal alcohol exposure has also been shown to alter a sexually dimorphic neocortical asymmetry found in normal control rats at birth (Zimmerberg and Reuter 1989). Alcohol exposure decreased body weight and total brain volume and had particularly severe growth-retarding effects on the anterior neocortex. In addition, FAE males exhibited a "feminized" anterior neocortical asymmetry; that is, the pattern of left-right anterior neocortical hemisphere differences of FAE males resembled that of control females.

The Sexually Dimorphic Nucleus

The sexually dimorphic nucleus of the preoptic area (SDN-POA) of the hypothalamus also seems vulnerable to the effects of in utero alcohol exposure in male rats. Ethanol exposure during the prenatal period (Barron, Tieman, and Riley 1988), during postnatal days 1–14 (Rudeen, Kappel, and Lear 1986), or during pre- and postnatal development (Rudeen, Kappel, and Lear 1986; Rudeen 1986) results in a significant reduction in the volume and average cell size of the SDN-POA in male rats but has no effect on nuclear volume or cell size in females. This reduction of SDN-POA volume is a specific effect of fetal ethanol exposure and not the result of reduced brain size or brain weight. Moreover, the SDN-POA seems particularly vulnerable to the effects of ethanol; nearby nuclei that are not sexually dimorphic—the nucleus of the anterior commissure (Barron, Tieman, and Riley 1988) and the nucleus accumbens septi (Rudeen 1986)—showed no differential effects of perinatal ethanol.

The mechanism by which perinatal alcohol exposure alters the adult SDN-POA volume is not known. The SDN-POA is normally larger in males than in females, and its development is known to be dependent on perinatal androgen levels (Gorski et al. 1978). Therefore, it is possible that ethanol-induced alterations in testosterone secretion, utilization, or metabolism mediated the change in SDN-POA volume. In support of this suggestion, Kelce, Ganjam, and Rudeen (1989) reported reduced testicular steroidogenic enzyme activity in newborn male rat pups after both prenatal ethanol exposure and acute exposure to ethanol at birth. In addition, it has been observed (Chen and Smith 1979; Parker et al. 1984; Rudeen, Kappel, and Lear 1986; Rudeen 1986) that differentiation of the external genitalia, which is partially dependent on androgen levels during the perinatal period, is also affected by in utero ethanol exposure, as will be discussed further below.

Neurochemical Effects

Differential effects of early postnatal ethanol exposure on brain catecholamine levels of males and females were reported by Kelly and Riley (1989). Increased norepinephrine levels were found in the hippocampus of females but not males exposed to ethanol on postnatal days

4–10; there were no differences among groups in norepinephrine content of the hypothalamus, brainstem, or septal area.

The Effects of Ethanol and Other Drugs on the Hypothalamo-pituitary-gonadal Axis

A number of studies have shown that perinatal exposure to alcohol or other drugs may alter perinatal levels of sex hormones as well as several parameters of sexual differentiation and development. Ethanol effects have been described at all ages studied, from prenatal/perinatal life through adulthood.

Pre- and Postnatal Sex Hormone Levels

In a recent study on fetal males, Udani et al. (1985) found that basal levels of plasma testosterone were similar in fetuses from ethanol-exposed, pair-fed, and chow-fed groups on day 18 of gestation. However, McGivern et al. (1988) reported that the testosterone surge found in control male fetuses on days 18 and 19 of gestation was absent in ethanol-exposed male fetuses. In vitro examination of fetal testes (McGivern et al. 1988) revealed that testes of ethanol-exposed males were insensitive to luteinizing hormone (LH) stimulation of testosterone secretion and, in response to ethanol, showed a suppression of testosterone secretion compared to a large increase in testosterone observed in control testes. In addition, at birth, there was a decrease in the number of Leydig cells in the testes and there were large vacuoles in the seminiferous tubules in ethanol-exposed males.

Decreased plasma testosterone levels and testicular enzyme (17α-hydroxylase/C17, 20-lyase) activity (Kelce, Rudeen, and Ganjam 1989), as well as decreased brain levels of dihydrotestosterone (Kakihana, Butte, and Moore 1980), were reported in newborn males exposed to ethanol pre- or perinatally. Moreover, ethanol exposure seems to attenuate the postnatal testosterone surge that occurs several hours after birth in normal control males (Redei and McGivern 1988). In other studies, the effects of prenatal ethanol on perinatal brain aromatase activity differed in males and females. McGivern, Roselli, and Handa (1988) reported that aromatase activity was significantly increased in the hypothalamus on gestation days 18 and 19 and in the preoptic area on postnatal day 1 in FAE males but not females. However, the elevation in hypothalamic aromatase activity in ethanol-exposed males began on day 18, when testosterone levels were not elevated over those observed on day 17, indicating that the increased aromatase activity was not induced by a testosterone substrate. The biological importance of this aromatase activation remains to be determined.

Hormone Responses in Prepubescent Rats

Fetal alcohol exposure may also differentially influence LH responses to clonidine and naloxone in prepubescent male and female rats. Normal males typically show a rise in plasma LH levels in response to clonidine but not naloxone, whereas females show an LH rise in response to naloxone but not clonidine. McGivern et al. (1986) found that, after fetal alcohol exposure, LH responses to both agents were altered. Both FAE and pair-fed males exhibited a significant LH response to clonidine, whereas control males showed no response. In contrast, clonidine produced no LH response in FAE or control females but produced a significant decrease in LH levels in pair-fed females. Naloxone, on the other hand, produced a significant LH increase in all three groups of females; in males, however, naloxone had no effect on FAE or control males but produced an LH decrease in pair-fed males.

Sexual Development and Differentiation

Parameters of sexual development may be altered in both males and females after prenatal ethanol exposure. A smaller anogenital distance, a marker for sexual differentiation, has been reported in FAE male (Chen and Smith 1979; McGivern 1987; Parker et al. 1984; Rudeen, Kappel, and Lear 1986) and female (Chen and Smith 1979; McGivern 1987) rats at birth. Interestingly, data indicate that, if anogenital distance is corrected for body length (Parker et al. 1984; Udani et al. 1985), alcohol-exposed males continue to show a reduction through the first two weeks of life; however, if anogenital distance is corrected for body weight, differences between ethanol-exposed male and female pups and controls are no longer evident. The issue of which is the more appropriate correction needs to be addressed (Graham and Gandelman 1986). A decreased anogenital distance in FAE males suggests a feminizing or demasculinizing effect of ethanol. The functional significance of a decreased anogenital distance in females remains to be determined.

Prenatal ethanol exposure results in delayed vaginal opening in female mice (Boggan, Randall, and Dodds 1979; Farry and Tittmar 1975) and rats (Esquifino, Sanchis, and Guerri 1986). In addition to this delay in sexual maturation, hormonal alterations persisting into adulthood have been reported in FAE females. Increased plasma pro-lactin and decreased plasma LH levels were found in ethanol-exposed females from weaning through 35 days of age, and it was suggested that these changes could contribute to the delay in vaginal opening (Esquifino, Sanchis, and Guerri 1986). By 40 days of age, FAE females no longer differed from controls in plasma LH levels; however, eleva-tions in plasma prolactin levels persisted into adulthood. In addition, Rudeen and Hagaman (1988) reported that FAE females seemed to show increased sensitivity to exogenous gonadotropins compared to controls. Thirty-day-old females were treated with pregnant-mare serum gonadotropin and human chorionic gonadotropin. Animals ex-posed to ethanol in utero showed greater ovarian stimulation than did controls, reflected in greater ovarian weights, more ova shed, more corpora lutea and antral follicles, and higher serum progesterone levels.

Hormone Responses in Adult Animals

Long-term differential effects of prenatal ethanol exposure on the pituitary-gonadal axes of males and females have also been reported. At both 55 and 110 days of age, males exposed to ethanol perinatally (gestation day 12 to postnatal day 10) had reduced weights of testes, prostate, and seminal vesicles compared to controls. (These differences persisted when organ weight was corrected for body weight.) In addi-tion, serum testosterone and serum LH levels were reduced in ethanol-exposed males compared to controls on day 55 but were increased to normal or near-normal levels by day 110 (Parker et al. 1984; Udani et al. 1985). A study by McGivern (1987) found that prenatal cimetidine (an H_2 receptor antagonist that also has antiandrogenic properties), given either alone or in combination with ethanol, produced a signifi-cant decrease in weights of seminal vesicles of adult males. However, in this study no long-term effects of ethanol or cimetidine on adrenal, testicular, or ovarian weights were observed. In contrast, Handa et al. (1985) found that both males and females exposed to ethanol in utero and then gonadectomized in adulthood had significantly reduced plasma LH levels compared to pair-fed control animals. In addition, a central dysregulation of LH secretion was observed. The phasic afternoon LH response to estrogen and progesterone priming was significantly re-duced in FAE females. In FAE males, the episodic pattern of LH secre-tion revealed reduced mean LH levels as well as a decreased pulse amplitude and frequency compared to those of pair-fed males. It is possible that changes in central regulation of LH secretion may be one factor underlying the changes in male sexual behavior reported after prenatal ethanol exposure. (Ethanol effects on sexual behavior will be discussed further in a subsequent section.)

Perinatal exposure to nicotine may similarly disrupt normal patterns of LH release in both male and female offspring during development (Meyer and Carr 1987). In control males and females, LH levels increased from 20 to 30 days of age and then decreased from 30 to 40 days of age. Nicotine exposure differentially altered this developmental pattern in males and females. These sex-related differences in the effects of nicotine depended both on dose and on duration of exposure (gestation only, lactation only, both gestation and lactation). Generally, LH levels in affected animals were elevated when compared to control values for animals of that sex and age. In addition, nicotine-exposed females had delayed vaginal opening, indicating delayed puberty.

The Effects of Ethanol and Other Drugs on the Hypothalamo-pituitary-adrenal Axis

There is now considerable evidence to indicate that alcohol consumption by pregnant female rats markedly alters the development and responsiveness of the hypothalamo-pituitary-adrenal axis of the offspring. Plasma, adrenal, and brain corticosterone levels are significantly elevated in ethanol-exposed pups at birth (Kakihana, Butter, and Moore 1980; Taylor, Branch, Cooley-Matthews, and Poland 1982; Taylor et al. 1986; Weinberg 1989). During the first 2–3 weeks of life, FAE pups show a blunted response to ethanol and morphine challenge (Taylor et al. 1986), as well as to ether, saline, and exposure to a novel environment (Weinberg 1989). During and after puberty, however, FAE offspring become hyperresponsive to stress, exhibiting enhanced pituitary-adrenal activation to certain neurogenic stressors, to intermittent footshock, to ether, and to challenges with drugs such as ethanol and morphine, compared to controls (Nelson et al. 1986; Taylor et al. 1983; Weinberg 1988; Weinberg and Gallo 1982).

The Adrenocortical Response to Stress

Studies have shown that prenatal or early postnatal ethanol exposure may differentially affect the hormonal responsiveness of males and females. In most studies to date, pituitary-adrenal hyperresponsiveness to stress has been found to be greater in ethanol-exposed females than in males. Weinberg (1988) examined adrenocortical activity in animals exposed to (1) restraint stress for 30 or 60 minutes or (2) to a novel cage that was empty or that had water available. Males prenatally exposed to ethanol were similar to pair-fed and control males in their response to the novel test cage, both with and without water available, and in their response to a one-hour period of restraint. Ethanol-exposed females, however, showed a smaller decrease in corticosterone than both pair-fed and control females when given the opportunity to drink water in the novel cage. Moreover, unlike females from both control groups, FAE females showed no significant decrease in corticosterone levels after 60 minutes of restraint. These data suggest that behavioral or psychological variables may be less effective in reducing or dampening the pituitary-adrenal response to stress in animals prenatally exposed to ethanol than in controls and indicate that females may be more vulnerable to this effect of prenatal ethanol than are males. Moreover, the deficits shown by the ethanol-exposed females during restraint stress and in the consummatory task provide evidence that hyperresponsiveness may be manifested not only by increased activation, but also by reduced inhibition or recovery of the pituitary-adrenal system toward basal levels after stress. This study was one of the first to demonstrate sex differences in adrenocortical responsiveness to stress after fetal ethanol exposure. However, it is important to note that, in most previous studies by Taylor and co-workers which demonstrated pituitary-adrenal hyperresponsiveness to stress in FAE animals (e.g., Taylor et al. 1981; Taylor, Branch, Liu, and Kokka 1982), only female offspring were tested.

Kelly et al. (1991) found that alcohol exposure during the early postnatal period in the rat, a period equivalent to the third trimester in the human with regard to brain development, also caused hyperresponsiveness of the hypothalamo-pituitary-adrenal axis in females but not males. In this study, pups were artificially reared and exposed to ethanol on postnatal days 4–10. Animals were then tested in adulthood for their response to a one-minute forced swim in 20°C water. Ethanol-exposed females showed significantly higher corticosterone levels than suckle and gastrostomy control females at 15, 45, and 60 minutes after stress. Ethanol-exposed males did not differ significantly from their controls.

In another study (Weinberg and Gallo 1982), it was shown that prenatal ethanol exposure may interact with postnatal handling experience to influence pituitary-adrenal activity. Pups from alcohol-exposed, pair-fed, and control treatment groups either were handled daily during the preweaning period or remained entirely undisturbed (nonhandled) and were then tested at 39 days of age for their response to the combined stress of ether and cardiac puncture. There were no sex differences in the plasma corticoid stress response of nonhandled animals from any of the three treatment groups. In handled animals, however, females prenatally exposed to alcohol showed a greater initial corticosterone response than did alcohol-exposed males, once again supporting the suggestion that pituitary-adrenal hyperresponsiveness occurs more often in FAE females than in FAE males.

Interestingly, a study by Weinberg (in press) demonstrated that, under certain conditions, pituitary-adrenal hyperresponsiveness to stress may be demonstrated in FAE males. The stressors examined in previous studies have typically been acute rather than chronic and/ or of relatively short duration. Therefore, a study was undertaken to examine adrenocortical activity in response to a more prolonged stressor. At 60–90 days of age, fetal alcohol-exposed, pair-fed, and ad libitum-fed (control) males and females were exposed to a four-hour period of restraint in plastic tubes that severely restricted movement, and a corticosterone time course was determined. All animals showed significant corticoid increases over the first hour of testing and a gradual return toward basal levels over the next three hours, although corticoids never completely returned to basal levels during the four-hour test. In addition, in contrast to previous data, FAE females were found to be similar to pair-fed and control females in their pattern of corticoid responsiveness. Ethanol-exposed males, however, were similar to pair-fed and control males in their initial response to stress but showed a prolonged corticoid activation over the four-hour test period. These data suggest that, under conditions of prolonged rather than short duration stress, adrenocortical hyperresponsiveness may be demonstrated in FAE males.

The Adrenocortical Response to Drugs

Prenatal alcohol exposure has also been shown to affect the adrenocortical response to naloxone and clonidine in both males and females (McGivern et al. 1986). Clonidine was shown to produce a corticosterone increase in normal rats of both sexes at 16 days of age. FAE males and females, however, showed no corticoid increase in response to clonidine. In contrast, naloxone significantly depressed corticoid levels of alcohol-treated males compared to their saline controls but did not differentially alter corticoid responses of alcohol-exposed females.

Zimmermann and colleagues (1974) demonstrated sex differences in adrenocortical responses to postnatal morphine exposure. They found that 78-day-old male rats treated with morphine from birth until day 21 showed significant increases in corticosterone levels in response to 20- or 40-mg/kg challenge doses of morphine, whereas females showed a significant steroid rise only in response to the 40-mg/kg challenge dose.

The Effects of Ethanol and Other Drugs on Behavior

A number of studies have shown that perinatal exposure to ethanol may alter both sexual behavior and noncopulatory sexually dimorphic behavior in both males and females.

Sexual Behavior and Maternal Behavior

Male rats exposed to ethanol in utero were found to be feminized in their sexual behavior, appearing less sexually motivated and impaired in performance. This was manifested by a decreased intromission frequency and an increased ejaculatory latency (Parker et al. 1984; Udani et al. 1985), as well as by increased lordosis responses (H'ard et al. 1985) compared to controls. Ethanol-exposed females showed no change in estrus cycles or in onset of vaginal estrus but were delayed in the onset of behavioral estrus (i.e., lordosis responses) and of regular behavioral estrus cycling (H'ard et al. 1985). Maternal behavior may also be adversely affected by in utero ethanol exposure. Induction of maternal behavior in virgin females by repeated exposure to young pups (Barron and Riley 1985), as well as nest building, retrieval, and other aspects of normal organized maternal behavior that occur after parturition (H'ard et al. 1984), have been shown to be impaired in females prenatally exposed to ethanol.

Saccharin Preference, Lashley III Maze, Rough and Tumble Play

Nonreproductive sexually dimorphic behaviors also seem to be highly sensitive to the effects of prenatal ethanol exposure. McGivern et al. (1984) reported on two behaviors, saccharin preference and performance in a Lashley III maze, that were altered by in utero ethanol exposure. In normal animals, females exhibit a greater preference for saccharin than do males, whereas males typically perform better than females in a Lashley III maze. Prenatal alcohol exposure, however, eliminated this sexual dimorphism in both behaviors; FAE males and females showed no difference in number of trials to reach criterion in the maze and showed similar intake of saccharin solution. (Indeed, at the 0.5% concentration the sexual dimorphism was reversed, with FAE males consuming more than FAE females.) In another study (McGivern, Holcomb, and Poland 1987), the administration of testosterone proprionate to pregnant, ethanol-consuming females could not counteract the feminizing effects of prenatal ethanol exposure on saccharin preference of their male offspring. Moreover, testosterone levels of FAE males at birth were not significantly lower than those of pair-fed males in this study. These data suggested that testosterone probably does not have a direct role in mediating this ethanol-induced feminization. It was proposed that saccharin preference may be organizationally dependent on estrogens during the prenatal period. In contrast to these data, Abel and Dintcheff (1986) found no evidence of altered sexual dimorphism in saccharin preference in animals tested at seven months of age. Several possibilities could account for these results: (1) There were differences in prenatal treatment methods. Abel and Dintcheff (1986) intubated pregnant dams twice daily during days 11–21 of gestation, whereas McGivern et al. (1984) gave alcohol via liquid diet from gestation day 7 through parturition. (2) There were differences in strain of rat and in age at time of testing. Long-Evans rats may be less vulnerable to these particular ethanol effects than are Sprague-Dawley rats, and there may be recovery from these deficits over time. (3) The animals were housed differently before testing (individual versus group housing).

Elimination of the typical sexual dimorphism in rough and tumble play by prenatal ethanol exposure has also been demonstrated (Meyer and Riley 1986). In contrast to normal juvenile males, young ethanol-exposed males were found to engage in rough and tumble play less often than did females.

Behavioral Laterality

The effects of prenatal ethanol exposure on behavioral laterality were assessed in several studies. In studies on juvenile (Zimmerberg and Riley 1986) and adult (Zimmerberg and Riley 1988) offspring, prenatal alcohol exposure decreased the degree of side preference similarly for both sexes. A sex difference was, however, noted in a study of behavioral laterality in neonatal (postnatal day 1) offspring (Zimmerberg and Reuter 1989). Newborn rats, like newborn humans, have marked postural asymmetries. There is a normal sex difference in tail bias (left, right, or neutral), with more females in the population having a left bias. Alterations in this tail bias have been associated with the prenatal hormonal milieu; for example, treating pregnant dams with testosterone reduces the percentage of female offspring with a left tail bias (Rosen et al. 1983). Prenatal alcohol exposure increased the percentage of males having a left tail bias, suggesting a "feminization" of the males. Among female neonates, both the ethanol-exposed and the pair-fed nutritional control group had a decreased percentage of left tail bias, suggesting a "masculinization" due to the stress/undernutrition of pair-feeding and not to a specific effect of alcohol.

Spatial Learning

A sex-dependent effect of prenatal alcohol exposure was also observed in a spatial learning task (Zimmerberg, Sukel, and Stekler 1991). Subjects were trained to alternate left and right turns in a T-maze to escape water. When exposed to alcohol prenatally, males, but not females, made more errors on the working memory component than did control subjects. These sex-dependent results were in contrast to the results of a food-rewarded operant alternation task, in which both males and females exposed to alcohol prenatally made more errors than did control subjects (Zimmerberg, Mattson, and Riley 1989). This discrepancy might be due to sex-dependent differences in the aversiveness of motivation (food deprivation versus cold water) or in the motoric demands of the testing situation (operant lever-pressing versus swim-escape). It does suggest that some tests may be more sensitive in detecting sex differences in outcome after prenatal drug exposure than are others.

Spatial learning ability may also be affected by postnatal ethanol exposure. A study of spatial navigation that used a Morris water maze (Kelly et al. 1988) reported deficits in performance in ethanol-exposed females but not males. These investigators used an artificial rearing procedure to expose rat pups to ethanol on postnatal days 4–10. One group received ethanol in a condensed manner, which caused cyclic blood alcohol levels with high peaks. A second group received alcohol in a uniform manner over the entire day. Condensed alcohol exposure during the early postnatal period resulted in a deficit in the ability of adult females to use distal cues for spatial navigation. Importantly, condensed alcohol exposure was shown to cause performance deficits of equal magnitude in juvenile males and females tested on this same task (Goodlett, Kelly, and West 1987). It was suggested that the differential permanency of the alcohol effect may be due to alterations of a still-developing neural system that was or would be sexually dimorphic in some manner, and the hippocampal formation was identified as the most likely structure mediating these effects. It seems that the neural substrate underlying performance in the Morris water maze (Kelly et al. 1988) must differ from that underlying performance in the water T-maze; alternatively, the time period of ethanol exposure may be critical. Early postnatal alcohol exposure has also been shown to produce greater deficits in female than in male weanlings tested in a passive avoidance task. Using the artificial rearing procedure to expose neonates from gestation day 26 to 32, Barron and Riley (1990) found that females exposed to a 6-g/kg ethanol dose required more trials to reach criterion during both acquisition and retention relative to all other groups.

The Morris water maze has also been used to assess possible deficits in response inhibition in FAE animals tested immediately after weaning (22–26 days of age). Differential effects of prenatal ethanol exposure on males and females have been found in some studies but not others. Blanchard, Riley, and Hannigan (1987) reported that, on day 3 of a four-day test, ethanol-exposed females took longer than controls to reach the platform, while ethanol-exposed animals of both sexes traveled greater distances than did controls. Furthermore, a test of reversal learning on day 4 revealed that spatial processing and not learning per se was impaired in FAE animals, with a greater effect in males than in females. In a subsequent study, however, although deficits in spatial navigation were again observed in ethanol-exposed offspring, no sex differences were found (Blanchard, Pilati, and Hannigan 1990).

Activity

Prenatal or early postnatal ethanol or other drug exposure can also alter spontaneous and drug-induced activity levels of males and females. Ethanol exposure in utero was found to eliminate the typical sexual dimorphism in open-field activity in animals tested at about three weeks of age. That is, ethanol-exposed males and females were both similar to female controls in locomotor activity (H'ard et al. 1985), suggesting that prenatal ethanol exposure may affect this aspect of behavior in males more than females. On the other hand, ethanol exposure on postnatal days 4–7 was found to increase open-field activity of females but not males tested at 30 days of age (females ambulated more and spent more time in the center of the field) (Grant, Choi, and Samson 1983).

Amphetamine-induced activity in animals tested at 28 days of age is altered by both prenatal ethanol and prenatal undernutrition (pair-feeding) as a function of sex and dose of drug (Blanchard, Hannigan, and Riley 1987). At a dose of 1.0 mg/kg, fetal ethanol-exposed males were similar in activity to control males, and both were more active than were pair-fed males. There were no differences among the three groups of females. At a dose of 2.0 mg/kg, FAE males were more active than were pair-fed and control males; FAE females showed a brief decrease in activity relative to controls and did not differ from pair-fed females.

Perinatal nicotine exposure may also differentially affect activity levels of males and females. Nicotine administered before mating and during pregnancy produced a reduction in rearing activity in male but not female offspring, compared to controls, when tested over 24-hour periods in the home cage (on days 25, 45, 60, and 85 of age) or when tested during a ten-minute exposure to an open field (at 60 days of age) (Peters and Tang 1982).

In another study (Holson et al. 1985), pregnant dams were given daily subcutaneous injections of *d*-amphetamine (0.5, 2.0, or 3.0 mg/kg) on gestation days 12–15. Of interest here is the fact that male but not female offspring from the high-dose mothers were significantly more active than were controls when tested over three days in a figure 8 maze. On the other hand, in this same study, when responses to auditory startle were tested as a measure of reactivity to stimulation (Holson et al. 1985), females exposed to the 3-mg/kg dose had an elevated startle response at postnatal days 47 and 120 but not at postnatal day 19, whereas males showed an elevated startle response at day 19 but not thereafter. In describing the complex array of behavioral effects obtained in their study, the authors concluded that the behavioral effects "have been subtle, inconsistent, and almost without exception sex-specific."

Finally, a series of experiments by Grimm and Frieder (1985) showed that exposure to diazepam or dietary monosodium glutamate during the prenatal or early postnatal period of rapid brain development may result in long-lasting behavioral changes in exposed offspring. Exposure to the same agent was shown to result in different behavioral consequences depending on the timing of the exposure. Moreover, male and female offspring were found to be differentially affected by the same agent at different periods of development. Diazepam exposure during the first two weeks of gestation or during either the second or third week only selectively impaired maze learning in males. In open-field activity, however, prenatal diazepam exposure eliminated sex differences observed in control animals (i.e., activity levels in drug-treated females were reduced to the level of males). Females exposed to diazepam during the third week of gestation showed more rearing during open-field testing than did drug-treated males or control females. Postnatal exposure to diazepam, on the other hand, increased open-field activity in males but not females and produced greater deficits in maze learning in females than in males. Prenatal exposure to monosodium glutamate decreased open-field activity in males more than in females and produced deficits in maze learning only in male offspring. Thus, in general, prenatal insults impaired the later performance of males but not females, whereas postnatal results seemed to impair the performance of animals of both sexes.

Analgesia

Perinatal exposure to drugs other than ethanol may also differentially alter behavior in male and female offspring. Zagon and McLaughlin (1982) examined the effects of maternal exposure to methadone during gestation and/or lactation on offspring sensitivity to pain. They found that both male and female methadone-exposed rats tested from weaning through 60 days of age showed increased analgesia compared to controls. At 90 and 120 days of age, however, methadone-exposed females appeared abnormally slow to respond to the hot plate, suggesting abnormally increased drug-induced analgesia.

Maze Learning

Neonatal opioid treatment (morphiceptin and D-ala D-leu enkephalin) alters maze learning in rats in a sex-dependent manner (de Avils and Martinez 1985). Testing in a complex maze at 25 days of age revealed that peptide-treated females made fewer errors than did peptide-treated males. It was also noted that opioid-treated females were lighter and opioid-treated males were heavier in body weight than controls.

The Collaborative Study

A Collaborative Behavioral Teratology Study was undertaken by investigators in several laboratories to assess the reliability and sensitivity of a variety of behavioral testing methods (Buelke-Sam et al. 1985). Pregnant animals in different laboratories were treated with varying doses of *d*-amphetamine sulfate or methylmercuric chloride. Of relevance here is the fact that sex differences in behavioral response levels were found, most notably in activity measures. In addition, males made more nose-poke responses than did females, whereas females tended to make more total correct responses in a discrimination learning task. The authors concluded that, in a screening situation, the potential for sex-dependent susceptibility to toxic insult should not be ignored and both sexes should be monitored. These investigators also stated that they found no evidence of greater female variability in behavior.

The Effects of Paternal versus Maternal Alcohol Exposure

Abel (1989) compared the effects of paternal and maternal alcohol consumption in two strains of rats upon their offspring. Long-Evans and Sprague-Dawley male rats were given liquid ethanol or control diets [35%, 17.5%, or 0% ethanol-derived calories (EDC)] for three to four weeks and were then bred with females of the same strain. Pregnant females, on the other hand, were exposed to one of these diet conditions beginning on gestation day 8. The effects upon the preweaning age offspring of the males and females differed. Paternal alcohol consumption was associated with decreased litter size, decreased testosterone levels, and a strain-related effect on offspring activity. Activity of offspring from Long-Evans males who consumed 35% and 17.5% EDC decreased, as did activity of offspring sired by the 17.5% EDC Sprague-Dawley males; however, activity increased for offspring of the 35% EDC Sprague-Dawley fathers. Neither postnatal mortality nor passive avoidance learning of the offspring was affected by alcohol consumption of the fathers. Offspring of the alcohol-treated females, however, had lower birth weights, lower body weights when weaned, increased postnatal mortality, and impaired passive avoidance learning. Interestingly, activity levels of the offspring of the females did not differ among the groups.

Gender-specific effects upon the offspring were not reported except with respect to sex ratio (male/female) differences. Sex ratios did not differ between the 0% EDC or ad libitum-fed males or females and their controls, nor were the main effects of paternal or maternal alcohol consumption or strain significant. Of interest, however, is the fact that, in the Sprague-Dawley rats, there was a higher sex ratio (male/female) among the offspring of the 35% EDC fathers compared to the 17.5% or 0% EDC fathers bred to 0% EDC mothers, a lower sex ratio for the 35% EDC males bred to 35% EDC mothers, and no significant sex ratio difference for males bred to 17.5% EDC females. Female offspring of the 35% EDC males seemed to be harmed more when the mothers were 17.5% or 0% EDC females, and male offspring were harmed more when both parents were exposed to 35% EDC alcohol.

Conclusions

The findings in the studies described here clearly demonstrate that male and female animal offspring may be differentially affected by perinatal exposure to a wide variety of drugs. In the studies described, the body weights of males seemed to be more adversely affected than those of females whether the exposure was to marijuana, naltrexone, nicotine, or morphine. On the other hand, postnatal exposure to alcohol produced a more dramatic effect on the brain weight of females than of males. Findings with respect to effects on specific brain structures, sexual development and differentiation, neuroendocrine function, or a variety of behaviors were much more varied; depending on the outcome variable examined, males seemed more vulnerable to certain treatments while females seemed more vulnerable to others.

At present, the underlying mechanisms for such differential effects have not been clearly delineated. What is clear, however, as was pointed out in the collaborative testing study by Judy Buelke-Sam and her colleagues (1985), is that the responses of both male and female rodents must be studied before one can accurately document the consequences of exposure to drugs early in life. Male and female offspring may be affected differently by the same agent at different periods in development or may show differential responsiveness depending on the parameters of the task or the type of challenge presented. By ignoring sex differences, we may underestimate or misinterpret the real effect of ethanol or other drugs on a particular system. Although not reviewed here, gender-specific effects have also been found when drugs have been given to adult rodents [e.g., diazepam (Pericic, Manev, and Lakic 1985), cocaine (Glick, Hinds, and Shapiro 1983), or amphetamine (Robinson, Becker, and Presty 1982)]. An understanding of sex differences in effects produced by perinatal exposure to drugs may well provide insight into how some of the actions of ethanol or other drugs may be mediated. (See chapter 7 for other gender-specific effects.)

GENDER-SPECIFIC FINDINGS FROM CLINICAL STUDIES

Although research findings in animal models of perinatal substance abuse suggest that there may be sex-dependent variations in outcome, an extensive review of the clinical data has proven problematic. Many clinical reports do not even identify the sex of the sample population or case. If sex is identified, it is typically used statistically as a covariate, not as an interactive factor. Therefore, the contribution of the sex of the offspring toward mean differences between exposed and nonexposed offspring in the dependent measure (e.g., head circumference, birth weight) is controlled for but not examined as an independent variable in its own right. The question we are left with is, Are sex-dependent differences in outcome rarely reported because there are none or because the right question is not being asked of the data?

The Possible Mechanisms

Should we have any expectation of sex-related differences in outcome? Two possible mechanisms for adverse effects of perinatal exposure to drugs of abuse suggest that sex differences may indeed exist. First, the drug could have differential effects on the male and female fetus/neonate. This would presuppose a sex-related difference in receptors or other substrates. There is certainly evidence that the vertebrate central nervous system can differ by sex (for a review see Fishman and Breedlove 1988). Males and females have been shown to differ in neuron morphology, the number of neurons, the degree of neural connectivity, and the concentrations of some neurotransmitters, receptors, and/or receptor binding in selected regions. There are also sex differences in steroid receptors in the brain. Thus, there may be substrate differences in the brain which might account for sex differences in the outcome of fetuses exposed to a neurotoxic agent during gestation, particularly differences in behavioral outcome.

A second possibility is that the teratological effects of the abused drug may be sex hormone dependent. Male and female fetuses produce different concentrations of different types of hormones; therefore, if the teratological outcome were mediated via these hormones, there would be apparent sex-related effects. A variation on this mechanism would be that sex hormones (either by concentration or type) have a protective effect on the fetus. Thus, one sex would be more affected than the other by prenatal substance abuse. Postnatal hormonal status also differs by sex. Male newborns experience a surge in serum testosterone on the first day of life and again at one month; prepubertal levels do not stabilize until four months of age. In contrast, female newborns experience high serum estrogen levels only during the first week of life. Both male and female neonates produce a similar total amount of growth hormone. However, the growth hormone "pulse" released for female neonates is more frequent and has a greater amplitude but also a shorter width than growth hormone "pulses" produced by male neonates (Hindmarsh and Brook 1988). Therefore, one might predict that any adverse effect associated with exposure to a drug of abuse during the perinatal period that was hormone dependent would exhibit a sex difference in outcome.

The Evidence of Sex-related Effects

Maternal Alcohol Consumption

The first reference to sex-dependent effects after perinatal drug exposure was in a brief note reporting that there seemed to be a greater number of female than male children being diagnosed with fetal alcohol syndrome (FAS),(Qazi and Masakawa 1976). These investigators commented that 8 of 11 of their FAS cases and 34 of 53 of other reported FAS cases were females. This excess of females was hypothesized to be caused by a greater mortality rate pre- or postnatally for males exposed to alcohol. Three years later, this question was reexamined by Abel (1979). In the case studies that he reviewed, there were more females (148 cases) than males (131 cases), but this difference was not statistically significant. The only subsequent mention of a sex difference in cases of FAS was in a study of 301 offspring of women enrolled in an alcoholism treatment center in Hungary (Vitez et al. 1984). These offspring were scored for symptoms and signs of FAS. Among the 25 children who scored the highest ("most typical") on the FAS scale used in this study, the authors reported a "conspicuous" male/female ratio of 18 boys to 7 girls. These children had been born to mothers who reported drinking more than 30 ml of ethanol daily during their pregnancies and whose fathers were also alcoholics. No differences in sex ratio were observed among children of alcoholic mothers who drank less ethanol or who abstained during their pregnancies. These results suggested that males might be at greater risk than females for more severe damage after high-dose alcohol exposure in utero.

More recently, the effects of moderate maternal drinking during the first trimester on fetal growth were reported to vary with the sex of the offspring (Little et al. 1986). In this study, 930 women were questioned about their alcohol consumption at their first prenatal visit (average of about 11 gestational weeks). Both male and female newborns from this sample population exhibited decreasing birth weight with increasing amounts of alcohol consumed during the week before the pregnancy was recognized. However, among women who reported drinking at least one drink a day during the week just before the first prenatal visit, there was a significant sex-by-alcohol interaction on birth weights. Male alcohol-exposed newborns in this group weighed an average of 225 g less than did nonexposed males, whereas alcohol-exposed females weighed only 25 g less. These results were interpreted as indicating that the male fetus may be more vulnerable to alcohol exposure late in the first trimester, even when the dose is moderate.

Another report of a sex difference in outcome after prenatal alcohol exposure was described by Landesman-Dwyer, Keller, and Streissguth (1978). In this study, infants born to mothers identified in pregnancy interviews as heavy drinkers exhibited significantly more body tremors than did infants born to moderate drinkers, who, in turn, had more body tremors than did infants born to infrequent drinkers and abstainers. Among the two heaviest maternal alcohol intake groups, male infants had more than twice as many body tremors as female infants. A parallel sex-by-alcohol interaction was also reported for the incidence of facial tremors. Again, male infants born to the two heaviest drinking groups had twice as much facial tremoring as had female infants in those groups. Other behavioral observations and neuropsychological tests conducted in this study did not reveal any sex differences. These authors suggested that males may be more vulnerable to a specific effect of alcohol on central nervous system control of body and facial movements.

Sex differences were not investigated systematically in the ten-year follow-up of 11 children who were the first to be diagnosed as having FAS (Streissguth, Clarren, and Jones 1985). However, this report does indicate that, at puberty, the four surviving females had attained normal weight for height. In contrast, the two males had not yet reached puberty and continued to be underweight for height. Again, these results suggest a more adverse effect on male offspring exposed to alcohol in utero. In comparison to the above studies, Spohr and Steinhausen (1987) conducted extensive pediatric, neurological, and psychiatric assessments of 54 children diagnosed with FAS and included sex as an interactive factor. They reported that sex did not significantly influence any of the results.

Maternal Smoking

Several studies investigating the effects of maternal smoking on fetal growth included contradictory sex-dependent effects. In the first brief report, Ravenholt and Levinski (1965) examined birth weight in 1,096 infants born to mothers who smoked regularly. In addition to birth weight deficits in offspring of both sexes, there was a negative correlation between the number of cigarettes smoked and the proportion of males among live offspring. This difference in sex ratio appeared in children of mothers who had smoked 2,000 to 3,999 cigarettes during the pregnancy and is suggestive of increased male mortality. In a subsequent study, Wertelecki, Hoff, and Zansky (1987) analyzed birth weights and lengths of 925 newborns whose mothers were enrolled in a large retrospective study. Male full-term neonates whose mothers smoked more than 10 cigarettes per day weighed 110 g less and were 1.1 cm shorter than male neonates born to nonsmoking mothers. Weight and length reductions in female neonates born to smoking mothers, in contrast, were not significantly different from those of female neonates born to nonsmoking mothers. Another study on the influence of maternal smoking (more than one cigarette per day during the pregnancy) concluded that decreased birth weight for male offspring was less dependent on the expression of fetal genes and more dependent on maternal environment (e.g., nicotine exposure) than for female offspring (Little and Sing 1987). In contrast to these studies, Davis (1977) examined the effect of maternal smoking on weight, length, and head circumference in 709 full-term infants and concluded that females were more severely affected than males after prenatal exposure to nicotine (15 or more cigarettes per day). Unfortunately, it is difficult to determine if sex was analyzed specifically as an interactive factor.

The Combined Effects of Smoking and Alcohol

Kariniemi and Rosti (1988) reported a sex difference in outcome in a study on the combined effects of maternal cigarette smoking and alcohol consumption on birth weight among 1,545 consecutive births. Maternal smoking (more than nine cigarettes per day) was significantly associated with reduced birth weight (about 200 g) in both sexes. Maternal alcohol consumption, however, was associated with reduced birth weight only in the female newborns (90 g reduction). Smoking and alcohol consumption did not interact. In this study, alcohol consumption was not quantified; the mothers were merely asked at admission whether they had consumed any alcohol during the current pregnancy.

The Indirect Evidence from Anthropological Morphometry

Physical anthropologists have been interested in the question of sexual dimorphism in size for some time (Hall 1982). According to Waddington's theory of canalization (conformity to growth patterns over time during development), females are better regulated in their growth patterns than are males. Thus, girls recover from conditions causing growth arrest (e.g., undernutrition, atomic bomb exposure) more quickly than do boys (Tanner 1978).

Inadequate Nutrition

Decreased sexual dimorphism (e.g., less difference in size between males and females) has been associated with undernutrition in human populations. Children of both sexes exhibit lags in height and weight gain and delays in maturation and puberty in response to diets deficient in proteins and/or calories. However, many studies in this field over the last 40 years suggested that boys are more severely affected by inadequate nutrition than are girls (e.g., Hall 1978; Stini 1969, 1972;

Stinson 1985). For example, male children in a chronically malnour-ished Columbian population had greater loss of adipose tissue and pro-tein stores, more decreased stature, and more delayed sexual and bone maturation than had girls (Stini 1972). Thus, a disproportionate effect on males results in a less sexually dimorphic population when there is chronic nutritional stress. In another study of the relationship between nutrition and birth weight and length in Peruvian newborns, boys were more affected by maternal nutritional status than were girls (Frisancho, Klayman, and Matos 1977). Conversely, several studies on the effects of nutritional supplementation during pregnancy reported that males responded more favorably with weight gain than did females (Mora et al. 1981; Stinson 1985).

The Critical Periods

Sex-dependent effects of drugs on growth may well depend on tim-ing; males and females may be passing through "critical periods" at different times. Males grow faster just before birth (34 weeks on) and just after birth than do females; weight velocity no longer differs by sex by one year of age (Lieberman 1982). Suggestive evidence that perinatal drug exposure could have sex-dependent effects because of sex differ-ences in maturational timing can be found in a study of the effect of environmental stress on growth. The heights of Japanese girls and boys from 1915 to 1971 were analyzed. There was less difference between the sexes in the slope of the adolescent growth spurt during the war years (1940–48) than either before or after that period of stress. How-ever, which sex was more affected by the stress depended on the matu-rational time table. Girls were more affected between 9 and 11 years of age, and boys were more affected between 13 and 14 years of age. These ages correspond to periods of more rapid growth, which differ between the sexes (L. M. Schell, personal communication).

Prenatal Hypoxia

Data from physical anthropologists also suggest that males may be more susceptible to prenatal hypoxia than are females. Measurements of birth weight and length of Bolivian newborns at different altitudes showed that only male infants were significantly lighter and shorter at high altitudes compared to low altitudes (Haas et al. 1982).

Prenatal Noise Exposure

Schell (1984) compared male and female birth weights and gestational lengths in 121 births to mothers exposed to high, moderate, and low levels of noise from airplane traffic during pregnancy. A high noise level (more than 99 dBA) was associated with decreased birth weight in females and shorter gestational length in males. The greater sensitivity to high noise levels in female fetal growth had also been noted by a previous study of aircraft noise (Knipschild, Meijer, and Salle 1981). Among 1,000 births studied, a greater percentage of low-birth-weight (less than 3,000 g) infants was born to mothers living in high airport noise areas than to those in low noise areas; this difference was mainly accounted for by female neonates (Knipschild, Meijer, and Salle 1981).

Other Indirect Evidence

Spontaneous Abortion and Postnatal Mortality

Studies on the effects of maternal factors on fetal growth have generally concluded that males are more severely affected than females (Stinson 1985). More males than females are spontaneously aborted, die from difficult births or maternal disease, and die during the first week of life.

The Susceptibility to Disease

At every gestational age, males have a greater incidence of respiratory distress syndrome (RDS) than do females (Rooney 1985). Ioffe and Chernick (1987) studied the incidence of RDS in infants born to alcoholic mothers. Male neonates had a greater incidence of RDS than had females, and young gestational age was associated with a greater incidence of RDS, as would be expected. Interestingly, infants born to binge or alcoholic mothers had a reduced incidence of RDS; there was no interactive effect of sex. Females also respond significantly better than males in clinical trials of glucocorticoid prevention of RDS (Collaborative Group on Antenatal Steroid Therapy 1981). One suggestion accounting for this sex difference is that androgens produced by the male neonate inhibit the production of surfactant (Nielson, Zinman, and Torday 1982). Males also predominate in incidences of mental retardation (Pauls 1979), developmental dyslexia (Finucci and Childs 1981), and nonstandard cerebral lateralization (Bryden 1981), conditions all thought to be associated with in utero damage to the developing fetal brain.

One report indicated that female infants have a higher rate of perinatal human immunodeficiency virus infection (vaginal delivery plus breast-feeding by seropositive mothers) than have males, and mortality rates were higher among female human immunodeficiency virus-positive infants compared to males (Italian Multicentre Study 1988).

The Composition of the Body

Outcome after perinatal drug abuse may be sex dependent because of differences in body composition between males and females. Female infants have more subcutaneous fat (about 5–10%) than male infants at all sites (Owen, Jensen, and Foman 1966). Throughout childhood and adolescence, boys have more fat-free weight and less fat mass than girls; by young adulthood, males have 15% adipose tissue by body weight while females have 27%, on average. Conversely, males have more body water than females (about 4% more intracellular water and 2% more total body water) than do females (Ross and Ward 1982). Sex differences in body composition could have pharmacokinetic significance. Given the same dose of drug, blood levels would be higher in females because the drug is more concentrated; brain levels would reflect blood levels. In postnatal alcohol exposure experiments, it seems that the peak blood alcohol level is more predictive of brain damage than is the total dose (Kelly, Pierce, and West 1987). However, some drugs may be more lipophilic than others and remain in the female neonate for a longer period. It would be interesting to examine sex differences in the pharmacokinetics of drugs of abuse in the neonate to determine whether some of the inconsistencies in the reports cited above can be partially explained by sex differences in body composition.

Conclusions

Although the data are still scarce and are sometimes conflicting, sex differences in outcome have been detected in offspring born to mothers engaging in substance abuse. Male fetuses and neonates seem, in general, to be more adversely affected than are females. Clearly, additional studies that directly address this question are necessary. We hope that this approach will shed light on some mechanisms of teratogenicity and will also prove useful for delineating therapeutic programs.

REFERENCES

Abel, E. L. 1979. Sex ratio in fetal alcohol syndrome. *Lancet* 2:105.
———. 1980. Fetal alcohol syndrome: Behavioral teratology. *Psychol Bull* 87:29–50.
———. 1981. Behavioral teratology of alcohol. *Psychol Bull* 90:564–58.
———. 1989. Paternal and maternal alcohol consumption: Effects on offspring in two strains of rats. *Alcohol Clin Exp Res* 12:465–70.
Abel, E. L., and Dintcheff, B. A. 1986. Saccharin preference in animals prenatally exposed to alcohol: No evidence of altered sexual dimorphism. *Neurobehav Toxicol Teratol* 8:521–23.
Abel, E. L., Dintcheff, B. A., and Day, N. 1980. Effects of marijuana on pregnant rats and their offspring. *Psychopharmacology (Berlin)* 71:71–74.
Barron, S., and Riley, E. P. 1985. Pup-induced maternal behavior in adult and juvenile rats exposed to alcohol prenatally. *Alcohol Clin Exp Res* 9:360–65.
———. 1990. Passive avoidance performance following neonatal alcohol exposure. *Neurotoxicol Teratol* 12:135–38.
Barron, S., Tieman, S. B., and Riley, E. P. 1988. Effects of prenatal alcohol exposure on the sexually dimorphic nucleus of the preoptic area of the hypothalamus in male and female rats. *Alcohol Clin Exp Res* 12:59–64.
Blanchard, B. A., Hannigan, J. H., and Riley, E. P. 1987. Amphetamine-induced activity after fetal alcohol exposure and undernutrition in rats. *Neurotoxicol Teratol* 9:113–19.
Blanchard, B. A., Pilati, M. L., and Hannigan, J. H. 1990. The role of stress and age in spatial navigation deficits following prenatal ethanol exposure. *Psychobiology* 18:48–54.
Blanchard, B. A., Riley, E. P., and Hannigan, J. H. 1987. Deficits on a spatial navigation task following prenatal exposure to ethanol. *Neurotoxicol Teratol* 9:253–58.
Boggan, W. O., Randall, C. L., and Dodds, H. M. 1979. Delayed sexual maturation in female C57BL/6J mice prenatally exposed to alcohol. *Res Commun Chem Pathol Pharmacol* 23:117–25.
Bryden, M. P. 1981. Sex-related differences in cerebral hemispheric asymmetry and their possible relation to dyslexia. In *Sex Differences in Dyslexia*, ed. A. Ansara, N. Geschwind, A. Galaburda, M. Albert, and N. Gartrell, 81–96. Towson, Md.: Orton Dyslexia Society.
Buelke-Sam, J., Kimmel, C. A., Adams, J., Nelson, C. J., Vorhees, C. V., Wright, D. C., St. Omer, V., Korol, A., Butcher, R. E., Geyer,

M. A., Holson, J. F., Kutscher, C. L., and Wayner, M. J. 1985.
Collaborative behavioral teratology study: Results. *Neurobehav Toxicol Teratol* 7:591–624.

Caldarone, B., and Kehoe, P. 1988. Neonatal naltrexone administration: Somatic and behavioral effects on the infant and adult rat. *Soc Neurosci Abstr* 14:31.

Chen, J. J., and Smith, E. R. 1979. Effects of perinatal alcohol on sexual differentiation and open-field behavior in rats. *Horm Behav* 13:219–31.

Collaborative Group on Antenatal Steroid Therapy. 1981. Effect of antenatal dexamethasone administration on the prevention of respiratory distress syndrome. *Am J Obstet Gynecol* 141:276–86.

Davis, D. P. 1977. Data cited by D. W. Smith. 1981. Maternal medications and drugs. In *Growth and Its Disorders*, 81–82. Philadelphia: W. B. Saunders.

de Avils, A., and Martinez, J. L., Jr. 1985. Sex-dependent effects of neonatally administered morphiceptin and D-ala D-leu enkephalin on maze learning in rats. *Behav Neural Biol* 44:393–402.

Esquifino, A. I., Sanchis, R., and Guerri, C. 1986. Effect of prenatal alcohol exposure on sexual maturation of female rat offspring. *Neuroendocrinology* 44:483–87.

Farry, K., and Tittmar, H. G. 1975. Alcohol as a teratogen: Effects of maternal administration in rats on sexual development in female offspring. *IRCS Med Sci Pharmacol Reprod Obstet Gynecol* 3:620–21.

Finucci, J. M., and Childs, B. 1981. Are there really more dyslexic boys than girls? In *Sex Differences in Dyslexia*, ed. A. Ansara, N. Geschwind, A. Galaburda, M. Albert, and N. Gartrell, 1–10. Towson, Md.: Orton Dyslexia Society.

Fishman, R. B., and Breedlove, S. M. 1988. Sexual dimorphism in the developing nervous system. In *Handbook of Human Growth and Developmental Biology*. Vol. 1, ed. E. Meisamo and P. S. Timiras, 45–57. Boca Raton, Fla.: CRC Press.

Frisancho, A. R., Klayman, J. E., and Matos, J. 1977. Influence of maternal nutritional status on prenatal growth in a Peruvian urban population. *Am J Phys Anthropol* 46:265–74.

Glick, S. D., Hinds, P. A., and Shapiro, R. M. 1983. Cocaine-induced rotation: Sex-dependent differences between left- and right-sided rats. *Science* 221:775–77.

Goodlett, C. R., Kelly, S. J., and West, J. R. 1987. Early postnatal alcohol exposure that produces high blood alcohol levels impairs development of spatial navigation learning. *Psychobiology* 15:64–74.

Gorski, R. A., Gordon, J. H., Shryne, J. E., and Southam, A. M. 1978. Evidence for a morphological sex difference within the medial preoptic area of the rat brain. *Brain Res* 148:333–46.

Graham, S., and Gandelman, R. 1986. The expression of ano-genital distance data in the mouse. *Physiol Behav* 36:103–4.

Grant, K. A., Choi, E. Y., and Samson, H. H. 1983. Neonatal ethanol exposure: Effects on adult behavior and brain growth parameters. *Pharmacol Biochem Behav* 18:331–36.

Grant, K. A., and Samson, H. H. 1982. Ethanol- and tertiary butanol-induced microcephaly in the neonatal rat: Comparison of brain growth parameters. *Neurobehav Toxicol Teratol* 4:315–21.

Grimm, V. E. 1984. A review of diazepam and other benzodiazepines in pregnancy. In *Neurobehavioral Teratology*, ed. J. Yanai, 153–62. Amsterdam: Elsevier Science Publishers.

Grimm, V. E., and Frieder, B. 1985. Differential vulnerability of male and female rats to the timing of various perinatal insults. *Int J Neurosci* 27:155–64.

Haas, J. D., Moreno-Black, G., Frongillo, G., Pabon, E. A., Pareja, L. G., Ybarnegaray, U. J., and Hurtado, G. L. 1982. Altitude and infant growth in Bolivia: A longitudinal study. *Am J Phys Anthropol* 59:251–62.

Hall, R. L. 1978. Sexual dimorphism for size in seven nineteenth-century Northwest Coast populations. *Hum Biol* 50:159–71.

———. 1982. *Sexual Dimorphism in Homo sapiens: A Question of Size*. New York: Praeger Publishers.

Handa, R. J., McGivern, R. F., Noble, E. S. P., and Gorski, R. A. 1985. Exposure to alcohol in utero alters the adult patterns of luteinizing hormone secretion in male and female rats. *Life Sci* 37:1683–90.

H'ard, E., Dahlgren, I. L., Engel, J., Larsson, K., Liljequist, S., Lindh, A. S., and Musi, B. 1984. Development of sexual behavior in prenatally ethanol-exposed rats. *Drug Alcohol Depend* 14:51–61.

H'ard, E., Engel, J., Larsson, K., Liljequist, S., and Musi, B. 1985. Effects of maternal ethanol consumption on the offspring sensory-motor development, ultrasonic vocalization, audiogenic immobility reaction and brain monoamine synthesis. *Acta Pharmacol Toxicol* 56:354–63.

Hindmarsh, P. C., and Brook, C. G. D. 1988. Hormonal control of infant growth in the first year. In *Fetal and Neonatal Growth*, ed. F. Cockburn, 195–210. New York: John Wiley.

Holson, R., Adams, J., Buelke-Sam, J., Gough, B., and Kimmel, C. A. 1985. Amphetamine as a behavioral teratogen: Effects depend on dose, sex, age and task. *Neurobehav Toxicol Teratol* 7:753–58.

Hull, E. M., Nishita, J. K., Bitran, D., and Dalterio, S. 1984. Prenatal dopamine-related drugs demasculinize rats. *Science* 224:1011–13.

Hutchings, D. E., Fico, T. A., and Dow-Edwards, D. L. 1989. Prenatal cocaine: Maternal toxicity, fetal effects and locomotor activity in rat offspring. *Neurotoxicol Teratol* 11:65–70.

Ioffe, S., and Chernick, V. 1987. Maternal alcohol ingestion and the incidence of respiratory distress syndrome. *Am J Obstet Gynecol* 156:1231–35.

Italian Multicentre Study. 1988. Epidemiology, clinical features, and prognostic factors of paediatric HIV infection. *Lancet* 2:1043–46.

Jones, K. L., and Smith, D. W. 1973. Recognition of the fetal alcohol syndrome in early infancy. *Lancet* 2:999–1001.

Jones, K. L., Smith, D. W., Ulleland, C. N., and Streissguth, A. P. 1973. Pattern of malformation in offspring of chronic alcoholic mothers. *Lancet* 1:1267–71.

Kakihana, R., Butte, J. C., and Moore, J. A. 1980. Endocrine effects of maternal alcoholization: Plasma and brain testosterone, dihydrotestosterone, estradiol and corticosterone. *Alcohol Clin Exp Res* 4:57–61.

Kariniemi, V., and Rosti, J. 1988. Maternal smoking and alcohol consumption as determinants of birth weight in an unselected study population. *J Perinat Med* 16:249–52.

Kelce, W. R., Rudeen, P. K., and Ganjam, V. K. 1989. Fetal rats exposed to alcohol in utero exhibit reduced testicular steroidogenic enzyme activity at birth. *Alcohol Clin Exp Res* 13:617–21.

Kellogg, C., Ison, J. R., and Miller, R. K. 1983. Prenatal diazepam exposure: Effects on auditory temporal resolution in rats. *Psychopharmacology (Berlin)* 79:332–37.

Kelly, S. J., Goodlett, C. R., Hulsether, S. A., and West, J. R. 1988. Impaired spatial navigation in adult female but not adult male rats exposed to alcohol during the brain growth spurt. *Behav Brain Res* 27:247–57.

Kelly, S. J., Mahoney, J. C., Randich, A., and West, J. R. 1991. Indices of stress in rats: effects of sex, perinatal alcohol and artificial rearing. *Physiol Behav* 49:751–56.

Kelly, S. J., Pierce, D. R., and West, J. R. 1987. Microencephaly and hyperactivity in adult rats can be induced by neonatal exposure to high blood alcohol concentrations. *Exp Neurol* 96:580–93.

Kelly, S. J., and Riley, E. P. 1989. Effects of alcohol exposure during the brain growth spurt on neurotransmitter levels in adult rats. *Alcohol Clin Exp Res* 13:319 (abstr).

Knipschild, P., Meijer, H., and Salle, H. 1981. Aircraft noise and birth weight. *Int Arch Occup Environ Health* 48:131–36.

Landesman-Dwyer, S., Keller, L. D., and Streissguth, A. P. 1978. Naturalistic observations of newborns: Effects of maternal alcohol intake. *Alcohol Clin Exp Res* 2:171–77.

Lemoine, P., Haronsseau, H., Borteyru, J-P., and Menuet, J-C. 1968. Les enfants de parents alcooliques; anomalies observés à propos de 127 cas. *Quest Med* 25:476–82.

Lieberman, L. 1982. Normal and abnormal sexual dimorphic patterns of growth and development. In *Sexual Dimorphism in Homo sapiens*, ed. R. L. Hall, 263–312. New York: Praeger Publishers.

Little, R. E., Asker, R. L., Simpson, P. D., and Renwick, J. H. 1986. Fetal growth and moderate drinking in early pregnancy. *Am J Epidemiol* 123:270–78.

Little, R. E., and Sing, C. F. 1987. Genetic and environmental influences on human birth weight. *Am J Hum Genet* 40:512–26.

McGivern, R. F. 1987. Influence of prenatal exposure to cimetidine and alcohol on selected morphological parameters of sexual differentiation: A preliminary report. *Neurotoxicol Teratol* 9:23–26.

McGivern, R. F., Clancy, A. N., Hill, M. A., and Noble, E. P. 1984. Prenatal alcohol exposure alters adult expression of sexually dimorphic behavior in the rat. *Science* 224:896–98.

McGivern, R. F., Holcomb, C., and Poland, R. E. 1987. Effects of prenatal testosterone propionate treatment on saccharin preference of adult rats exposed to ethanol in utero. *Physiol Behav* 39:241–46.

McGivern, R. F., Poland, R. E., Noble, E. P., and Lane, L. A. 1986. Influence of prenatal ethanol exposure on hormonal responses to clonidine and naloxone in prepubescent male and female rats. *Psychoneuroendocrinology* 11:105–10.

McGivern, R. F., Raum, W. J., Salido, E., and Redei, E. 1988. Lack of prenatal testosterone surge in fetal rats exposed to alcohol: Alterations in testicular morphology and physiology. *Alcohol Clin Exp Res* 12:243–47.

McGivern, R. F., Roselli, C. E., and Handa, R. J. 1988. Perinatal aromatase activity in male and female rats: Effect of prenatal alcohol exposure. *Alcohol Clin Exp Res* 12:769–72.

Martin, J. C., and Becker, R. F. 1971. Effects of maternal nicotine absorption or hypoxic episodes upon appetitive behavior of rat offspring. *Dev Psychobiol* 4:133–47.

Meyer, D. C., and Carr, L. A. 1987. The effects of perinatal exposure to nicotine on plasma LH levels in prepubertal rats. *Neurotoxicol Teratol* 9:95–98.

Meyer, L. S., and Riley, E. P. 1986. Social play in juvenile rats prenatally exposed to alcohol. *Teratology* 34:1–7.

Middaugh, L. D., Simpson, L. W., Thomas, N. T., and Zemp, J. W. 1981. Prenatal maternal phenobarbital increased reactivity and retards habituation of mature offspring to environmental stimuli. *Psychopharmacology (Berlin)* 74:349–52.

Mora, J. O., Sanchez, R., DeParedes, B., and Herrera, M. G. 1981. Sex related effects of nutritional supplementation during pregnancy on fetal growth. *Early Hum Dev* 5:243–51.

Nelson, L. R., Taylor, A. N., Lewis, J. W., Poland, R. E., Redei, E., and Branch, B. J. 1986. Pituitary-adrenal responses to morphine and footshock stress are enhanced following prenatal alcohol exposure. *Alcohol Clin Exp Res* 10:397–402.

Nielson, H. C., Zinman, H. M., and Torday, J. S. 1982. Dihydrotestosterone inhibits fetal rabbit pulmonary surfactant production. *J Clin Invest* 69:611–16.

Owen, G. M., Jensen, R., and Foman, S. 1966. Sex-related differences in total body water and exchangeable chloride during infancy. *J Pediatr* 60:858–68.

Parker, S., Udani, M., Gavaler, J. S., and Van Thiel, D. H. 1984. Adverse effects of ethanol upon the adult sexual behavior of male rats exposed in utero. *Neurobehav Toxicol Teratol* 6:289–93.

Pauls, D. L. 1979. Sex effect on the risk of mental retardation. *Behav Genet* 9:289–95.

Pericic, D., Manev, M., and Lakic, N. 1985. Sex differences in the response of rats to drugs affecting GABAergic transmission. *Life Sci* 36:541–47.

Peters, D. A., and Tang, S. 1982. Sex-dependent biological changes following prenatal nicotine exposure in the rat. *Pharmacol Biochem Behav* 17:1077–82.

Pierce, D. R., and West, J. R. 1986. Alcohol-induced microencephaly during the third trimester equivalent: Relationship to dose and blood alcohol concentration. *Alcohol* 3:185–91.

Qazi, Q. H., and Masakawa, A. 1976. Altered sex ratio in fetal alcohol syndrome. *Lancet* 2:42.

Ravenholt, R. T., and Levinski, M. J. 1965. Smoking during pregnancy. *Lancet* 1:961–62.

Redei, E., and McGivern, R. 1988. Attenuation of postnatal testosterone surge and decreased response to LH in fetal alcohol exposed males. *Alcohol Clin Exp Res* 12:341.

Riesenfeld, A. 1985. Growth-depressing effects of alcohol and nicotine in two strains of rats. *Acta Anat (Basel)* 122:18–24.

Riley, E. P., Lochry, E. A., and Shapiro, N. R. 1979. Lack of response inhibition in rats prenatally exposed to alcohol. *Psychopharmacology (Berlin)* 62:47–52.

Robinson, T. E., Becker, J. B., and Presty, S. K. 1982. Long-term facilitation of amphetamine-induced rotational behavior and striatal dopamine release produced by a single exposure to amphetamine: Sex differences. *Brain Res* 253:231–41.

Rooney, S. A. 1985. The surfactant system and lung phospholipid biochemistry. *Am Rev Respir Dis* 131:439–60.

Rosen, G. D., Berrebi, A. S., Yutzey, D. A., and Denenberg, V. H. 1983. Prenatal testosterone causes a shift of asymmetry in neonatal tail posture of the rat. *Dev Brain Res* 9:99–101.

Ross, W. D., and Ward, R. 1982. Human proportionality and sexual dimorphism. In *Sexual Dimorphism in Homo sapiens*, ed. R. L. Hall, 317–59. New York: Praeger Publishers.

Rudeen, P. K. 1986. Reduction of the volume of the sexually dimorphic nucleus of the preoptic area by in utero ethanol exposure in male rats. *Neurosci Lett* 72:363–68.

Rudeen, P. K., and Hagaman, J. 1988. Ovarian stimulation by exogenous gonadotrophins in fetal ethanol-exposed immature rats. *Experientia* 44:714–15.

Rudeen, P. K., Kappel, C. A., and Lear, K. 1986. Postnatal or in utero ethanol exposure reduction of the volume of the sexually dimorphic nucleus of the preoptic area in male rats. *Drug Alcohol Depend* 18:247–52.

Samson, H. H. 1986. Microcephaly and fetal alcohol syndrome: Human and animal studies. In *Alcohol and Brain Development*, ed. J. R. West, 167–83. New York: Oxford University Press.

Schell, L. M. 1984. The effects of chronic noise exposure on human prenatal growth. In *Human Growth and Development*, ed. J. Borms, R. Hauzpie, A. Sand, C. Susanne, and M. Hebbelnick, 125–29. New York: Plenum Press.

Shaywitz, B. A., Griffith, G. G., and Warshaw, J. B. 1979. Hyperactivity and cognitive deficits in developing rat pups born to alcoholic mothers: An experimental model of the expanded fetal alcohol syndrome (EFAS). *Neurobehav Toxicol* 1:113–22.

Smith, R. F., Mattran, K. M., Kurkjian, M. F., and Kurtz, S. L. 1989. Alterations in offspring behavior induced by chronic prenatal cocaine dosing. *Neurotoxicol Teratol* 11:35–38.

Sonderegger, T., O'Shea, S., and Zimmermann, E. 1979. Progeny of male rats addicted neonatally to morphine. *Proc West Pharmacol Soc* 22:137–39.

Spear, L. P., Kirstein, C. L., Bell, J., Yoottanasumpun, V., Greenbaum, R., O'Shea, J., Hoffman, H., and Spear, N. E. 1989. Effects of prenatal cocaine exposure on behavior during the early postnatal period. *Neurotoxicol Teratol* 11:57–64.

Spohr, H. L., and Steinhausen, H. 1987. Follow-up studies of children with fetal alcohol syndrome. *Neuropediatrics* 18:13–17.

Stini, W. 1969. Nutritional stress and growth. *Am J Phys Anthropol* 31:417–26.

————. 1972. Reduced sexual dimorphism in upper arm muscle circumference associated with protein-deficient diet in a South American population under nutritional stress. *Am J Phys Anthropol* 36:341–52.

Stinson, S. 1985. Sex differences in environmental sensitivity during growth and development. *Yearbook Phys Anthropol* 28:123–47.

Streissguth, A. P., Barr, H. M., Martin, D. C., and Darby, B. L. 1986. The fetal alcohol syndrome as a model for the study of the behavioral teratology of alcohol. In *Developmental Behavioral Pharmacology*. Vol. 5, ed. N. A. Krasnegor, D. B. Gray, and T. Thompson, 265–91. New Jersey: Lawrence Erlbaum Associates.

Streissguth, A. P., Clarren, S. K., and Jones, K. L. 1985. Natural history of the fetal alcohol syndrome: A ten-year follow-up of eleven patients. *Lancet* 2:85–92.

Streissguth, A. P., Landesman-Dwyer, S., Martin, J. C., and Smith, D. W. 1980. Teratogenic effects of alcohol in humans and laboratory animals. *Science* 209:353–61.

Streissguth, A. P., and Randels, S. P. 1989. Long-term effects of fetal alcohol syndrome. In *Alcohol and Child/Family Health*, ed. G. Robinson. In press.

Tanner, J. M. 1978. *Foetus into Man: Physical Growth from Conception to Maturity*. Cambridge, Mass.: Harvard University Press.

Taylor, A. N., Branch, B. J., Cooley-Matthews, B., and Poland, R. E. 1982. Effects of maternal ethanol consumption on basal and rhythmic pituitary-adrenal function in neonatal offspring. *Psychoneuroendocrinology* 7:49–58.

Taylor, A. N., Branch, B. J., Kokka, N., and Poland, R. E. 1983. Neonatal and long-term neuroendocrine effects of fetal alcohol exposure. *Monogr Neural Sci* 9:140–52.

Taylor, A. N., Branch, B. J., Liu, S. H., and Kokka, N. 1982. Long-term effects of fetal ethanol exposure on pituitary-adrenal response to stress. *Pharmacol Biochem Behav* 16:585–89.

Taylor, A. N., Branch, B. J., Liu, S. H., Wiechman, A. F., Hill, M., and Kokka, N. 1981. Fetal exposure to ethanol enhances pituitary-adrenal and temperature responses to ethanol in adult rats. *Alcohol Clin Exp Res* 5:237–45.

Taylor, A. N., Branch, B. J., Nelson, L. R., Lane, L. A., and Poland, R. E. 1986. Prenatal ethanol and ontogeny of pituitary-adrenal responses to ethanol and morphine. *Alcohol* 3:255–59.

Udani, M., Parker, S., Gavaler, J., and Van Thiel, D. H. 1985. Effects of in utero exposure to alcohol upon male rats. *Alcohol Clin Exp Res* 9:355–59.

Vitez, M., Koranyi, G., Conczy, E., Rudas, T., and Czeizel, A. 1984. A semiquantitative score system for epidemiologic studies of fetal alcohol syndrome. *Am J Epidemiol* 119:301–8.

Weinberg, J. 1985. Effects of ethanol and maternal nutritional status on fetal development. *Alcohol Clin Exp Res* 9:49–55.

———. 1988. Hyperresponsiveness to stress: Differential effects of prenatal ethanol on males and females. *Alcohol Clin Exp Res* 12:647–52.

———. In press. Prenatal ethanol effects: sex differences in offspring stress responsiveness. *Alcohol.*

———. 1989. Prenatal ethanol exposure alters adrenocortical development of offspring. *Alcohol Clin Exp Res* 13:73–83.

Weinberg, J., and Gallo, P. V. 1982. Prenatal ethanol exposure: Pituitary-adrenal activity in pregnant dams and offspring. *Neurobehav Toxicol Teratol* 4:515–20.

Weinberg, J., Nelson, L. R., and Taylor, A. N. 1986. Hormonal effects of fetal alcohol exposure. In *Alcohol and Brain Development*, ed. J. R. West, 310–42. New York: Oxford University Press.

Wertelecki, W., Hoff, C., and Zansky, S. 1987. Maternal smoking: Greater effects on males, fetal tobacco syndrome. *Teratology* 35:317–20.

West, J. R., Dewey, S. L., Pierce, D. R., and Black, A. C., Jr. 1984. Prenatal and early postnatal exposure to ethanol permanently alters the rat hippocampus. In *Mechanisms of Alcohol Damage in Utero*, Ciba Foundation Symposium No. 105, ed. M. O'Connor, 8–25. London: Pitman Books.

West, J. R., Hamre, K. M., and Cassell, M. D. 1986. Effects of ethanol exposure during the third trimester equivalent on number in rat hippocampus and dentate gyrus. *Alcohol Clin Exp Res* 10:190–97.

West, J. R., Hamre, K. M., and Pierce, D. R. 1984. Delay in brain growth induced by alcohol in artificially reared rat pups. *Alcohol* 1:213–22.

West, J. R., Hodges, C. A., and Black, A. C., Jr. 1981. Prenatal exposure to ethanol alters the organization of hippocampal mossy fibers in rats. *Science* 211:957–60.

Zagon, I. S., and McLaughlin, P. J. 1982. Analgesia in young and adult rats perinatally exposed to methadone. *Neurobehav Toxicol Teratol* 4:455–57.

Zimmerberg, B., Mattson, S., and Riley, E. P. 1989. Impaired alternation performance in rats following prenatal alcohol exposure. *Pharmacol Biochem Behav* 32:293–99.

Zimmerberg, B., and Reuter, J. M. 1989. Sexually dimorphic behavioral and brain asymmetries in neonatal rats: Effects of prenatal alcohol exposure. *Dev Brain Res* 46:281–90.

Zimmerberg, B., and Riley, E. P. 1986. Side preference in rats exposed to alcohol prenatally. *Neurobehav Toxicol Teratol* 8:631–35.

———. 1988. Prenatal alcohol exposure alters behavioral laterality of adult offspring in rats. *Alcohol Clin Exp Res* 12:259–63.

Zimmerberg, B., and Scalzi, L. V. 1989. Commissural size in neonatal rats: Effects of sex and prenatal alcohol exposure. *Int J Dev Neurosci* 7:81–86.

Zimmerberg, B., Sukel, H. L., and Steckler, J. D. 1991. Spatial learning of adult rats with fetal alcohol exposure: Deficits are sex-dependent. *Behav Brain Res* 42:49–56.

Zimmermann, E., Branch, B., Taylor, A. N., Young, J., and Pann, C. N. 1974. Long-lasting effects of prepubertal administration of morphine in adult rats. In *Narcotics and the Hypothalamus*, ed. E. Zimmermann and R. George, 183–96. New York: Raven Press.

Zimmermann, E., and Sonderegger, T. 1980. A syndrome of drug-induced delay of maturation. In *Biogenic Amines in Development*, ed. H. Parvez and S. Parvez, 591–606. Amsterdam: Elsevier/North-Holland.

3

Risk Factors for Alcohol-related Birth Defects: Threshold, Susceptibility, and Prevention

Robert J. Sokol, M.D., and Ernest L. Abel, Ph.D.

ALCOHOL is now widely recognized as a human teratogen capable of producing a wide range of anomalies from spontaneous abortion to behavioral abnormalities in the absence of physical malformations. Current appreciation of alcohol's teratogenicity followed the seminal articles by Jones and Smith and their colleagues (Jones et al. 1973; Jones and Smith 1973) and their coining of the term *fetal alcohol syndrome* to describe a cluster of anomalies (Jones and Smith 1973), since confirmed to occur in many children born to alcoholic women. In 1980, the Fetal Alcohol Study Group of the Research Society on Alcoholism proposed three specific criteria for the diagnosis of fetal alcohol syndrome (FAS):

- Pre-or postnatal growth retardation, or both
- Facial anomalies, including microphthalmia, a long and indistinct or absent philtrum, low-set and posteriorly rotated ears, and a flattened nasal bridge
- Indications of central nervous system dysfunction, including varying degrees of mental retardation

To merit a diagnosis of FAS, an individual must exhibit traits from each of these three categories. There is no single pathognomonic physical or behavioral characteristic. The occurrence of only one or two of the three diagnostic features has been previously referred to as *partial fetal alcohol syndrome* or *fetal alcohol effect*. Currently, a recommended term is *alcohol-related birth defects*.

Fetal alcohol syndrome is estimated to occur in 1.9 per 1,000 births in the United States and in about 25 per 1,000 children born to alcoholics (Abel and Sokol 1987). Estimates for alcohol-related birth defects are highly variable. Based on several epidemiological studies, we estimated the average minimal occurrence at about 3.1 per 1,000 for the total population and 90 per 1,000 for alcohol-abusing women (Abel 1984). We also estimated that about 5% of all congenital anomalies may be due to prenatal alcohol exposure (Sokol 1981). If substantiated, this would mean that a considerable number of birth defects previously attributed to "unknown origin" are caused by one of the most widely used substances in the world.

We recently estimated the economic impact of fetal alcohol syndrome in the United States. Based on an estimate of about 7,000 patients with FAS born each year in the United States (Abel and Sokol 1987) and on the costs of treating the problems of low birth weight, malformations, and mental retardation associated with these cases, we estimated an annual cost of $321 million (Abel and Sokol 1987). We also found that FAS is now the leading known cause of mental retardation in the Western world (Abel and Sokol 1987) and may account for as much as 11% of the annual cost for all mentally retarded institutionalized residents in the United States (Abel and Sokol 1987). Incidentally, the treatment costs for all FAS-related problems are about 100 times greater than the federal funding for FAS research necessary for the development of cost-effective early identification and prevention strategies.

FACTORS CONTRIBUTING TO THE TERATOGENICITY OF ALCOHOL

Alcohol alone is not always sufficient for teratogenicity. Other factors must be present for teratogenic effects to occur. Among the major risk factors that we have identified as contributing to alcohol's teratogenic effects are excessive drinking producing heavy exposure (probably at critical periods), black race, and increased maternal age/parity (Sokol et al. 1987; Abel and Dintcheff 1985).

Excessive Drinking

All studies of drinking during pregnancy rely on the patients' self-reported information about consumption. Detailed recall of drinking behavior is likely to be inaccurate, however, especially in the case of heavy drinkers, who may underreport their drinking or be unable to recall drinking patterns accurately. Estimates of alcohol consumption may vary from one to eight ounces, depending on how the questions about drinking behavior are posed (Rosett et al. 1983). There is also the problem of summarizing drinking throughout pregnancy by means of some simple statistic, such as number of drinks or ounces of absolute alcohol per day. Most people do not "standardize" their drinks. Except in the case of beer (where the container is the premeasured amount), a "drink" can vary considerably.

Patterns of drinking can also vary widely. If drinking does not occur every day (and it seldom does), the number of "drinks per drinking day" will be much higher than the average drinks per day. For example, a woman who drinks every other day would consume 4 drinks per drinking day but only an average of 2 drinks per day; a binge drinker who drank 14 drinks per drinking day once a week would also average only 2 drinks per day.

Jones and Smith (1984) reported one of the few comparisons of drinking patterns as they relate to FAS. Pregnant women were divided into three groups. One group consisted of women who binged one to three times during their first trimester (the time most likely to give rise to the physical anomalies associated with FAS). A second group was made up of women who drank regularly and heavily during this period. The third group consisted of women who drank lightly. None of the binge drinkers and light drinkers delivered children with FAS, whereas FAS was seen in children born to the chronic heavy drinkers. These results suggest that steady heavy drinking is a more important risk factor for FAS than is intermittent intake.

The Threshold for FAS

Based on our ongoing epidemiological studies (Sokol et al. 1987), we estimated the threshold for FAS at six drinks per day. We arrived at this threshold by first identifying 25 cases of FAS out of 1,290 prospectively studied pregnancies. We then tested the hypothesis that higher intake leads to FAS by dividing the pregnancies into five exposure groups consisting of no drinks, some but less than two drinks per day, etc., up to six or more drinks per day. We found no significant increments in risk for FAS at levels of less than six drinks per day. Considerably less than 10% of the study group and about 1% of the total population under study were drinking at or above this amount.

The Threshold for Specific Adverse Outcomes

Maternal drinking during pregnancy considerably increases the risk of spontaneous abortion. Some studies report as much as a twofold increase (Kline et al. 1980). However, this may be true only for women who are heavy drinkers (Sokol 1981). In nonhuman primates, pregnant animals abort more frequently only after being given alcohol at levels causing a blood alcohol concentration of 0.2 g/100 ml (200 mg/dl) or above (e.g., Clarren, Bowden, and Astley 1987; Scott and Fradkin 1982). A 140-lb woman would have to consume about eight drinks to produce this blood alcohol concentration (American Council on Alcoholism, n.d.).

Progressively less severe effects than abortion would include fetal alcohol syndrome and isolated alcohol-related birth defects. As previously noted, we estimated the threshold for FAS at six drinks. Specific effects ought to occur at lower alcohol doses, which are imbibed by higher proportions of the population. Thus, about 1% of the population drinks enough to cause FAS (Sokol et al. 1987), whereas we have estimated that 3.5% of the population drinks enough to increase the risk of birth defects significantly (Ernhart et al. 1987). This estimate is reasonably close to that of Mills and Graubard (1987), who found that the risk for isolated anatomical birth defects in association with prenatal alcohol exposure was limited to the top 2.9% of their very large sample of 32,870 conceptuses.

A threshold has now been reported for the craniofacial anomalies seen in connection with FAS (Ernhart et al. 1987). To estimate this threshold, 1,284 neonates from the Cleveland Prospective Study were examined without knowledge of maternal drinking histories. We were able to detect a threshold for increased craniofacial abnormalities when mothers consumed more than four drinks per day, with no effect attributable to alcohol consumption below this level of embryonic exposure ("no effect zone"). This level of drinking was noted in only 2% of the study population.

The most consistent effect of prenatal alcohol exposure is decreased birth weight. The average birth weight of children born with FAS is about 2,000 g, compared to a median birth weight of 3,300 g for all infants in the United States. Low birth weight (< 2,500 g) and, in particular, intrauterine growth retardation are of concern because they are generally associated with an increased risk of neurological abnormalities.

Decreases in birth weight due to prenatal alcohol exposure may occur in the absence of FAS. Little (1977) reported that such decreases were related to the dose of alcohol. However, alcohol abusers in Little's study could have accounted for most of the observed relationship. Kuzma and Sokol (1982) found that consumption of 1.5 drinks per day did not result in a statistically significant decrease in birth weight. Examination of the contribution of various beverages suggested that a small proportion (3%) of beer drinkers who were frequent drinkers gave birth to children with reduced birth weight. At present, a threshold for decreased birth weight is still unknown.

Havlicek, Childiaeva, and Chernick (1977) found electroencephalographic (EEG) hypersynchronies so prominent in the delta and theta frequencies that they were able to identify 20 out of 22 infants born to alcoholic mothers on the basis of EEG patterns alone. Chernick, Childiaeva, and Joffe (1983) also noted that "this increase in [EEG] amplitude was in several instances of such magnitude that amplification had to be reduced by half." Such hypersynchronous EEG patterns were also noted by Majewski and colleagues (1976) and represent a possible end point for which thresholds can be determined as well as a marker for early detection of neural damage in children with the FAS, which would otherwise go undetected until the children were aged 8–10 years.

The Continuum of Reproductive Casualty

During the course of our examinations of thresholds for the effect of prenatal alcohol exposure, we are using the concept of a "continuum of reproductive casualty." The basis of this application of the concept is that alcohol has different influences on offspring depending on the amount of exposure. To appreciate this relation, one must first determine the lowest exposure that may yield an adverse outcome and then delineate the range of adverse outcomes. From our own studies and those in the literature, we had concluded that spontaneous abortion is related to the consumption of alcohol at amounts that produce blood alcohol levels of at least 0.2 g/100 ml (Abel and Sokol 1989) during the first trimester. As noted above, this blood alcohol level is associated with the consumption of about eight drinks per day, which occurs in much less than 2% of our patient population. Spontaneous abortion, of course, constitutes a very severe alcohol-related birth defect, with failure of the pregnancy to progress beyond the first trimester. Our estimate of the rarity of drinking at a level sufficient to cause abortion is reasonably consistent with other estimates in the literature (Sokol et al. 1977; Harlap and Shiono 1980; Kline et al. 1980). Most likely, the threshold for FAS is slightly lower (six drinks per day) and is exceeded somewhat more frequently; the thresholds for isolated alcohol-related birth defects are lower still but are still relatively rarely exceeded—perhaps by 3–5% of pregnant women.

It is reasonable to conclude that, for the outcomes evaluated, a limited proportion of the population is at risk—the very heaviest drinkers. However, our estimates and concepts must be tempered by our awareness of denial and maternal underreporting, especially among the women who drink most heavily.

Because of denial, actual alcohol intake is probably much higher than the levels reported by the abusive drinker—the individual most likely to be at risk for giving birth to a child with alcohol-related birth defects. To examine this issue more closely, Ernhart et al. (1988) obtained self-reported drinking levels at the time of the first prenatal visit and at 4–5 years after giving birth. Retrospective drinking reports were highly correlated with in-pregnancy reports. For 41% of the women, however, the retrospective reports gave higher amounts than those obtained during the pregnancy. Especially noteworthy was the fact that the retrospective report was a better predictor of alcohol-related birth defects than was the in-pregnancy report. This improved predictive validity suggests that the reports of more drinking were more accurate. Furthermore, the higher the Michigan Alcohol Screening Test (MAST) score, the greater the underreporting. Consequently, the risk to the fetus of what might appear to be "two drinks a day" is probably the result of much higher intake.

A study using the "bogus pipeline" points to the same conclusion. With this technique, the patient is told that her verbal or written response may be independently checked by laboratory tests of her blood or urine. Using this technique, Lowe et al. (1986) found that 14% of pregnant patients admitted drinking when asked to complete a questionnaire only, whereas 27% said that they drank if they were asked to complete a questionnaire and were told that laboratory tests would also be conducted to verify their responses.

Genetic Susceptibility

Although fraternal twins are presumably exposed to the same level and duration of alcohol, one of the twins may be more severely affected than the other by prenatal alcohol exposure (Christoffel and Salafsky 1975; Santolya et al. 1978). Such occurrences point to genetically determined differences in prenatal susceptibility to alcohol's effects in utero.

Genetically determined rates of alcohol absorption, metabolism, and elimination are also a factor. Chernoff (1980), for instance, found that differences in rates of fetal anomalies in different strains of mice were directly related not to the amount of alcohol consumed by pregnant mothers, but to the blood alcohol levels attained after the same amount of alcohol was consumed. Although this has not been directly studied in the human being, it is possible that two women might consume the same amount of alcohol but develop very different blood alcohol levels, leading to very different levels of exposure of their conceptuses.

Other than clinical reports in twins, there is currently little in the literature concerning susceptibility to alcohol-related birth defects in humans. With regard to intrauterine growth retardation and FAS, our studies have found that the risk to the black fetus is seven times higher than that to the white fetus. With regard to alcohol-related birth defects, we were able to detect a lower threshold for blacks than whites. Analyzed dose for dose above the threshold, there were approximately twice as many alcohol-related birth defects in blacks as in whites. Furthermore, in this analysis the alcohol-by-race interaction term was statistically significant. Finally, many other factors were tested in these analyses, including many patient characteristics, nutrition, and exposure to other drugs, with no significant findings.

In assessing genetic susceptibility factors, future studies must evaluate not only the genes themselves, but also their expression. The first question, of course, will be, "which genes?" There is some current work on the genes controlling alcohol dehydrogenase isoenzymes. Acetaldehyde dehydrogenase isoenzymes should also be addressed. Perhaps the most promising genetic area regarding alcohol metabolism will focus on genes controlling the microsomal ethanol-oxidizing system. This is the inducible alcohol metabolic pathway and, hence, would constitute an interesting approach to the evaluation of genetic tolerance. Equally important may be evaluation of the genes controlling central nervous system characteristics (e.g., membrane constitution). Susceptibility may be due to innate sensitivity of the organism to exposure to differing alcohol levels. With the availability of gene amplification techniques, a true genetic marker for susceptibility to alcohol-related birth defects may well become available for clinical application.

A final thought concerning genetic susceptibility involves the potential for retrospective ascertainment of cases. In other words, an individual's genes are constant. Thus, a very good strategy might be to study affected and unaffected offspring, given that it is possible to obtain reasonable estimates of their prenatal alcohol exposure. This would constitute a classic case-control study design, but one using very sophisticated genetic technology.

Maternal Age/Parity

Later-born children of alcoholic mothers tend to be more severely affected by prenatal alcohol exposure than are those born earlier (Abel 1988; Fitze, Spahr, and Pescia 1978; Majewski 1978; Manzke and Grosse 1975). This suggests that either increased parity or increased maternal age increases the risk of fetal alcohol effects.

Parity can adversely influence reproductive outcome because it is associated with (1) an increased risk for congenital anomalies among women aged 35 and older (Taffel 1978), (2) an increase in low birth weight for parity of four or more (U.S. National Center for Health Statistics 1980), and (3) a possible decrease in nutritional support for the conceptus due to an increase in uterine collagen and elastin content with an ensuing decreased blood supply (Robertson and Manning 1974; Woessner 1963). In terms of maternal age, the conceptus of a women over 35 years of age is at increased risk for spontaneous abortion, congenital anomalies, low birth weight, and postnatal mortality (Butcher and Page 1981; Chamberlain and Kasahara 1971; Talbert and Blatt 1978). Such parity- and/or age-related factors could conceivably interact with alcohol to place the conceptus at greater risk for fetal alcohol effects.

The influence of maternal parity and age on fetal alcohol effects was previously examined in the rat. Maternal age was identified as a critical variable in alcohol's effects during pregnancy (Abel and Dintcheff 1985). On the other hand, parity per se was not a major factor influencing alcohol's effects on the conceptus (Abel and Dintcheff 1984).

These results raise additional questions about how maternal age potentiates the effects of fetal alcohol exposure. We previously showed that increased age is associated with increased blood alcohol concentrations in pregnant rats (Church et al 1990). It is likely that higher blood alcohol concentrations increase the risk to the fetus (for review, see Abel 1984).

PREVENTION: THE BOTTOM LINE

The most rational and cost-effective way of reducing alcohol-related birth defects is prevention. About 30% of adult American women are abstinent or drink so little as to be considered abstinent. Most of the remaining 70% drink only occasionally, and most of these will not realize that they are pregnant until well into their first trimester. It is prudent to discuss drinking habits during prenatal visits, but even more prudent to alert women who are intending to become pregnant to the potential dangers of alcohol consumption. If warnings about alcohol and pregnancy are delayed until the first prenatal visit, some women who do not receive prenatal care may not receive any such notices.

Broad media coverage on the dangers of drinking has proven successful from an information standpoint but has failed to have the desired effect. For example, in one survey 90% of those questioned showed an awareness of the harm that drinking during pregnancy could do to their babies, but 75% considered three or more drinks per day to be safe for their developing infants (Little et al. 1981). Other studies showed that, despite public education efforts, the proportion of women drinking an average of at least two drinks per day had remained relatively constant over the preceding six years (Streissguth et al. 1980). This group very probably represents the most vulnerable population of the development of fetal alcohol effects; if so, mass media efforts to warn women of the dangers of drinking during pregnancy have, for the most part, been preaching to the converted.

A viable alternative for prevention is to raise the issue in the clinic or physician's office and to attempt to help patients decrease alcohol consumption before and during pregnancy. This has already been implemented in a number of cities in the hope that pregnancy outcomes for many women will improve (Rosett et al. 1978; Sokol and Judge 1983). A major difficulty with this approach is the need to educate and train health care personnel to identify alcohol abuse in their patients. Sokol provided one strategy for such determinations (Sokol, Martier, and Ager 1989). This involves indirectly probing for alcohol use and related problems by imbedding pertinent questions in the overall history taking, rather than pointedly asking the patient questions about volume and frequency of drinking, an approach often frustrated by patient denial, especially when there is a drinking problem.

When patients indicate that they can consume three or more drinks at a time without feeling "high," the physician should be alerted to the possibility of tolerance. If the patient becomes irritable or defensive when questioned about drinking behavior, this is also suggestive of underlying alcohol abuse. In both cases, a more detailed history taking is warranted. If it appears that the patient does indeed have an alcohol problem, repeating the suggestion to stop, or at least decrease drinking, during later prenatal visits, along with follow-up questions about drinking, may help her to attain abstinence or at least to cut down significantly on her drinking during pregnancy. This seems to be an effective way of aiding women whose fetuses may be at risk.

We believe that the sine qua non for preventing alcohol-related birth defects requires identification of the at-risk group. This in turn requires a clear definition of that group based on information from threshold and susceptibility studies. Many questions concerning the potential for early identification of women at risk remain. The literature in this particular area is distinctly limited. Many more studies involving the development and application, as well as testing for transportability and validity, of questionnaires and biochemical markers are needed. Will it be possible to develop a clinical/genetic profile of patients at risk to facilitate the focusing of prevention efforts? Can the affected embryo/fetus be detected early enough in pregnancy to support appropriate clinical decision making? Ultrasound technology, with the use of high-resolution vaginal probes, is advancing rapidly. Abnormal facial features, genito-urinary development, and other anomalies might be detectable during the late first or early second trimester.

Although somewhat beyond the purview of this review, it is important to comment that, even given the ability to identify a group for whom we might focus prevention efforts, there is little available to tell us what might constitute an appropriate set of prevention efforts for women of reproductive age. One research opportunity at the time of this writing (early 1989) would be to look at the effect of the new law on labeling from the perspectives of what women know and also of any change in behavior, particularly among heavy-drinking women (i.e., risk-drinkers). In addition, we need to look carefully at the physician's office/gynecology clinic/antenatal clinic as an environment for focused prevention.

The final crucial step toward an effective prevention strategy is very likely a prospective randomized clinical trial of early identification and intervention. The outcome measure of interest might initially be evidence of decreased alcohol intake periconceptionally and through-out gestation. Ideally, one would like to see evidence of improved pregnancy outcome. When one considers the relative rarity of reliably documented alcohol-attributable abnormality in offspring, however, the potential for a clinical trial with infant outcome as the primary outcome measure seems limited. Nonetheless, clinical trials will be necessary, along with studies of transportability and, finally, of the overall effect of such prevention interventions on the national prevalence of fetal alcohol syndrome and alcohol-related birth defects.

ACKNOWLEDGMENTS

The research reported in this chapter was supported in part by grants from the National Institute on Alcohol Abuse and Alcoholism (AA 05631, 06999; P50 AA07606).

REFERENCES

Abel, E. L. 1984. *Fetal Alcohol Syndrome and Fetal Alcohol Effects.* New York: Plenum Press.

Abel, E. L. 1988. Fetal alcohol syndrome in families. *Neurobehav Toxicol Teratol* 10:1–2.

Abel, E. L., and Dintcheff, B. A. 1984. Factors affecting the outcome of maternal alcohol exposure: I. Parity. *Neurobehav Toxicol Teratol* 6: 373–77.

———. 1985. Factors affecting the outcome of maternal alcohol exposure: II. Maternal age. *Neurobehav Toxicol Teratol* 7: 263–66.

Abel, E., and Sokol, R. J. 1987. Incidence of fetal alcohol syndrome and economic impact of FAS-related mental retardation. *Drug Alcohol Depend* 19: 51–70.

Abel, E., and Sokol, R. J. 1989. Alcohol consumption during pregnancy: The dangers of moderate drinking. In ed. H. W. Goedde and D. E. Agarwal, *Alcoholism: Biomedical and Genetic Aspects*, 228–39. New York: Pergamon Press.

American Council on Alcoholism. n.d. *Know Your Limits.* Towson, Md.

Butcher, R. L., and Page, R. D. 1981. Introductory remarks: Environmental and endogenous hazards to the female reproductive system. *Environ Health Perspect* 38:35–37.

Chamberlain, J. C., and Kasahara, M. 1971. Influence of maternal age and parity on fetal mortality and congenital abnormalities induced in rats. *Growth* 35:213–20.

Chernick, V., Childiaeva, R., and Joffe, S. 1983. Effects of maternal alcohol intake and smoking on neonatal electroencephalogram and anthropometric measurements. *Am J Obstet Gynecol* 146:41–47.

Chernoff, G. F. 1980. The fetal alcohol syndrome in mice: Maternal variables. *Teratology* 22:71.

Christoffel, K. K., and Salafsky, I. 1975. Fetal alcohol syndrome in dizygotic twins. *J Pediatr* 87:963–67.

Church, M. W., Abel, E. L., Dintcheff, B. A., and Matyjasik, C. 1990. Maternal age and blood alcohol concentration in the pregnant Long-Evans rat. *J Pharmacol Exp Ther* 253:192–99.

Clarren, S. K., Bowden, D. M., and Astley, S. 1987. Pregnancy outcomes after weekly oral administration of ethanol during gestation in the pig-tailed macaque (*Macaca nemestrina*). *Teratology* 35:345–56.

Ernhart, C. B., Morrow-Tlucak, M., Sokol, R. J., and Martier, S. 1988. Underreporting of alcohol use in pregnancy. *Alcohol Clin Exp Res* 12:506–11.

Ernhart, C., Sokol, R. J., Martier, S. S., Moron, P., Nader, O., Ager, J. W., and Wolfe, A. 1987. Alcohol teratogenicity in the human: A detailed assessment of specificity, critical period and threshold. *Am J Obstet Gynecol* 156:33–39

Fitze, F., Spahr, A., and Pescia, G. 1978. Familienstudie zum problem des embryofotalen alkoholsyndroms (Fetal alcohol syndrome: Follow-up of a family). *Schweiz Rundsch Med Prax* 67:1338–54.

Harlap, S., and Shiono, P. 1980. Alcohol, smoking and incidence of spontaneous abortions in the first and second trimester. *Lancet* 2:173–76.

Havlicek, U. Childiaeva, R., and Chernick, U. 1977. EEG frequency spectrum characteristics of sleep states in infants of alcoholic mothers. *Neuropediatrie* 8:360–73.

Jones, K. L., and Smith, D. W. 1973. Recognition of the fetal alcohol syndrome in early infancy. *Lancet* 2:999–1001.

———. 1984. Study shows maternal alcohol binges may not hurt the fetus. *Med World News* 25:102–21.

Jones, K. L., Smith, D. W., Streissguth, A. P., and Myrianthopoulos, N. C. 1973. Patterns of malformation in offspring of chronic alcoholic women. *Lancet* 1:1267–71.

Kline, J., Shrout, P., Stein, A., Susser, M., and Warburton, D. 1980. Drinking during pregnancy and spontaneous abortion. *Lancet* 2:176–80.

Kuzma and Sokol, R. J. 1982. Maternal drinking behavior and decreased intrauterine growth. *Alcohol Clin Exp Res* 6:396–402.

Little, R. E. 1977. Moderate alcohol use during pregnancy and decreased infant birthweight. *Am J Public Health* 67:1154–56.

Little, R. E., Grathwohl, H. L., Streissguth, A. P., and McIntyre, C. 1981. Public awareness and knowledge about the risks of drinking during pregnancy in Multhomah County, Oregon. *Am J Public Health* 71:312–14.

Lowe, J. B., Windsor, R. A., Adams, B., Morris, J., and Reese, V. 1986. Use of bogus pipeline method to increase accuracy of self-reported alcohol consumption among pregnant women. *J Stud Alcohol* 47:173–75.

Majewski, F. 1978. Uber schadigende einflusse des alkohol auf die nachkommen (The damaging effects of alcohol on offspring). *Nervenarzt* 49:410–16.

Majewski, F., Bierich, J., Loeser, H., Michaelis, R., Leiber, B., and Bettecker, F. 1976. Diagnosis and pathogenesis of alcohol embryopathy: Report of 68 cases. *Munich Med Wochenschr* 118:1635–41.

Manzke, H., and Grosse, F. R. 1975. Inkomplettes und Komplettes des Alkoholsyndrome: Bei drei Kindern einer Trinkerin (Incomplete and complete alcohol syndrome: Three children of a female drinker). *Med Welt* 26:709–12.

Mills, J., and Graubard, B. 1987. Is moderate drinking during pregnancy associated with an increased risk for malformation? *Pediatrics* 80:309–14.

Robertson, W. B., and Manning, P. J. 1974. Elastic tissue in uterine blood vessels. *J Pathol* 112:237–43.

Rosett, H. L., Ouellette, E. M., Weiner, L., and Owens, E. 1978. Therapy of heavy drinking during pregnancy. *Obstet Gynecol* 51:41–46.

Rosett, H. L., Weiner, L., Lee, A., Zuckerman, B., Dooling, E., and Oppenheimer. 1983. Patterns of alcohol consumption and fetal development. *Obstet Gynecol* 61:539–46.

Santolya, J. M., Martinez, G., Gorostiza, E., Alzpiri, J., and Hernandez, M. 1978. Alcoholismo fetal *Drogalcohol* 3:183–93.

Scott, W. J., and Fradkin, R. 1982. The effects of prenatal alcohol in cynomolgus monkeys. *Teratology* 29:49–56.

Sokol, R. J. 1981. Alcohol and abnormal outcomes of pregnancy. *Can Med Assoc J* 125:143–48.

Sokol, R. J., Ager, J., Martier, S., Debanne, S., Ernhart, C., Kuzma, J., and Miller, S. 1987. Significant determinants of susceptibility to alcohol teratogenicity. *Ann NY Acad Sci* 477:87–102.

Sokol, R. J., Ernhart, C., Ager, J., and Martier, S. 1987. Embryonic

susceptibility to anatomic alcohol-related birth defects (ARBD).
Alcohol Clin Exp Res 11:212.

Sokol, R. J., and Judge. 1983. Drug abuse in pregnancy. In *Current Therapy in Obstetrics and Gynecology*, ed. E. J. Quelligan, 74–77. Philadelphia: W. B. Saunders.

Sokol, R. J., Martier, S., and Ager, J. 1989. The t-ace questions: Practical prenatal detection of risk-drinking. *Am J Obstet Gynecol* 160:863–70.

Sokol, R. J., Rosen, M., Stojkow, J., and Chik. L. 1977. Clinical application of high risk scoring on an obstetric service. *Am J Obstet Gynecol* 128:652–61.

Streissguth, A. P., Barr, H. M., Martin, D. C., and Herrman, C. S. 1980. Effects of maternal alcohol, nicotine and caffeine use during pregnancy on infant mental and motor development at 8 months. *Alcohol Clin Exp Res* 4:152–64.

Taffel, S. 1978. *Congenital Anomalies and Birth Injuries among Live Births: United States, 1973–1974.* Washington, D. C.: U. S. Department of Health, Education and Welfare. DHEW Publication (PHS) 79–1909.

Talbert, L. M., and Blatt, P. M. 1978. Disseminated intravascular coagulation in obstetrics. *J Clin Obstet Gynecol* 22:889–900.

U.S. National Center for Health Statistics. 1980.

Woessner, J. F., 1963. Age-related changes of the human uterus and its connective tissue framework. *J Gerontol* 18:220–26.

4

Clinical Considerations Pertaining to Adolescents and Adults with Fetal Alcohol Syndrome

Robin A. LaDue, Ph.D., Ann P. Streissguth, Ph.D., and Sandra P. Randels, M.S.N.

PRENATAL substance abuse can produce a multitude of long-range, serious effects on offspring. This book reviews the research findings on many teratogenic substances and their effects on laboratory animals and human subjects. The purpose of this chapter is to demonstrate how one teratogen, alcohol, affects the lives of children and adults who were exposed in utero. Although alcohol has been clearly established as a teratogenic drug with particular effects on the central nervous system (CNS), the long-term clinical consequences in terms of individual psychopathology and social maladjustment are only recently being recognized.

In this chapter we draw on our clinical experience with fetal alcohol syndrome over a 15-year period and on our recent study of adolescents and adults. We show why it is important to identify the basic CNS deficits in the individual patient to facilitate the most efficacious environmental interventions. We also show how diagnostic and psychological test results are used in evaluating cognitive and adaptive functioning and obtaining needed services for patients manifesting the long-term consequences of prenatal alcohol exposure.

The data in this paper derive from a study of 92 patients with fetal alcohol syndrome (FAS) and fetal alcohol effects (FAE) with a mean age of 18.4 years (age range, 12–42). The sample was 77% American Indian, 20% white, and 3% black. The racial characteristics of the sample reflect the original recruitment policies and are not representative of the prevalence of FAS in these populations. FAS occurs in all racial groups according to the proportion of alcohol-abusing mothers (Majewski, Bierich, and Seidenberg 1978; May et al. 1983).

DIAGNOSTIC CONSIDERATIONS

A diagnosis of FAS is given when prenatal alcohol consumption is confirmed and the child has a cluster of three characteristics: growth deficiency, certain dysmorphic features, and CNS deficits. It is now recognized that there are partial and less severe manifestations of alcohol damage that are probably related to variations in dose, timing, and individual factors, but which are not necessarily as unique to prenatal alcohol exposure as is FAS. These partial effects are frequently termed possible *fetal alcohol effects* (FAE) (Clarren 1981). Although one cannot say with certainty in the case of patients with FAE that the symptoms are necessarily caused only by alcohol, recognition of the organic nature of the deficits can be extremely useful in developing treatment programs.

The growth deficiency typical of FAS encompasses both height and weight. It is of prenatal onset, and postnatal "catch-up" does not usually occur, at least for height. Some girls with FAS gain weight during adolescence, but boys tend to remain thin throughout adolescence (Streissguth, Clarren, and Jones 1985).

The facial features commonly seen in FAS (fig. 4.1) include short palpebral fissures (eye slits), a low nasal bridge, epicanthal folds, a flat midface, an indistinct philtrum, microcephaly, a thin upper vermillion, and a small chin (Jones and Smith 1973; Jones et al. 1973). Other abnormalities noted include congenital eye defects, such as strabismus, ptosis, and optic nerve hypoplasia (Stromland 1985), minor ear anomalies, and posteriorly rotated ears (Smith 1982), as well as dental malocclusions, malformations, and misalignments of the secondary teeth. Many of the craniofacial features noted above stay relatively constant over time, but changes do occur at puberty. The most notable of these are growth of the nose and lower jaw, less flattening of the nasal bridge, and more prominent dental abnormalities (figs. 4.2–4.4).

Joint anomalies, altered palmar creases, minor genital anomalies, and heart defects are also noted. The heart defects are less observable with increasing age. Other physical problems seen in adolescent and adult patients include scoliosis and gait and hip abnormalities.

The third characteristic for diagnosing FAS is CNS deficits. These deficits include small brain size (manifested through microcephaly), brain malformation, delayed development, mental retardation, and learning disabilities, as well as fine motor tremor, hyperactivity, and

FACIES IN FETAL ALCOHOL SYNDROME

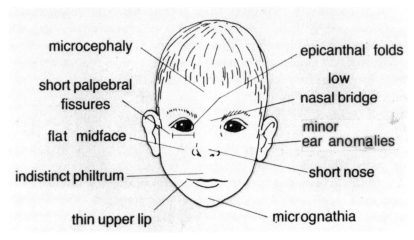

microcephaly

short palpebral fissures

flat midface

indistinct philtrum

thin upper lip

epicanthal folds

low nasal bridge

minor ear anomalies

short nose

micrognathia

Figure 4.1. Common facial characteristics in children with fetal alcohol syndrome. The characteristics on the left are those most frequently seen; those on the right are less specific.
Source: Little and Streissguth 1982.

poor attention span. With the exception of hyperactivity, these problems persist over time. As the patient gets older, hyperactivity evolves into problems of easy distractibility, inability to attend to relevant data, and inability to ignore irrelevant information (Streissguth, Clarren, and Jones 1985).

IQ and Achievement

Standardized IQ tests [the Wechsler Intelligence Test for Children-Revised (n = 82) and the Wechsler Adult Intelligence Scale-Revised (n = 67) were administered to the patients in the present study. For these analyses, we combined the scores for patients with FAS and FAE.

The mean IQ for these patients was 70, but the range was broad (20–108). As the cut-off for developmental disability services is usually an IQ of 69 or below, only 46% of this group would qualify for such services on the basis of IQ scores alone. This is a major problem because the cognitive problems manifested by these patients also occur

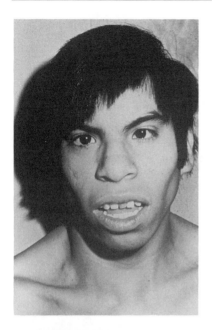 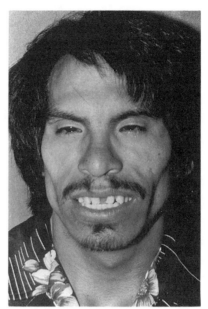

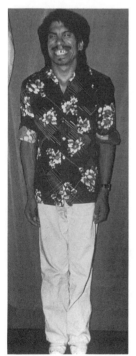

Figure 4.2. A man with fetal alcohol syndrome at age 19 (left) and at age 30 (right and below left). Note the long arms; short, lean stature; and coarser features in adulthood.
Sources: Streissguth, Herman, and Smith 1978 (a); Streissguth and LaDue 1987 (b, c).

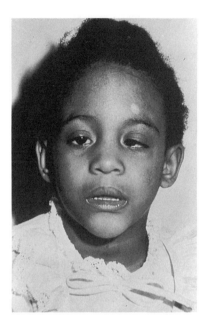
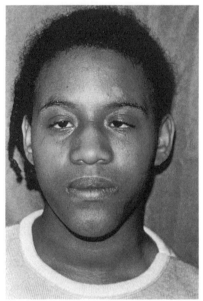

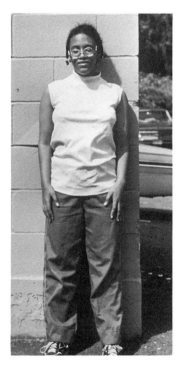

Figure 4.3. A patient with fetal alcohol syndrome at age 3 years 9 months (left) and at age 14 years 2 months (right and below left). Note the persistence across ages of the short palpebral fissures, hypoplastic philtrum, strabismus, and ptosis; the increased growth of the nose and mandible at the later age; and the short, stocky stature often associated with puberty in girls with fetal alcohol syndrome.

Sources: Jones et al., 1973 (a); Streissguth, Clarren, and Jones 1985 (b, c).

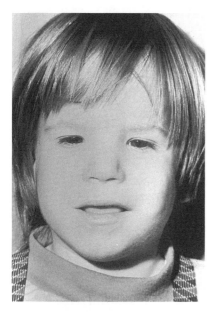 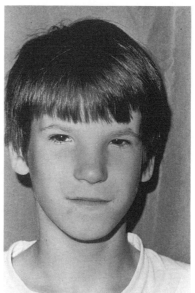

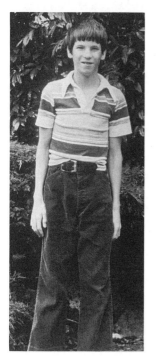

Figure 4.4. A patient with fetal alcohol syndrome at age 2 years 6 months (left) and at age 12 years 2 months (right and below left). Note the short, lean prepubertal stature of young adolescent boys with fetal alcohol syndrome.
Sources: Jones et al., 1973 (a); Streissguth, Clarren, and Jones 1985 (b, c).

in those with an IQ over 69 and can require special services to amelio-rate. The mean Verbal IQ for the group was 65, and the mean Perfor-mance IQ was 79. The higher Performance IQ score is consistent with the clinical picture presented by patients with FAS. The Performance subtests require less abstracting ability and less short-term memory (except Coding) and are more tactile than the Verbal subtests. The more abstract the task and the more memory needed (e.g., the Similari-ties and Arithmetic subtests), the poorer these patients perform. Ab-stracting and memory deficits are manifested in many areas, affecting not only academic performance, but also daily living skills.

The discrepancy between Performance and Verbal IQ scores is often used as a measure of CNS dysfunction. A significant proportion of the sample (33%) had a Performance IQ minus Verbal IQ discrepancy of 20 points or more. This difference was seen in both FAS and FAE patients, indicating a consistent pattern of CNS damage and consequent dysfunction for both diagnostic groups.

The Peabody Picture Vocabulary Test-Revised was administered to measure receptive language levels. The mean standard score was 60, indicating more difficulty in the area of receptive language than in gen-eral intelligence.

It is frequently thought that IQ scores are a fairly accurate predictor of academic achievement. However, the data from the current study do not fully support this contention. The Wide Range Achievement Test-Revised (WRAT-R) was used to measure Reading, Spelling, and Arithmetic. (The Reading subtest consists of letter and word recogni-tion and does not measure reading comprehension.) The mean standard scores were 71 for Reading, 72 for Spelling, and 64 for Arithmetic. Thus, we see that, for patients with FAS/FAE, Arithmetic achievement is considerably below what one would predict from their IQ scores, while Spelling and Reading are in the predicted range. This low Arith-metic score is another manifestation of the underlying difficulty with memory and abstraction that we note clinically.

Adaptive Functioning

Clinical observations and caretaker reports document social and adaptive functioning as the areas of most concern. Adaptive functioning was measured with the Vineland Adaptive Behavior Scales (VABS), which were filled out during an interview with the caretaker. The VABS yield standard scores (SS) and age equivalents (AE) for communication, daily living, and socialization skills. An overall adaptive behavior score and a maladaptive behavior score are also given. Data were obtained on a subset of 54 patients who had the same mean IQ as the full sample.

The Communication Domain

The Communication Domain measures written or verbal communication skills, as well as expressive and receptive interactions. The mean SS for the sample was 51, far below the IQ and achievement scores. Although the mean age of these patients was 17.3 years, their mean age *level* on the Communication Domain was 8.1 years.

The Daily Living Skills Domain

The Daily Living Skills Domain evaluates items such as hygiene, household tasks, use of money and time, and job skills. These tasks are more repetitive and concrete than those in the Communication and Socialization domains. As with the Verbal and Performance subtests on the IQ tests, patients with FAS did better on tasks requiring less abstracting ability. For the sample, the mean SS and AE scores on the VABS in the Daily Living Skills Domain were 60 and 9.2 years, respectively. As with the Arithmetic scores, IQ is not an accurate predictor of daily living skills for these patients.

The Socialization Domain

The Socialization Domain of the VABS includes interpersonal skills and the ability to follow social rules and conventions. The skills needed to perform well in these areas are more abstract and subtle than those needed in the first two domains. As might be expected, the SS and AE scores are lower than in the Communication and Daily Living Skills domains. The overall sample had a mean SS of 53 and a mean AE of 6.9 years.

The Adaptive Behavior Composite Score

The Adaptive Behavior Composite Score of the VABS is an average of all three domains and is quite useful in predicting long-term functional abilities of patients with FAS. The sample had a mean composite SS of 50 and a mean AE of 8.0 years. The pattern of deficits of these patients is the same regardless of mean chronological age (17.3

years overall). IQ scores are not an accurate predictor of adaptive functioning and may be misleading in many cases. Regardless of age, IQ, diagnosis, socioeconomic background, level of education, or sex, these patients do not function at a level that allows independent living or self-sufficiency.

Maladaptive Behavior

Maladaptive Behavior is another important dimension evaluated by the VABS. The behaviors in this area include a spectrum from less severe behaviors (such as temper tantrums) to severely maladaptive behaviors (such as self-abusive, stereotypic, and self-destructive behaviors). Maladaptive behavior scores are classified according to three levels of severity: nonsignificant (low), intermediate (medium), and significant (high). The level of maladaptive behavior in patients with FAS/FAE is very high. The majority (58%) of them exhibited significant maladaptive behaviors. Poor concentration and attention were the items most frequently noted as problems (77% of patients); other frequently observed problem behaviors included compulsivity, stubbornness, teasing, and dependency (table 4.1; fig. 4.5).

Psychosocial Functioning

A primary area of concern has been the myriad of personal and social difficulties manifested by both FAS and FAE patients. The maladaptive behavior questions on the VABS are helpful in quantifying these difficulties. To give a more complete picture of the psychosocial functioning of affected patients, we developed the Symptom Checklist, which we administered to the caretakers of 88 patients, supplemented with data from the medical records. The symptoms most characteristic of adolescents and adults with FAS/FAE were attentional deficits (80%), memory problems (73%), and hyperactivity (72%). The findings are summarized in table 4.2.

Another area covered by the Symptom Checklist was the patient's background. Factors of specific interest were neglect, physical abuse, and sexual abuse. Overall, 86% of the patients had been neglected at some point in their lives, 52% had a history of physical abuse, and 35% had a history of sexual abuse. Valid data are difficult to obtain retrospectively; these figures may represent minimal estimates as there was often not a single caretaker who had known the patient across the life-span.

Table 4.1. Percentage of Patients with FAS/FAE with Specific
Maladaptive Behaviors from the Vineland Adaptive Behavior Scales

Behavior	
1. Has poor concentration and attention	77
2. Withdraws	62
3. Is too impulsive	57
4. Is overly dependent	53
5. Teases or bullies	53
6. Exhibits extreme anxiety	51
7. Is stubborn or sullen	50
8. Lies, cheats, or steals	49
9. Is negativistic or defiant	43
10. Cries or laughs too easily	42
11. Shows lack of consideration	42
12. Has poor eye contact	40
13. Is overly active	40
14. Exhibits excessive unhappiness	38
15. Expresses thoughts that are not sensible	38
16. Avoids school or work	34
17. Rocks back and forth while sitting or standing	33
18. Has temper tantrums	28
19. Is unaware of what is happening in immediate surroundings	27
20. Runs away	26
21. Is truant from school or work	25
22. Bites fingernails	25
23. Intentionally destroys own or another's property	25
24. Engages in inappropriate sexual behavior	21
25. Exhibits extremely peculiar mannerism or habits	20
26. Exhibits a sleep disturbance	19
27. Is too physically aggressive	19
28. Swears in inappropriate situations	19
29. Exhibits an eating disturbance	17
30. Sucks thumb or fingers	15
31. Exhibits tics	15
32. Grinds teeth during day or night	15
33. Has excessive or peculiar preoccupations with objects or activities	15
34. Displays behaviors that are self-injurious	15
35. Uses bizarre speech	12
36. Wets bed	6

Note: For all patients (N = 54); mean age = 17.3 years; age range = 15 to 33
years; mean IQ = 71.

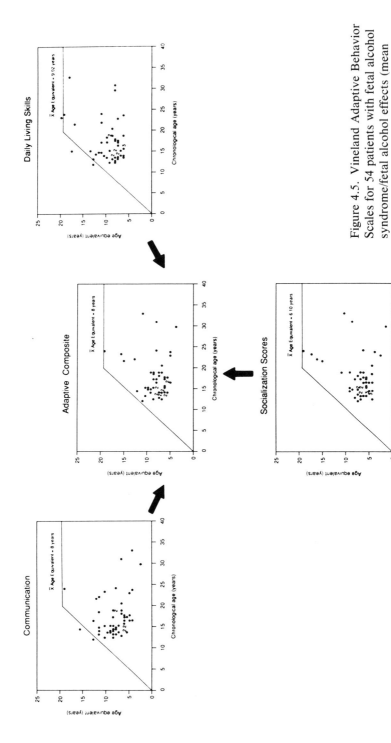

Figure 4.5. Vineland Adaptive Behavior Scales for 54 patients with fetal alcohol syndrome/fetal alcohol effects (mean chronological age 17 years).
Source: Streissguth et al. 1991.

Table 4.2 Symptom Checklist: Problems Reported for Patients with
Fetal Alcohol Syndrome/Fetal Alcohol Effects

Problem	*n*	FAS/FAE	Males	Females
Attention deficit	73	80%	80%	78%
Memory problems	74	73	70	78
Hyperactivity	67	72	75	65
Child neglect	80	86	83	91
Physical abuse	60	52	46	60
Sexual abuse	52	35	19	57
Sexually inappropriate with people	75	31	38	18
Sexually inappropriate with animals	72	6	9	0
Legal problems with sexual misconduct	68	13	20	4
Pregnancy/fathered a child	68	10	3	19
Truancy	68	53	52	54
School suspension	54	32	32	30
School dropout	56	29	29	29
School expulsion	53	9	15	0
Drug abuse	73	25	26	22
Alcohol abuse	76	36	45	21
Petty larceny	68	28	27	30
Grand larceny	69	4	7	0
Vandalism	62	27	32	21
Drunk driving	70	23	23	22
Lying	49	57	57	58
Stealing	63	35	41	27
Temper tantrums	62	60	63	55
Disobedience	72	64	67	58
Defiance of authority	57	46	46	46
Seizure disorder	62	10	6	15

Note: *n* = the appropriate sample size for each question. It was not possible
to obtain valid data on all questions for all patients because of discontinuities
in their caretaking environments.

The third area addressed by the Symptom Checklist dealt with the sexual behavior of the patients. As our patients matured, caretakers expressed increasing concern about sexually inappropriate behavior and possible exploitation. Sexually inappropriate behavior with people was reported for 31% of the patients. Male patients were more likely than females to be involved in sexually inappropriate behavior (38% versus 18%). These gender differences are consistent with concerns expressed clinically by patient caretakers.

The incidence of sexual misconduct leading to legal problems was higher in this population than might have been anticipated, with 13% of our patients being charged with some type of violation. Again, males (20%) were far more likely to have such complaints lodged against them than were females (4%). Males, as anticipated, were more sexually aggressive than females. However, female patients were still at risk for sexual problems such as exploitation or promiscuity. Nineteen percent of our female patients had had children, but only one male was known to have fathered a child.

School attendance and behavior were also explored by the checklist. A majority (53%) of our sample had truancy problems. Interestingly enough, this truancy rate was almost identical for both sexes. Given the academic difficulties experienced by these patients, the school dropout rates were surprisingly low—29% for the entire sample. As with truancy problems, there was no difference by sex. Many of the caretakers and teachers described disruptive classroom behavior on the part of patients with FAS/FAE, but the suspension and expulsion rates were lower for this sample than we anticipated: 32% and 9%, respectively. No gender difference was noted for suspension, but all of those expelled from school were male.

Drug and alcohol use and abuse were of concern to us, given the high risk for substance abuse among the offspring of alcoholic patients. In terms of drug abuse, 25% of our patients reported past or current problems. Alcohol abuse, not surprisingly, was reported at a higher level, with 36% of the patients acknowledging alcohol abuse. We found no significant gender differences in terms of drug use, but males abused alcohol at a higher rate than females.

Socially inappropriate behavior has sometimes led to legal problems among our patients with FAS/FAE. The Symptom Checklist included questions about problems with shoplifting or petty larceny, grand larceny, vandalism, and drunk driving. The rate for petty larceny was 28%, and that for grand larceny was 4%. For petty larceny, no gender difference was noted. For grand larceny, however, the three patients involved were all male. Twenty-seven percent of our patients had been involved in the destruction of property. The drunk driving rate was high (23%), given that only one of our patients was known to have a driver's license.

The final area of the Symptom Checklist addressed inappropriate social and personal behaviors, such as lying, stealing, temper tantrums, disobedience, and defiance of authority. A surprisingly high percentage of patients (57%) were described as having problems with lying. Many times the "lying" seemed to be the patient simply choosing whichever version of events came to mind. It is often difficult for these patients to separate fact from fantasy. Stealing was observed in 35% of affected patients. Temper tantrums were also reported at a high level, 60% of all patients regardless of sex or age. Problems with disobedience were reported at a rate of 64%. Problems with defiance of authority were seen in 46% of our patients. Clearly, the social and behavioral problems so frequently described in younger patients with FAS do not disappear, and new problems emerge with physical maturation.

FOUR CASE HISTORIES

The following four case studies (two males, two females; two patients with FAS, two with FAE) illustrate the cognitive, academic, and social deficits seen in patients with FAS/FAE and show how the environment can help or hinder these patients in reaching their full potential.

Case 1

Patient 1 is an 18-year-old, single woman of Canadian Indian and white descent. She was born to alcoholic parents and has a diagnosis of FAS. She has small palpebral fissures, small eyes, and a history of growth deficiency in height, weight, and head circumference. She was described as being quite delayed in reaching her developmental milestones: walking occurred at 24 months, talking in sentences at 3½ years, and toilet training at 4 years.

Her early years were marked by repeated bouts with pneumonia and other respiratory problems, as well as recurrent otitis media. She also had frequent urinary tract infections found to be caused by kidney and ureter problems. These difficulties were corrected through surgery. At present, she appears well nourished and healthy.

The life history of patient 1 is very similar to that of most patients with FAS. She was placed in foster care at six months of age because of neglect by her biological mother. She has never had any contact with her biological father. At age 4, her biological mother attempted to retrieve her from the foster family and give her to the maternal grandparents living on the reservation. It was this attempt that prompted her foster family to adopt her.

Her adoptive family consists of two parents and their grown children. The family has often taken in foster children, particularly those who are disadvantaged or handicapped. The parents are retired and in their 60s. During the past two years, the care of patient 1 and her disruptive behavior have become too difficult for the parents to handle, and she is now in an adult care facility.

Before her current placement, her adoptive parents had established a structured routine at home and had worked closely with her teachers to help develop her academic and living skills. They encouraged her to help out with chores and to be an active participant in family life. The parents had hopes of their daughter being able to "grow up and have babies," yet they would not let her boil water for fear of her hurting herself. This conflict between wanting her to have a normal life and the reality of her deficits is a common problem for the caretakers of patients with FAS.

Patient 1 has been described as being disruptive and attention seeking, as well as stubborn and manipulative. She has little awareness of the appropriateness or consequences of her behavior. As she reached adolescence and sexual maturity, her adoptive parents became concerned about possible sexual exploitation. She talked to strangers and responded to others' suggestions without regard to the possible consequences and despite repeated admonitions from her teachers and parents. These behaviors are what led to the adult group-home placement.

Patient 1 has poor socialization skills and is easily influenced by others. She is more comfortable around younger children and adults than with her age mates. She is unable to structure her own time or to set reasonable limits. The group home where she now resides provides structure and clear guidelines to which she has responded in a very positive fashion. She can now take care of her own hygiene and also help with household and cooking tasks. She has remained in close contact with her adoptive parents and spends one month each summer with them.

Between the ages of seven and nine, patient 1 received complete psychological and psychiatric evaluations. The results of these tests indicated that she had a borderline IQ with specific learning disabilities, poor short-term memory and concentration, auditory and perceptual problems, distractibility, poor motor skills, hyperactivity, lack of persistence, poor socialization skills, and emotional deprivation in early infancy. She was given a tentative diagnosis of FAS at this time.

When we examined patient 1 at age 14, she had a Weschler Intelligence Scale for Children-Revised (WISC-R) Full-Scale IQ of 65, a Verbal Scale IQ of 64, and a Performance Scale IQ of 69. Thus, as an adolescent, her intellectual functioning was in the mildly retarded range, although her general physical appearance, sociable manner, and conversational skills would not indicate to the casual observer the degree of her intellectual handicap. The school, however, recognized her as a slow learner, and she was placed in special education classes. At age 14, the WRAT revealed reading (Word Recognition) skills at the sixth grade level, spelling skills at the 6.7 grade level, and arithmetic skills at the kindergarten level. Thus, we can see that her reading and spelling skills were at a higher level than would be predicted from her IQ (WRAT standard scores of 85 and 90, respectively), while her arithmetic skills were far worse. Unfortunately, a Reading Comprehension score was not obtained.

The Vineland Adaptive Behavior Scale was administered at age 16. She functioned as predicted by her IQ score in the Communication Domain (standard score, 67; age equivalent, 10 years 4 months) and the Daily Living Skills Domain (SS = 65, AE = 10 years). However, she functioned far below expectations on both the Socialization Domain (SS = 50, AE = 6 years 1 month) and the overall Adaptive Behavior Composite (SS = 56, AE = 8 years 10 months). Her maladaptive behavior was at the "intermediate" level.

The pattern of academic achievement and adaptive functioning displayed by patient 1 is typical of many patients with FAS. Their often adequate performance on the rote aspects of word recognition and spelling failed to reveal their difficulty in basic comprehension and problem solving. A low arithmetic score, both in absolute terms and in relation to word recognition and spelling, is also customary. In patients with

FAS, the arithmetic score often serves as a marker for their current level of abstract thinking and problem solving. Although patient 1 reads and writes at the sixth grade level, she has considerable difficulty organizing her life and very poor judgment. Thus, she does not function as one would predict for a person with sixth grade reading skills.

It is likely that patient 1 is going to continue to need a structured living situation for the remainder of her life. She is capable of holding a job such as a nurse's aide or cook's helper, but she is not able to manage her own finances nor to live independently. Despite the special services and the excellent adoptive and residential placements she has had, patient 1, at the age of 18, continues to show many of the physical, cognitive, and social deficits associated with FAS in adolescents and adults.

Case 2

Patient 2 is a 23-year-old, single, white man with a diagnosis of FAS. He has one older brother who also has been diagnosed as having FAS. Patient 2 was born to a chronic alcoholic mother; he has had little or no contact with his biological father. He was placed temporarily in foster care at age 5 when his mother had tuberculosis and in permanent foster care with the same family after his biological mother died when he was 10 years old. He has remained with this family throughout his life.

Patient 2 was growth deficient for height, weight, and head circumference during childhood and continues to be so in early adulthood. He has the facial features commonly associated with FAS, as well as hand and other abnormalities (e.g., clinodactyly and pectus excavatum). He had respiratory problems during early childhood, as well as tuberculosis meningitis at age 3. His IQ scores have been consistent, ranging from a low of 68 at age 14 to a high of 76 at age 15. His IQ score on the last evaluation (age 20) was 67. His current IQ scores are close to what is usually expected from patients with FAS and are in the borderline to mildly retarded range.

He was in special education all during his schooling and received additional vocational training after graduation from high school. His achievement scores on the WRAT-R are consistent with expectations based on IQ. At age 20 his Reading score was at the 6.2 grade level, with a standard score of 79; his Spelling score was at grade 5.2, with a standard score of 77; and his Arithmetic score was at grade 5.0, with a standard score of 81 (a higher Arithmetic score than we find with most FAS patients).

Compared to his level of academic achievement, patient 2 had rather low scores on the VABS. At age 20 he had a Communication Domain AE of 6 years 5 months, with a standard score of 30. His score on Daily Living Skills was higher (AE = 8 years 4 months; SS = 54), but his Socialization scores were quite low (4 years 2 months, with a standard score of 27). His social skills and judgment were consistent with those of a 6-year-old child. His overall Adaptive Behavior score was 6 years 4 months, with a standard score of 34. Patient 2's Maladaptive Behavior score was at the "significant" level.

His poor performance on these tests is strongly reflected in his personal life. At age 20, patient 2 was charged with indecent liberties for molesting an 8-year-old foster sister. He was placed on probation and received special therapy.

Patient 2's appearance is that of a fairly normal young man, leading people to perceive him as far more functional than is actually the case. His foster parents have been very consistent in their expectations and awareness of their son's needs. They have encouraged him to go on to vocational training and to work. However, he tends to lose interest in his jobs rapidly and to be easily distracted. He is quite sociable but without a sense of direction. He has had some work experience as a janitor and chef's aid and, at last report (age 21), was working as an aide on a bus for a charity organization. His job consists of helping handicapped people on and off buses. He continues to live next door to his adoptive mother and has girl friends. No additional reports of grossly inappropriate sexual behavior have been received. When he tried to live on his own, he was unsuccessful because of his inability to structure his life and manage his own affairs. It is highly unlikely that he will ever be able to function independently despite general academic functioning at the fifth to sixth grade level. Plans for a group placement when his foster family can no longer care for him are under consideration.

Case 3

Patient 3 is a 14-year-old American Indian boy with FAE. He was the third of five children born to alcoholic parents. All of the children have been removed from the care of the biological parents because of neglect and placed in foster care. Parental rights were formally terminated by the tribe. Patient 3 was first described as FAE at age 7 because of his growth deficiency for height and weight and his microcephaly. He lacks the usual FAS dysmorphology. He was hospitalized during his first years of life for pneumonia, bronchitis, and failure to thrive. At present, no health problems are reported, although he remains growth deficient and microcephalic.

Little is known of patient 3's early development. At age three he was placed in a group home because of abandonment by his biological parents. Group home and early school reports describe him as being shy, emotionally deprived in early childhood, and having a tendency to display temper tantrums. Reports also indicate that he needed constant supervision and had difficulties setting limits on his own behavior.

Patient 3 was moved from the group home to a single foster family four years ago, at age ten. He shares the home with one of his older biological brothers, his foster mother and father, and a younger foster sister. The home is warm but structured, with a great deal of nurturance and guidance. His foster mother seems to have a good sense of what her son needs emotionally and academically. When he first came to live with the family, he displayed temper tantrums and cried frequently. The family approached these issues with love and firmness. None of these behaviors is a problem at this time.

Patient 3 seems to enjoy school and has been in part-time special education classes. IQ scores have remained stable over time, with a Full-Scale IQ of 88, which represents the low normal range of intelligence, at age 14. He has a Verbal IQ of 78, and a Performance IQ of 102. His standard score and age equivalency score on the Peabody Picture Vocabulary Test-Revised were 69 and 8 years 7 months, respectively. His academic achievement, despite special services, is lower than expected based on his IQ scores. His standard score and grade equivalency score on the WRAT-R were, respectively: Reading, 74 and 3.3; Spelling, 76 and 4.7; and Arithmetic, 66 and 4.7.

Patient 3's adaptive behavior scores on the VABS were also lower than those of his age mates and, again, were lower than might be expected from his diagnosis and IQ scores. His standard scores and age equivalent scores on the VABS at age 14 were, respectively: Communication, 70 and 9 years; Daily Living Skills, 56 and 7 years 7 months; Socialization, 63 and 7 years 2 months and Adaptive Behavior Composite, 58 and 7 years 11 months. His score on Maladaptive Behavior was at the "significant" level.

Patient 3 appeared somewhat shy but behaved appropriately when evaluated at age 14. His verbal skills were low, but he did not seem to be easily distracted or to have a significant memory problem. The more serious problems in his life have appeared during times of change. He has responded well to structure and love. One of the more positive aspects of his foster home is the encouragement that he has received for developing his social skills. He has several close friends, one of whom was at the same group home.

One of the crucial items that should be noted in this case is his lower level of academic and adaptive functioning despite his higher IQ. It seems that he is at or close to his academic ceiling. In spite of living in an excellent foster home, his adaptive functioning is low. He may be able to maintain employment in a semiskilled or even skilled job, if enough structure and support are provided. However, he is unable to handle his own finances or to set his own behavioral limits. These problems are likely to make it difficult for him to function in a totally independent fashion despite an IQ score in the normal range.

Case 4

Patient 4 is an 18-year-old, single woman who has FAE. She was the last of six children born to an alcoholic mother. The biological mother has had little contact with her; the biological father is deceased.

Patient 4 was placed in a series of foster homes between birth and age five because of her mother's continuing alcoholism, abuse, and neglect. She was then adopted and did fairly well until preadolescence. The adoptive family consisted of the mother and two older brothers. The adoptive mother had consistently been employed and provided a stable, warm, and caring environment, even moving to a small town to provide a less dangerous setting for her daughter's development.

In early childhood, patient 4 was growth deficient for height and weight and was microcephalic. By age eight, she was no longer growth deficient for weight but remained so for height and head circumference. In adolescence, she has the appearance of being slightly obese; she lacks the more obvious facial features associated with FAS.

Her IQ score has dropped from 99 at age 6 to 86 at age 14. The results from her last evaluation (at age 14) showed her Reading level at grade 7, her Spelling skills at grade 7½, and her Arithmetic skills at grade 5. She was placed in special education classes, but the school wanted to mainstream her because of her success in the special education program. Mainstreaming was not successful because of behavioral and academic problems. Her general comportment and school performance deteriorated markedly after the cessation of special education classes.

Despite IQ scores in the normal to low normal range, neither her academic achievement nor her adaptive functioning has been at the expected level. She is several years behind her age mates in both areas. At age 14, her scores on the Vineland Adaptive Behavior Scales placed her Communication skills at age 7 years 7 months, with a standard score of 51; her Daily Living skills at 7 years 3 months, with a standard score of 50; and her Socialization abilities at age 4 years 2 months, with a standard score of 43. Her overall Adaptive Behavior score was 6 years 4 months, with a standard score of 45. Her Maladaptive Behavior was at the "significant" level.

The deficits shown on patient 4's test results are consistent with the concerns noted by her adoptive mother, including impulsive and sexually provocative behavior, as well as poor judgment and a refusal to help out around the house. Of major concern has been her inappropriate and sexually aggressive behavior toward her adoptive brothers. At age 16 she began running away from home, cutting school, and living on the streets, coming home only for food. She finally ran away to live with a married relative, who has young children. Her biological family, however, has had many problems and is quite unstable. One of her sisters is involved with drugs and prostitution; another is mentally retarded and has cerebral palsy. After a year in a new school, she again dropped out and was last known to be living with a friend and the friend's mother for a short period of time. She has a child whom she is unable to care for and also has been institutionalized for mental problems.

Patient 4 and her adoptive mother attempted counseling before she left home. They began counseling because of the numerous fights they were having and because of patient 4's suicide attempts and depression. The adoptive mother had made her daughter the top priority in her life and felt frustrated and saddened by the problems her daughter was having. The mother was in the process of locating a temporary home for her daughter when she ran away.

Patient 4's behavior deteriorated despite the support and encouragement provided in the adoptive home. Her poor judgment, coupled with sexually aggressive behavior, put her at high risk for exploitation and her subsequent pregnancy. It is difficult to determine the causes of the poor outcome with this patient, but they are undoubtedly multiple. It seems likely that late placement in a stable home left many emotional scars that normal mothering could not overcome. Furthermore, the school's refusal to place patient 4 in special education classes resulted in a frustrating and difficult school experience. The crucial factor seems to have been her removal from special education classes, where she had done well.

PSYCHIATRIC AND SOCIAL IMPLICATIONS

The first two sections of this chapter outline the deficits seen in patients with FAS and provide four case histories to illustrate the effects of such deficits. This section focuses at a more general level on the emotional and social implications of FAS and how these are influenced by the patient's environment. As previously detailed, the academic, social, and cognitive functioning of these patients is impaired, regardless of diagnosis, IQ, or residential placement.

The most salient problems experienced by patients with FAS result from the CNS damage due to prenatal alcohol exposure. These include impulsivity, poor judgment, poor social skills, difficulty in organizational skills, and difficulty in recognizing and setting boundaries. In day-to-day living, those patients in tightly structured homes with vigilant parents were able to minimize but not prevent or eradicate problems.

Some of our older adolescent and adult patients with FAS/FAE are living in shelters or low income housing. Others are wandering from relative to relative, and still others are in dysfunctional and/or alcoholic homes. It is these latter patients who are having the worst time. Many of them seem to be decompensating emotionally or to have other mental disorders. The question of dual diagnosis should be addressed in relation to patients with FAS/FAE, particularly as they mature.

We see these older patients having difficulty communicating their needs, being self-sufficient, maintaining their own hygiene, and applying for and receiving social services. Many, if not most, of these patients have a great deal of difficulty relating to their age mates in an appropriate fashion. They are often made the center of jokes at school, are easily led and manipulated by others, and, as adults, are frequently at risk for social, sexual, and financial exploitation.

A major concern for the caretakers of our female patients is the high risk of sexual abuse and/or pregnancy. These young women usually have little sense of protecting their bodies or of how to avoid potentially dangerous situations. We have had several reports of them talking to strange men, being sexually provocative, and being involved in other behavior that could lead to problems. These behaviors persist despite caretakers repeatedly telling them not to behave this way. Women with FAE often look fairly "normal" and do not give the appearance of being handicapped. Thus, they seem to be in control of their lives when they really are not.

In our study, six women and one man are known to have had children. Four women are on one Indian reservation. One is married but wanders in and out of the marriage and provides only sporadic child care. Her husband refused to give up the baby and is raising him. The second woman and her child are living with an aunt. We have no information on who is raising the child. We do have information indicating that the mother is abusing alcohol and other drugs. The third woman is married and apparently doing adequately in the marriage and with child care. The fourth woman is a divorced mother of two and is a chronic alcoholic as well as being transient. The father cares for the children. The other two women and one man live in an urban area. One of these women is single. One of her children has been adopted, and she has had one abortion. She is now caring for one child on her own and is pregnant again. She is 21 years old, and her caseworker keeps in close contact with her. The other woman is 18 years old and has one child. Our one known male parent had been living with his girlfriend, a mildly retarded young woman, and their baby. They were in close contact with his foster parents. They have recently separated, and the mother is caring for the child.

Given our patients' difficulty in raising children and the likelihood of a second generation being impaired if mothers with FAS abuse alcohol during pregnancy, the issue of birth control is critical. Until recently, there have been almost no practical options for these patients. Many are not responsible enough to use a diaphragm or to take the pill. Sterilization is a very controversial issue and one that must be approached with sensitivity and care. Depo-Provera (medroxyprogesterone 17-acetate; The Upjohn Co.) is in use with some of our most dysfunctional patients and has proven to be a viable option. One promising option is Norplant, a progesterone implant that lasts for five years. A major drawback, however, to the use of Norplant is the current cost of $500. It is hoped that the social services system will take a proactive approach and provide funds for this important method of birth control. Accessible pregnancy terminations should also be among the choices available to patients with FAS who do not wish to have children.

Many of our higher-functioning patients (IQ > 80) are aware of their deficits, some to the point of understanding that the deficits were caused by their mothers' drinking during pregnancy. These patients start to rebel in their teens when this awareness manifests itself. They see that they are not doing as well in school as their age mates and are falling behind academically, they find themselves isolated from these age mates, and they are unable to compete successfully in any realm of daily living. Among these patients, we see increased levels of depression, anger, suicidal ideation, antisocial behavior, and drug and alcohol use.

Our patients with FAE seem to be particularly at risk for more academic and social problems and fewer services. Frequently, these patients are normal or nearly normal in their physical appearance. A higher IQ, sometimes in the normal range, leads to greater expectations on the part of teachers and caretakers. Despite a higher IQ, the pattern of cognitive and social deficits is the same as in those patients with FAS. In some areas (e.g., neglect, school truancy and dropout, alcohol abuse, petty larceny, and pregnancy), patients with FAE are experiencing more difficulties than are those with FAS.

Ill and aging foster and adoptive parents are other environmental problems that threaten the home life of these patients as they mature. Foster and adoptive parents who have successfully parented younger children may have difficulty with the changing demands of mentally handicapped adults, especially if the parents are already in their 60s, as is often the case. Communities must provide appropriately sheltered environments, such as supervised group homes, and must aid the smooth transition from family living to group-home life. It is clear from this study that most patients with FAS and many with FAE will be unable to live normal, independent lives in our complex society. Continued protection by the community will be necessary for those whose adoptive and foster families are unable to continue with their care.

It is our sense that patients with FAS and particularly those with FAE are "dropping through the service gap" at an alarmingly high rate for a myriad of reasons. As previously noted, many of these patients "appear" normal and have IQ scores far higher than the cutoff rate for developmentally disabled services. They are less likely to have been placed in foster or adoptive care at an early age and are far less likely to be receiving services for adult developmentally disabled patients.

"Insight" therapy has had limited success with patients with FAS/FAE. A more instructive, practical, daily living approach, which helps to teach the patient to respond appropriately, make healthy choices, and avoid dangerous situations, is far more useful. However, in situations where there is depression, antisocial behavior, and drug use, we strongly recommend professional intervention and support, preferably by therapists experienced with handicapped adolescents and adults. Additionally, we find that support and respite care are valuable for the caretakers of these patients. Many patients and families make effective use of a "case manager," who helps them access community resources, provides crisis intervention, and acts as a "sounding board" for problem situations. Many of these interactions can be carried out by telephone, although regular appointments are useful for some patients.

In accessing community services, psychiatric diagnoses are often useful adjuncts to the diagnosis of FAS/FAE, particularly for patients with IQ scores within the normal or dull-normal range. Many of our patients with FAS and FAE fit the diagnostic criteria for attention deficit disorder with hyperactivity and for conduct disorders. Some of our older and more functional patients meet the criteria for a major affective disorder, particularly depression. Unfortunately, an increasing number of these patients are also beginning to fall in the category of substance use disorders (e.g., alcohol dependence). Until fetal alcohol syndrome is more widely recognized as a cause of adult and developmental disabilities, the psychiatric sequelae should, at the very least, be criteria for these patients to receive special services, particularly an appropriate, structured, safe residential placement.

SUMMARY AND RECOMMENDATIONS

Prenatal alcohol exposure resulting in FAS is now identified as the major known cause of mental retardation in this country (Abel and Sokol 1987). However, mental retardation per se is not the only problem facing these patients as they mature. Their attention deficits, poor judgment, and impulsivity continue into adolescence and adulthood, often creating major obstacles to employment and stable living. IQ scores alone do not accurately predict school success or long-term independent functioning. Academic, language, and social problems are not just childhood problems for these patients. Depression, pregnancy, and alcohol abuse present new problems during the adolescent years and into adulthood.

A study such as ours provides no information on children of alcoholic mothers who have no characteristics of FAS. Furthermore, as our study was clinically based rather than population based, it is biased toward the inclusion of patients with problems. Thus, although it seems likely that there are patients with FAS/FAE who have successfully found their niches in society as productive citizens, they are less likely to be seen in a clinically based study such as this one. Systematic evaluation of such patients might provide further insight into effective intervention strategies.

Most of the homes in which patients in this study lived provided nurturance, guidance, careful monitoring, and structure. Even in these homes, these patients with FAS experienced significant social and legal difficulties. Although a positive environment can minimize problems and an unstructured environment puts patients with FAS at even higher risk, a good home does not always prevent the psychosocial difficulties experienced by so many of these patients, particularly those who remained several years in alcoholic households as young children.

Prevention is certainly the desirable goal in terms of birth defects; however, certain intervention strategies can improve the quality of life for affected patients. Patients with FAS/FAE usually continue to need protective environments even as older adolescents and adults. In particular, they need structured but nurturant residential placements, which provide careful and constant monitoring of the patients' time; placement in jobs meeting the patients' skill level; and therapy for patients and caretakers to help set reasonable expectations and to deal with issues as they arise. Unfortunately, such placements are extremely rare.

The emphasis on IQ as a criterion for special services should be transferred to measures of adaptive functioning. Other specific recommendations and actions that we have found helpful include the following: formal and complete psychological and physical evaluations beginning at an early age and continuing at key ages through adulthood; proper school placement with close contact between school personnel and the family to help implement behavioral management programs; the development of a case management approach with one person coordinating all services and developing needed resources; the availability of safe, chaperoned leisure activities; and the development of a program of respite care for caretakers. FAS is a birth defect with life-long consequences that affect every aspect of functioning. We hope that, with appropriate recognition of their specific cognitive deficits and special needs, the quality of life for these patients and their families can be improved.

ACKNOWLEDGMENTS

This work was partially supported by a contract from the Indian Health Service (243-87-0047) to Ann P. Streissguth. The assistance of Carol Giunta, Pam Phipps, Meg Bridewell, Anne Garing, and Annie Gage is gratefully acknowledged.

REFERENCES

Abel, E. T., and Sokol, R. J. 1987. Incidence of fetal alcohol syndrome and economic impact of FAS-related anomalies. *Drug Alcohol Depend* 19:51–70.

Clarren, S. K. 1981. Recognition of fetal alcohol syndrome. *JAMA* 245:2436–39.

Jones, K. L., and Smith, D. W. 1973. Recognition of the fetal alcohol syndrome in early infancy. *Lancet* 2:999–1001.

Jones, K. L., Smith, D. W., Ulleland, C. N., and Streissguth, A. P. 1973. Pattern of malformation in offspring of chronic alcoholic mothers. *Lancet* 1:1267–71.

Little, R. E., and Streissguth, A. P. 1982. Alcohol, pregnancy, and the fetal alcohol syndrome. In *Alcohol Use and Its Medical Consequences: A Comprehensive Teaching Program for Biomedical Education.* Project Cork of Dartmouth Medical School (Slide/teaching unit available from Milner-Fenwick, Inc., 2125 Greenspring Drive, Timonium, Md. 21093).

Majewski, F., Bierich, J. K., and Seidenberg, J. 1978. The incidence and pathogenesis of alcohol embryopathy. *Monatsschr Kinderheilkd* 126:284–85.

May, P. A., Hymbaugh, K. J., Aase, J. M., and Samet, J. M. 1983. Epidemiology of fetal alcohol syndrome among American Indians of the Southwest. *Soc Biol* 30:374–87.

Smith, D. W. 1982. *Recognizable Patterns of Human Malformation*. 3d ed. Philadelphia: W. B. Saunders.

Streissguth, A. P., Aase, J. M., Clarren, S. K., Randels, S. P., LaDue, R. A., and Smith, D. F. 1991. Fetal alcohol syndrome in adolescents and adults. *JAMA* 265:1961–67.

Streissguth, A. P., Clarren, S. K., and Jones, K. L. 1985. Natural history of the fetal alcohol syndrome: A ten-year follow-up of eleven patients. *Lancet* 2:85–92.

Streissguth, A. P., Herman, C. S., and Smith, D. W. 1978. Intelligence, behavior, and dysmorphogenesis in the fetal alcohol syndrome: A report on 20 patients. *Pediatr* 92:363–67.

Streissguth, A. P., and LaDue, R. A. 1987. Fetal alcohol: Teratogenic causes of developmental disabilities. In *Toxic Substances and Mental Retardation*. ed. S. R. Schroeder, 1–32. Washington, D. C.: American Association on Mental Deficiency.

Stromland, K. 1985. Ocular abnormalities in the fetal alcohol syndrome. *Acta Ophthamol [Suppl] (Copenh)* 171:63.

5

Paternal Exposure to Alcohol

Ernest L. Abel, Ph.D.

ALCOHOL is now recognized as the leading known cause of mental retardation in the Western world (Abel and Sokol 1987). Almost all of the research examining risk factors and mechanisms of action contributing to alcohol's effects on the conceptus has focused on maternal alcohol consumption. This chapter surveys recent evidence that paternal alcohol exposure also contributes to the prenatal effects of alcohol.

THE HISTORICAL BACKGROUND

Two major errors have firmly entrenched themselves in the historical bowels of research on fetal alcohol syndrome. The first is that the ancient Hebrews, Greeks, and Romans were well aware of the damaging effects of alcohol on the conceptus. The second is that they attributed these effects to maternal alcohol consumption. Since this review is primarily concerned with paternally transmitted effects, I have focused on this aspect of the historical record.

Among the earliest unequivocal references to possible prenatal effects of alcohol are two passages in the *Talmud* (Cohen 1965). In tractate *Sabbath* (80b), Rabbi Nachman stated that Rabbi Bibi's daughter was hirsute and had to be treated with a depilatory: "As for R. Bibi who drank strong liquor," he explains, "his daughter required pasting over; [but] as for us, who do not drink strong liquor, our daughters do not require such treatment." The same anecdote is repeated in tractate *Moed Katon* (9b) and, in a footnote to this passage, the commentator explains that alcohol causes hair to grow.

The only other instance where alcohol-induced teratogenicity is mentioned in the rabbinical literature is in chapter 52a of *Kallah Rabbathi*, which says that children conceived during intoxication will be demented. In this passage, however, the damage is clearly attributed to maternal drunkenness.

Although Robert Burton's *Anatomy of Melancholy* (1621) cited several Greek and Roman writers as being aware of the damaging effects of drinking during pregnancy, Burton fabricated his references (Burton 1977). For example, he quoted Aristotle's *Problemata* (4.2) on the damaging effects of maternal drinking: "foolish, drunken, or harebrained women (for) the most part bring forth children like unto themselves, morose and lanquid" (p. 213) and Aulius Gellius' *Attic Nights* on the effects of paternal drinking: "if a drunken man get a child, it will never likely have a good brain" (p. 213), but neither the *Problemata* nor *Attic Nights* contains any such statements.

The closest Burton (1977) comes to reporting any statements of this sort accurately is his quotation from Plutarch that "one drunkard begets another," which he assigns to Plutarch's *Symposiacs* (1.5). No such remark is made in *Symposiacs*, but in his *Education of Children* (ch. 3) Plutarch mentions paternal drinking: "children whose fathers have chanced to beget them in drunkenness are wont to be fond of wine, and to be given to excessive drinking."

Bruton is not the only writer whose creative inventions continue to be cited. In the clinical report in which Jones and Smith (1973) coined the term "fetal alcohol syndrome," they cited an anecdote concerning Carthaginian weddings which continues to be repeated but also has no historical basis. The point of the anecdote is an alleged law forbidding bridal couples to drink wine. I was able to trace this anecdote through Haggard and Jellinek's classic *Alcohol Explored* (1942) to a 1784 German translation of a Swedish text on alcohol. The author of this book in turn may have relied on Plato, who talked about a Carthaginian law forbidding soldiers on the march from drinking wine and then mentioned others who should not drink, among them "any man or woman—when proposing to procreate children." The reason, Plato explained much later, is that "when drunk, a man is clumsy and bad at sowing seed and is likely to beget unstable and untrusty offspring, crooked in form and character" (*Laws* 6:775).

Another anecdote that appears to be a modern invention but that nevertheless has crept into the literature on fetal alcohol syndrome concerns the misshapen Vulcan, the Roman god of fire and metal working. According to this recently invented myth, Vulcan's lameness was due to the fact that his father, Zeus, conceived him while he was drunk

(Green 1974). This anecdote was likewise probably adopted from Haggard and Jellinek (1942), who in turn probably adopted it from a paper written toward the end of the nineteenth century whose source is unknown (Abel 1984).

To sum up, the ancient Greeks or Romans were not aware of any dangers associated with maternal drinking during pregnancy. These writers were all men, and they were interested only in the effects of alcohol on themselves and other men.

In France, Claude Quillet, a French physician of the mid 1600s, wrote a poem entitled "Callipaedia: or the Art of Begetting Beautiful Children," in which he too focused on the adverse effects of paternal drinking:

> Remember how once Bacchus fluster'd came,
> And hot with Wine compress'd the Cyprian Dame:
> Folding the Goddess in his drunken Arms,
> Glowing he kiss'd and rioted in Charms:
> The crude warm seed thus immaturely wrought,
> A foul, obscene disfigur'd Daughter brought,
> The gout her Name, of pale and squallied face.
> [Quoted by Watson (1951)]

There were sporadic statements about the effects of prenatal alcohol exposure during the Middle Ages, especially in the 1700s during the "gin epidemic," but these statements had little lasting influence. By the middle of the twentieth century, the tide had turned and most writings on the subject belittled the possibility of such an influence. For example, in their influential book, *Alcohol Explored*, Haggard and Jellinek (1942) wrote that "germ cells do not have nerves, they do not become intoxicated, and they are injured by alcohol only when it is present in concentrations far higher than those causing death from failure of respiration—concentrations which are strong enough to be 'germicidal.' Thus, in a sense, the body protects the germ cells; it is sacrificed before they can be injured." Haggard and Jellinek's book was published in 1942 and summed up scientific opinion on the issue of prenatal alcohol damage at the time. Two years later, Oswald Avery and his coworkers (Avery, MacLeod, and McCarty 1944) found that deoxyribonucleic acid (DNA) was the vehicle for hereditary transmission. Had they written their book after this time, Haggard and Jellinek may have been more circumspect in their conclusions.

It was not until 1973 that interest in prenatal alcohol exposure was once again aroused (Jones and Smith 1973). For the most part, nearly all subsequent attention has been devoted to maternal rather than paternal routes of exposure. However, the latter route is now once again beginning to receive attention.

MALE AND FEMALE DRINKING PATTERNS

In every age group the percentage of men who drink is considerably higher than the percentage of women who drink and there are more "heavy" drinkers (consumption of five or more drinks per occasion at least once per week) among men than women (Secretary of Health and Human Services 1987). In general, about 14% of men in the United States consume two or more drinks a day compared to 3–4% of women (Secretary of Health and Human Services 1987).

Assortive mating for alcoholism, however, is also higher among women than among men. For example, Jacob and Bremer (1986) determined that about 34% of all alcoholic women are married to alcoholic men, whereas 12% of all alcoholic men are married to alcoholic women. Hall, Hesselbrock, and Stabenau (1983) reported even higher disparities: 26% of male alcoholics they studied had an alcoholic spouse, whereas 69% of female alcoholics had an alcoholic for a husband.

A retrospective examination of clinical case reports of fetal alcohol syndrome revealed that in only 36 of 358 cases was the father even mentioned. Of these cases, however, 29 (81%) fathers were identified as alcoholic (Abel 1983).

These paternal-maternal comparisons indicate that (1) paternal alcohol consumption is considerably higher than maternal consumption; (2) many women who drink excessively are married to men who also drink excessively, whereas the converse is not necessarily so; and (3) the overwhelming majority of women who give birth to children with fetal alcohol syndrome probably have mates who are also alcoholic. Collectively, these results imply that studies examining the effects of maternal drinking in offspring are probably "confounded" by paternal drinking. The implication is that some of the effects attributed to maternal exposure may actually be a consequence of paternal drinking.

THE COMPOUNDS TESTED FOR PATERNAL INFLUENCE

Since the possibility of a paternally mediated effect often raises considerable skepticism, I have provided a partial summary of studies examining this contribution for agents and conditions other than alcohol (table 5.1).

The purpose of this summary is twofold. First, it indicates that other researchers have been exploring this formidable terrain, and second, it indicates that, despite problems in finding a mechanism to account for paternally mediated effects, they seem to occur.

Since such tests require large numbers of animals and considerable time, space, and effort, it is not surprising that more such studies have not been conducted. This is, of course, a biased sample because "negative" results are usually not reported. These studies also differ markedly in their methodological vigor.

THE STUDIES EXAMINING PATERNAL ALCOHOL EFFECTS

Relevant studies involving paternal alcohol exposure are listed in table 5.2. These have been divided into those examining physical parameters such as dominant lethal mutations, sex ratios, malformations, and birth weight and those examining behavioral end points. In general, there is little evidence that paternal alcohol exposure significantly affects physical parameters. Effects on dominant lethal mutations are equivocal. A study by Little and Sing (1987) is worth noting, however, because it documents decreased birth weight in conjunction with human paternal alcohol consumption during the month of conception.

Studies from our laboratory (Abel and Lee 1988; Abel and Tan 1988) and from Gladys Friedler's laboratory (Friedler and Meadows 1987; Meadows, Schmidt, and Friedler 1987) suggested that paternal alcohol consumption may affect the behavior of rodent and murine offspring. An early study by Pfeifer, Mackinnon, and Seiser (1977) also reported behavioral changes in rat offspring associated with paternal alcohol consumption, but this report appeared only in abstract form, with few details given as to procedures or results. On the other hand, Nelson, Brightwell, and Burg (1985) did not observe any significant changes associated with paternal inhalation of alcohol vapor.

Since this is such a controversial area of research, we have been especially concerned about possible sources of confounding and inconclusive findings due to methodological shortcomings noted by Randall et al. (1982) in their critique of work in this area. Accordingly, we have incorporated into our overall treatment/test paradigms the following efforts to decrease the uncertainty of results:

- Large numbers of animals per group
- Three concentrations of alcohol plus nontreated control
- Use of two different species (rat and mouse)
- Daily administration of alcohol for minimum of one cycle of spermatogenesis
- Pair-feeding to control for caloric influences
- Several behavioral tests
- Testing at different ages

After conception, fathers are removed from mothers and never come in contact with offspring. Therefore, those changes that we see in offspring sired by alcohol-consuming fathers can only be due to some effect of alcohol on the sperm that fertilized mothers.

Since the protocol for both our rat and mouse studies is almost identical, I will briefly describe our basic procedures and will mention minor variations only where they are relevant.

Male rats and mice are assigned to one of four groups. One group is given free access to a liquid alcohol diet supplemented with vitamins and minerals. Two other groups are given similar isocaloric diets in which maltose-dextrin is substituted for a portion of the alcohol-related calories. For rats, the ad libitum alcohol group consumes a diet containing 35% ethanol-derived calories (EDC), whereas the two other groups receive diets containing 17.5% or 0% EDC. For mice the three diet concentrations are 20%, 10%, and 0% EDC. Animals in the two lower-alcohol groups are pair-fed to those in the higher-alcohol group. A fourth group of nontreated animals is fed laboratory chow as a further control for possible effects of diet restriction associated with pair-feeding. In virtually none of our tests have offspring of those animals fed laboratory chow differed significantly from offspring of the 0% EDC fathers.

Our behavioral test procedures are identical to those that we use to test offspring of animals born to mothers that consumed alcohol during pregnancy (e.g., Abel 1979; Abel 1982). The most consistent effect on offspring behavior associated with paternal alcohol exposure that we

Table 5.1   Agents Other than Alcohol Associated with the Paternal Transmission of Effects to Offspring

Agent/Cause	Species	Type of Effect	Reference
Anesthesia	Human	Congenital anomalies	American Society of Anesthesiologists 1974 Tomlin 1979 Cohen et al. 1975, 1980
Cyclophos-phamide	Rat	Behavior	Adams, Fabricant, and Legator 1981
	Rat	Behavior	Adams, Fabricant, and Legator 1982
	Rat	Behavior	Auroux and Dulioust 1985
	Rat	Behavior	Auroux et al. 1986
	Rat	Malformation	Jenkinson, Anderson, and Gangolli 1987
	Rat	Neurochemistry	Hsu and Adams 1987
	Rat	Malformation	Trasler, Hales, and Robaire 1985
Lead	Rat	Behavior	Brady, Herrera, and Zenick 1975
	Rabbit	Birth weight	Cole and Bachhaber 1914
	Guinea pig	Birth weight Postnatal growth retardation	Weller 1915
	Rat	Birth weight	Stowe and Goyer 1971
X-ray	Human	Cancer	Graham et al. 1966
	Mouse	Sperm	Hugenholtz and Bruce 1983
Thalidomide	Rabbit	Malformation	Lutwak-Mann 1964
Opiates	Rat	Birth weight	Joffe et al. 1976
	Rat	Neonatal and postnatal weight	Smith and Joffe 1975
	Mouse	Birth weight	Friedler 1974
	Rat	Postnatal weight	Sonderegger, O'Shea, and Zimmerman 1979
	Mouse	Behavior	Friedler and Wheeling 1979
Anesthetic gases	Human	Malformations	Cohen et al. 1975
	Human	Malformations	Knill-Jones, Newman, and Spence 1975
Vinyl chloride	Human	Spontaneous abortions	Infante et al. 1976
Chemotherapy	Human	Congenital malformations	Senturia, Peckham, and Peckham 1985 Li and Jaffe 1974 Li et al. 1979 Green, Fine, and Li 1982 Rustin et al. 1984

Table 5.1 (*Continued*)

Agent/Cause	Species	Type of Effect	Reference
Hydrocarbons	Human	Cancer	Fabia and Thuy 1974
			Peters, Preston, and Yu 1981
			Zack et al. 1980
			Kantor et al. 1979
			Hakulinen, Salonen, and Teppo 1976
			Hemminki et al. 1981
			Kwa and Fine 1980
			Hicks et al. 1984
Marijuana	Rat	Altered sex ratios	Fried and Charlebois 1979
	Mouse	Fertility of male offspring	Dalterio, Steger, and Bartke 1984
Stress (immobility)	Mouse	Postnatal mortality Postnatal body weight Behavior	Sirtori 1971
Age	Human	Down's syndrome	Stene and Stene 1978
	Human	Down's syndrome	Stene et al. 1981
	Human	Down's syndrome	Matsunaga et al. 1978
	Human	Achondroplasia	Murdoch et al. 1970
	Human	Achondroplasia	Stevenson 1957
	Human	Apert's syndrome	Bland 1960
	Human	Apert's syndrome	Erickson and Cohen 1974
	Human	Marfan's syndrome	Murdoch, Walker, and McKusick 1972
	Human	Crouzon's syndrome	Jones et al. 1975
	Human	Cleidocranial dysostosis	Jones et al. 1975
	Human	Treacher Collins' syndrome	Jones et al. 1975
	Human	Waardenburg syndrome	Jones et al. 1975
	Human	Neurofibromatosis	Borberg 1951
	Human	Tuberous sclerosis	Borberg 1951
Agent Orange	Human	Malformations	Erickson et al. 1984a, 1984b
			Nelson et al. 1979
Electromagnetic fields	Human	Cancer	Spitz and Johnson 1985

Source: Abel and Tan 1988.

Table 5.2 Summary of the Effects of Paternal Alcohol consumption on Offspring

Type of Effect	Species	Highest Dose	Duration (Days)	Effect	Reference
Dominant lethal	Mouse	20% EDC	42	−	Abel and Moore 1987
mutation/	Mouse	About 1.6 g/kg	3	+	Badr and Badr 1975
litter size					
	Rat	25% EDC	28	−	Bennett, Sorette, and Greenwood 1982
	Rat	30% in water	35	−	Chauhan et al. 1980
	Rat	10% Alc in water	15	+	Klassen and Persaud 1979
	Rat	20% Alc in water	60	+	Mankes et al. 1982
	Mouse	8% in water	100	+	Pfeifer, Mackinnon, and Seiser 1977
	Mouse	30% EDC	28	−	Randall et al. 1982
	Rat	30% in water	100	+	Tanaka, Suzuki, and Armina 1982
Sex ratio	Mouse	32% EDC	28	+	Anderson et al. 1981
	Rat	25% EDC	21	−	Bennett, Sorette, and Greenwood 1982
	Rat	10% Alc diet	15	−	Klassen and Persaud 1979
	Rat	30% in water	42	−	Leichter 1986
	Mouse	30% EDC	28	−	Randall et al. 1982
Malformations	Mouse	32% EDC	28	−	Anderson et al. 1981
	Rat	25% EDC	21	−	Bennett, Sorette, and Greenwood 1982
	Rat	0.6 g/kg	49	−	Cake and Lenzer 1985
	Rat	10% Alc diet	15	−	Klassen and Persaud 1979
	Rat	30% in water	42	−	Leichter 1986
	Rat	20% in water	60	−	Mankes et al. 1982
	Mouse	30% EDC	28	−	Randall et al. 1982
	Human	≥2 drinks/day	?	−	Little and Sing 1987
Fetal birth	Mouse	20% EDC	42	−	Abel and Moore 1987
weight/length	Mouse	32% EDC	28	+	Anderson et al. 1981
	Rat	25% EDC	21	−	Bennett, Sorette, and Greenwood 1982
	Rat	0.6 g/kg	49	−	Cake and Lenzer 1985
	Rat	10% in diet	15	+	Klassen and Persaud 1979
	Rat	30% in water	42	−	Leichter 1986
	Rat	20% in water	60	+	Mankes et al. 1982
	Mouse	30% EDC	28	−	Randall et al. 1982
	Rat	30% in water	10	+	Tanaka, Suzuki, and Armina 1982
	Human	≥2 drinks/day	?	+	Little and Sing 1987

Table 5.2 (*Continued*)

Type of Effect	Species	Highest Dose	Duration (Days)	Effect	Reference
Behavior	Mouse	3.5 g/kg twice daily	8.5	+	Friedler and Meadows 1987
	Rat	16,000-ppm inhalations	7 hr/day for 7 weeks	−	Nelson et al. 1979
	Rat	8% in water	100	+	Pfeifer, Mackinnon, and Seiser 1977
	Mouse	20% EDC	50	+	Abel and Lee 1988
	Rat	35% EDC	50	+	Abel and Tan 1988

Source: Abel and Tan 1988.

have observed is a *decrease* in activity (figs. 5.1 and 5.2). Since it was possible that the changes in activity we observed were transitory, we examined activity at 20 and 24 days of age in mice. The decreased activity occurred at both ages, as shown in figure 5.2.

This effect on activity was surprising because it is opposite to the increased activity in offspring associated with maternal alcohol exposure which we (Abel 1982) and others (e.g., Bond and DiGuisto 1977; Martin et al. 1978; Riley, Shapiro, and Lochry 1979) have reported. Further evidence for the reliability of our finding with paternal alcohol was a third study that we conducted in mice in which we gave alcohol to fathers for only 25 days. As shown in figure 5.2 ($d_{24}B_1$), activity was still decreased in animals sired by fathers who consumed the higher alcohol diets.

A second reason for our surprise was that several studies have shown that children of fathers who were alcoholics were hyperactive (Goodwin et al. 1975; Morrison and Stewart 1971). We can only guess at the reasons for this difference between the animal and human data. One, of course, is that rats and mice are affected differently by paternal alcohol consumption before birth. This is hardly a satisfying possibility, since it implies two different mechanisms in rodents and humans.

A second is that some strains of rats and mice may react differently to paternal alcohol exposure. Preliminary data from our laboratory in fact indicate that paternal alcohol exposure results in a dose-related increase in activity in Sprague-Dawley rats compared to a decrease in Long-Evans rats.

A third possibility is that the effects on activity are related to the cha-

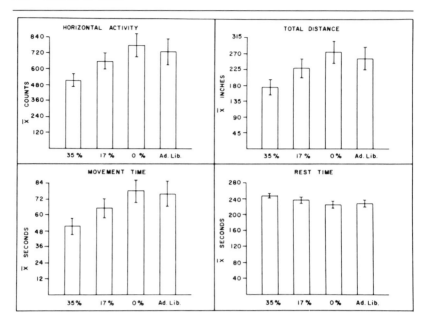

Figure 5.1. The effects of paternal alcohol consumption in rats on the activity of offspring at 20 days of age (mean ± SE). Fathers consumed alcohol at 35%, 17%, or 0% EDC for a minimum of 53 days.
Reprinted with permission from *Neurotoxicology and Teratology*, volume 10, Abel and Tan, Effects of paternal alcohol consumption on pregnancy outcome in rats. Copyright 1988, Pergamon Press.

otic postnatal environment in which the children of alcoholics are raised. This possibility would be difficult to address by animal experimentation.

A fourth possibility is that hyperactive children are also exposed to alcohol by their mothers. This possibility is supported by the similarity of these behavioral effects to those seen in conjunction with maternal exposure.

The other behavioral measures that we have examined have proven less consistent and do not exhibit dose/response relations. For example, we have found changes in spontaneous alternation in rats and mice sired by fathers consuming an alcohol diet for 25 days but not in offspring of rats who consumed the diet for 50 days. We also did not observe deficits in passive avoidance learning in rats sired by fathers that consumed alcohol (Abel and Tan 1988), but we did observe such changes in mice. Interestingly, these mice required fewer trials to learn a passive avoidance task (Abel and Lee 1988).

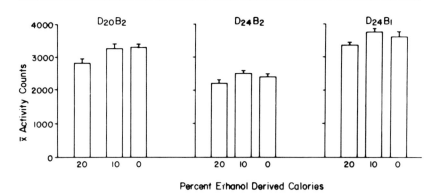

Figure 5.2. Mean (± SE) activity counts for mice sired by males consuming liquid alcohol diets containing 20%, 10%, or 0% ethanol-derived calories. $D_{20}B_2$: 20-day-old offspring sired by fathers consuming alcohol for at least 56 days. $D_{24}B_2$: 24-day-old offspring sired by fathers consuming alcohol for at least 56 days. $D_{24}B_2$: 24-day-old offspring sired by fathers consuming alcohol for only 25 days.
Reprinted with permission from *Neurotoxicology and Teratology*, volume 10, Abel and Tan, Effects of paternal alcohol consumption on pregnancy outcome in rats. Copyright 1988, Pergamon Press.

Another interesting finding in mice is a dose-dependent reduction in serum testosterone levels in male mice sired by alcohol-consuming fathers (Abel and Lee, in press).

THE SPERM ABNORMALITIES ASSOCIATED WITH ALCOHOL CONSUMPTION

One of the conceptual difficulties associated with experiments of the type just described is how these changes are mediated. The obvious candidate is the genetic material in sperm.

One indication of germ cell damage in males is a change in sperm morphology, count, or motility. Several genes control sperm morphology; thus far, at least ten such genes have been identified in mouse sperm (e.g., Beatty 1970; Krzanowska 1976). Abnormal sperm shape does not necessarily reflect abnormal chromosomal complement (Wyrobek, Heddle, and Bruce 1975) but may reflect more subtle damage to one or more genes occurring before meiosis (Beatty 1970). In this regard, several investigators (e.g., Lester and Van Thiel 1977; Nagy et al. 1986; Semczuk 1978), as well as our laboratory (Abel and Moore

1987), have reported alcohol-induced changes in sperm morphology, count, or motility.

Increases in alcohol-induced aneuploidy in spermatogonia have also been reported in mice and rats (Alvarez 1985; Hunt 1987; Il'inskikh et al. 1978) but not in hamsters (Daniel and Roane 1987). Since spermatocytes with incomplete pairing of homologous chromosomes rarely produce viable sperm (Hunt 1987), paternal alcohol exposure should not be associated with decreased implantations. However, if sperm are viable, conception could occur.

Alcohol or its metabolite have also been examined in various mammalian mutagenicity assays, especially sister chromatid exchange. Positive effects on human lymphocytes in vitro (Ristow and Obe 1978) and in hamster ovary cells (Obe and Ristow 1977) have been noted. Alvarez, Cimino, and Pusateri (1980) and Czajka, Tucci, and Kaye (1980) also reported an alcohol augmentation of bromodeoxyuridine-induced sister chromatid exchanges in mice embryos, but alcohol alone had no significant effect on the frequencies of sister chromatid exchange (Alvarez, Cimino, and Pusateri 1980). Koike (1985), however, reported a dose-related increase in the frequency of abnormal cells (gaps or breaks) in mouse fetuses whose mothers had consumed alcohol before and during pregnancy. Although the biological consequences of sister chromatid exchanges are not fully understood, mutagenic substances cause elevations of sister chromatid exchanges at concentrations that do not produce gross chromosomal aberrations (Latt 1981). Since sister chromatid exchanges represent reciprocal interchanges of DNA between chromatids at homologous loci, sister chromatid exchanges are regarded as a sensitive means of detecting DNA damage possibly resulting in teratogenicity (Latt 1981).

THE MECHANISM OF ACTION

To account for the effects of paternal alcohol exposure on offspring, I have hypothesized that the mechanism of action involves damage to sperm DNA by free oxygen radicals and related oxygen species, similar to the processes by which alcohol causes lipid peroxidation in the liver (e.g., Shaw and Jayatilleke 1987).

Oxygen is one of biology's enigmas. On the one hand, it is essential for cellular energy production, metabolism, resistance to infection, etc. On the other, it represents a major source of cellular toxicity.

The toxic potential of oxygen became very apparent clinically when retrolental fibroplasia, a disorder in premature infants, was traced to hyperoxygenation of premature infants experiencing pulmonary insufficiency or respiratory distress syndrome. Subsequent studies indicated that oxygen's toxicity arises from its oxygen free radical or related reduction products. These are molecules or molecular fragments with unpaired electrons (Slater 1984) that bind covalently to cellular macromolecules like DNA, causing cytotoxic effects including mutagenesis, carcinogenesis, teratogenesis, and necrosis (Kocsis et al. 1986).

Free oxygen radicals are produced, although at relatively low levels, even when intra- and extracellular oxygen content is relatively low. Although there are many enzyme systems that generate free oxygen radicals in vivo (e.g., xanthine oxidase and aldehyde oxidase), the following discussion will focus only on the enzymatic process involved in cellular respiration.

During the course of cellular respiration, O_2 acts as an electron "sink" because molecular oxygen has a greater affinity for electrons than any other substance in the respiratory chain. However, during this respiratory electron transfer, the electron "leakage" rate (Levine and Kidd 1985) is about 2–4% (Forman and Boveris 1982), which results in the generation of possible reactions such as this:

$$O_2 + 4e^- + 4H^+ \rightarrow 2H_2O \qquad (5.1)$$

Equation 5.1 represents the textbook version of the final reaction in the respiratory chain. However, electrons are not transferred in pairs. There is a sequential rather than simultaneous transfer of individual electrons so that initially a superoxide radical (O_2) is formed, which is then propagated until, finally, it is terminated, as shown below:

$$O_2 + e^- \longrightarrow \cdot O_2^- \text{ (superoxide anion radical)} \qquad (5.2)$$
$$2 \cdot O_2^- + 2H^+ \longrightarrow O_2 + H_2O_2 \text{ (hydrogen peroxide)} \qquad (5.3)$$
$$H_2O_2 + e^- + H^+ \longrightarrow H_2O + \cdot OH \text{ (hydroxyl radical)} \qquad (5.4)$$
$$\cdot OH + e^- + H^+ \longrightarrow H_2O \qquad (5.5)$$

Since electrons have a high affinity for oxygen, the first electron transfer results in superoxide. Other activated species then occur as additional electrons are captured. As superoxide is a weak oxidant, it is likely that superoxide itself is only a precursor for cellular toxicity. Likewise, H_2O_2 also has a low toxicity of its own. However, hydrogen peroxide may acquire another electron and go through the reaction shown in equation (5.4),or hydrogen peroxide may combine with super-oxide to form hydroxyl free radical ($\cdot$HO) via the Haber-Weiss reaction [equation (5.8)]. This reaction needs a heavy metal for catalysis, as shown in equations (5.6) and (5.7):

$$Fe^{3+} + \cdot O_2^- \longrightarrow Fe^{2+} + O_2 \tag{5.6}$$

$$Fe^{2+} + H_2O_2 \longrightarrow \cdot OH + Fe^{3+} + OH^- \tag{5.7}$$

$$H_2O_2 + \cdot O_2^- \longrightarrow \cdot OH + OH^- + O_2 \tag{5.8}$$

The hydroxyl radical is the most reactive free radical produced in biological systems (Grisham and McCord 1986).

Because these oxygen species are potentially damaging, intrinsic mechanisms have evolved to protect cells against them. The first line of defense is superoxide dismutase (McCord and Fridovich 1969), which converts superoxide to oxygen and hydrogen peroxide. Superoxide dismutase is found in cells throughout the body, especially in liver and blood. The higher the superoxide production the greater the cell's superoxide dismutase production (Fridovich 1983). Protection against hydrogen peroxide is provided by the catalase and peroxidase enzymes contained in vesicles and by glutathione peroxidase contained in the cytoplasm. These enzymes convert H_2O_2 to H_2O and O_2. Catalase and peroxidase are found in most cells. However, catalase is especially found in liver, whereas peroxidase is especially found in sperm. The hydroxyl radical, however, is the most reactive of free radicals produced in biological systems (Grisham and McCord 1986) and the most difficult to eliminate.

Under normal aerobic conditions, superoxide dismutase, catalase, and glutathione peroxidase are able to remove these reactive intermediates. These enzymes receive additional assistance from small-molecular-weight radical scavengers such as ascorbate, α-tocopherol, and β-carotene.

However, when the steady-state levels of either superoxide or hydrogen peroxide are elevated due to conditions that either increase oxygen radical generation or inhibit the enzymes or scavengers that remove them, the protective function of these enzymes and scavengers may be inadequate to prevent these oxygen species from damaging cells. One such factor is alcohol.

A noteworthy consequence of chronic alcohol consumption is increased generation of superoxide (Boveris et al. 1983), hydrogen peroxide (Lieber and DeCarli 1970), and hydroxyl radicals[3] (Dicker and Cederbaum 1987) as a consequence of metabolism of alcohol by the microsomal ethanol-oxidizing system (MEOS), which is a part of the cytochrome P_{450} system located in the endoplasmic reticulum. MEOS is generally less involved in alcohol metabolism than is alcohol dehydrogenase, except at high blood alcohol levels.

During the course of metabolism by MEOS, molecular oxygen is split. Hydrogen from the reduction of NADPH combines with one of the oxygen ions to form a water molecule; the other oxygen atom becomes the intermediate superoxide radical (Boveris et al. 1983). Superoxide then combines with alcohol and oxidizes it to its metabolite, acetaldehyde, producing NADP+ and water in the process. During the course of this conversion, hydrogen peroxide is generated (Lieber and DeCarli 1970; Thurman 1973). The rate of H_2O_2 production is also increased as a result of chronic alcohol exposure due to microsomal NADPH oxidase (Boveris et al. 1983; Klein et al. 1983; Lieber and DeCarli 1970). Also contributing to the generation of free oxygen species is an increase in the iron content in microsomes caused by chronic alcohol consumption (Krikun and Cederbaum 1986). Thus, in addition to the Haber-Weiss reaction, ·OH radicals can also be generated by the Fenton reaction as a result of chronic alcohol consumption (Dicker and Cederbaum 1987; Klein et al. 1983; Krikun, Lieber, and Cederbaum 1984; Shaw, Jayatilleke, and Lieber 1984). Although alcohol is a "scavenger" of ·OH radicals (Cederbaum, Dicken, and Cohen 1978), thereby providing some protection against tissue damage, the scavenging may occur too slowly to prevent interaction of ·OH with biological membranes or other cellular components because the reaction of ·OH with most organic compounds is among the most biologically reactive processes in the body (Grisham and McCord 1986).

Another major scavenger of free radicals is glutathione, but levels of glutathione are decreased in alcoholics (Shaw et al. 1981), thereby reducing that protection.

EXAMPLES OF DAMAGE DUE TO FREE RADICALS GENERATED BY ALCOHOL

Free radical-induced lipid peroxidation was described in detail by Aust and Svingen (1982). As a result of such peroxidation, the lipid part of the cell membrane will degenerate and disintegrate, protein-bound sulfhydryl groups will be oxidized to disulfides, cleavage of DNA may then occur, followed by entry of calcium cells into the cell or leakage from intracellular sites. Increases in such cellular levels of calcium are a universal feature of cell death (Schane et al. 1979).

Lipid peroxidation has frequently been hypothesized as a mechanism for alcohol-induced liver damage (e.g., Shaw et al. 1981). Shaw and Jayatilleke (1987) showed that acetaldehyde initiated lipid peroxidation in a concentration-dependent manner, and this was enhanced in the presence of ferritin. Peroxidation was inhibited by a chelator of iron and by superoxide dismutase, but neither catalase nor dimethyl sulfoxide (a scavenger of ·OH) had any effect. Because superoxide dismutase, catalase, or dimethyl sulfoxide did not block peroxidation, ·OH could not be responsible for peroxidation in this system (Taylor and Townsley 1986). The most likely possibility is that hepatic lipid peroxidation results from acetaldehyde-generated superoxide acting in concert with ferritin iron (Shaw and Jayatilleke 1987).

The Damage to Sperm

Many studies have shown that lipid peroxidation occurs spontaneously in mammalian sperm of many species, including humans. The oxygen species responsible for these effects are superoxide and H_2O_2. Interestingly, the threshold for peroxidation in human sperm is about eightfold lower than that in mouse sperm (Alvarez et al. 1987) because of the lower activity of glutathione peroxidase and superoxide dismutase in human sperm (Alvarez and Storey 1984).

Lipid peroxidation in sperm could be due to either alcohol or acetaldehyde. Although there is little alcohol dehydrogenase activity in testes or accessory organs, alcohol is converted to acetaldehyde in adipose tissue homogenates (Scheig 1971). Since seminal vesicles and sperm contain large amounts of lipids (Polaska, Syner, and Zameveld 1976; White, Darin-Bennett, and Poulos 1976), acetaldehyde may be generated in situ. Generation of alcohol-induced free radicals in testes or accessory organs could thus contribute to the lipid peroxidation that occurs in sperm by placing additional demands on the peroxidases and dismutases that convert these radicals.

The Damage to DNA

Oxidative DNA damage has been implicated in both cytotoxicity (Kappus 1987) and mutagenicity (Levin et al. 1982). Different nucleotides seem to be more susceptible than others to oxidation. For instance, hydrogen peroxide attacks pyrimidines preferentially over purines (Sangelsdorff and Lutz 1987), and cytosine seems to be preferred over thymine (Sangelsdorff and Lutz 1987).

In addition to the formation of reactive oxygen species, the metabolism of alcohol can lead to the formation of covalent adducts between nucleotides and acetaldehyde. During its metabolism, acetaldehyde is reduced and looks for electrons, which are available on DNA nucleotides. Preliminary studies in Djuric's laboratory (Z. Djuric and E. L. Abel, unpublished observations) showed that acetaldehyde reacts with all four nucleotides but reacts with purines (guanine and adenine) faster than with pyrimidines (thymine and cytosine). However, the products are not stable. Deoxyguanosine reacts to completion with acetaldehyde at −20°C after 48 hours of incubation. If the mixture is heated to 37°C for 4 hours, however, half of the product disappears and deoxyguanosine is reformed.

As a preliminary examination of possible alcohol-related damage to sperm DNA, we looked for some way to characterize such damage. In 1984, Schwartz and Cantor described a pulsed-field gel electrophoresis technique for fractionating large DNA molecules. Conventional techniques for DNA fractionation allow for resolution of DNA fragments of only 20 kilobase pairs (Kbp) because of the shearing that DNA experiences in a unidirectional electrical field as it moves through the pores in the agarose gel. The shearing occurs because DNA molecules larger than 50 Kbp must distort their shape as they pass through the pores, which are not linear; they cannot do so in a unidirectional applied field without fragmenting. With pulsed-field techniques, sequences of DNA molecules of up to 10 Mbp (10,000 Kbp) can be obtained (Anand 1986) because, in the pulsed-field gel, the regular changes in the applied electrical field force the DNA molecules to change orientation and allow them to move through the gel [the smallest human chromosome contains about 30 Mpb (Anand 1986)]. In the pulsed field, each DNA molecule spends time reorienting and migrating. Since smaller molecules will take less time to reorient, mobility is a function of size domain. Size is measured by comparison with the mobility of molecular-weight size standards such as bacteriophage lambda. Results are then visualized using ethidium bromide staining or special blotting procedures.

In our laboratory, sperm are removed from the epididymis and minced with a razor blade. The tissue is suspended in a buffer (10 mM

Tris, 100 mM NaCl, 1 mM EDTA—TNE) that breaks all membranes but leaves nuclei intact. After various extractions, DNA is isolated and its concentration in a sample is determined. Equal amounts of DNA are then placed into the pulsed-field gel for approximately 24 hours at 225 V, which switches direction every 20 seconds. The gel is then stained with ethidium bromide, destained in distilled water, and photographed under ultraviolet light.

From our initial and probably naive perspective, we assumed that if alcohol was altering DNA, the alteration would show up as a difference in molecular weight which might be revealed by the pulsed-field gel technique. Since we did not have any expectations as to where such change might occur, we felt that the most reasonable approach would be to examine the largest fragments of DNA possible.

Our preliminary results show that DNA of alcohol-treated males migrated further than DNA of pair-fed controls. Examination of the DNA suggests that there is about a 50-Kpb difference between the two samples. Although we cannot attribute any meaningful biological interpretation to this observation, it does suggest that alcohol may indeed have altered genomic DNA in some way and that this alteration may be responsible for our behavioral observations.

ACKNOWLEDGMENTS

The preparation of this chapter and the research described herein were supported by grants from the National Institute on Alcohol Abuse and Alcoholism (AA 06999 and P50 AA07606). I thank Rebecca Barnett-Hagan for editing and typing.

REFERENCES

Abel, E. L. 1979. Prenatal effects of alcohol on adult learning in rats. *Pharmacol Biochem Behav* 10:239–43.

———. 1982. In utero alcohol exposure and developmental delay of response inhibition. *Alcohol Clin Exp Res* 6:369–76.

———. 1983. *Marihuana, Tobacco, Alcohol and Reproduction.* Boca Raton, Fla.: CRC Press.

———. 1984. *Fetal Alcohol Syndrome/Fetal Alcohol Effects.* New York: Plenum Press.

Abel, E. L., and Lee, J. 1988. Paternal alcohol exposure affects offspring behavior but not body or organ weights in mice. *Alcohol Clin Exp Res* 12:349–55.

Abel, E. L., and Moore, C. 1987. Effects of paternal alcohol consumption in mice. *Alcohol Clin Exp Res* 11:533–35.

Abel, E. L., and Sokol, R. J. 1987. Incidence of fetal alcohol syndrome and economic impact of FAS-related anomalies. *Drug Alcohol Depend* 19:51–70.

Abel, E. L., and Tan, S. E. 1988. Effects of paternal alcohol consumption on pregnancy outcome in rats. *Neurotoxicol Teratol* 10:187–92.

Adams, P., Fabricant, J., and Legator, M. S. 1981. Cyclophosphamide-induced spermatogenic effects detected in the F_1 generation by behavioral testing. *Science* 211:80–82.

———. 1982. Active avoidance behavior in the F_1 progeny of male rats exposed to cyclophosphamide prior to fertilization. *Neurobehav Toxicol Teratol* 4:531–34.

Alvarez, J. G., and Storey, B. T. 1984. Lipid peroxidation and the reactions of superoxide and hydrogen peroxide in mouse spermatozoa. *Biol Reprod* 30:833–41.

Alvarez, J. G., Touchstone, J. C., Blasco, L., and Storey, B. T. 1987. Spontaneous lipid peroxidation and production of hydrogen peroxide and superoxide in human spermatozoa. *J Androl* 8:338–48.

Alvarez, M. R. 1985. Aneuploidy in male germ cells induced by alcohol ingestion. *Gamete Res.* 12:165–70.

Alvarez, M. R., Cimino, L. E., Jr., and Pusateri, T. J. 1980. Induction of sister chromatid exchanges in mouse fetuses resulting from maternal alcohol consumption during pregnancy. *Cytogenet Cell Genet* 28:173–80.

American Society of Anesthesiologists. 1974. Occupational disease among operating room personnel: A national study. *Anesthesia* 41:321–40.

Anand, R. 1986. Pulsed field gel electrophoresis: A technique for fractionating large DNA molecules. *Trends Genet* 2:278–83.

Anderson, R. A., Furby, J. E., Oswald, C., and Zaneveld, L. J. D. 1981. Teratological evaluation of mouse fetuses after paternal alcohol ingestion. *Neurobehav Toxicol Teratol* 3:117–20.

Auroux, M. R., and Dulioust, E. M. 1985. Cyclophosphamide in the male rat: Behavioral effects in the adult offspring. *Behav Brain Res* 16:25–36.

Auroux, M. R., Dulioust, E. M., Nawar, N. Y., and Yacoub, S. G. 1986. Antimitotic drugs (cyclophosphamide and vinblastine) in the male rat: Deaths and behavioral abnormalities in the offspring. *J Androl* 7:378–86.

Aust, S. D., and Svingen, B. A. 1982. The role of iron in enzymatic lipid peroxidation. In *Free Radicals in Biology*, ed. W. A. Pryor, 1–25. New York: Academic Press.

Avery, O. T., MacLeod, C. M., and McCarty, M. 1944. Studies on the chemical nature of the substance inducing transformation of pneumococcal types: Induction of transformation by a desoxyribonucleic acid fraction isolated from pneumococcus type III. *J Exp Med* 79:137–58.

Badr, F. M., and Badr, R. S. 1975. Induction of dominant lethal mutation in male mice by ethyl alcohol. *Nature* 253:134–36.

Beatty, R. A. 1970. The genetics of the mammalian gamete. *Biol Rev* 45:73–119.

Bennett, A. L., Sorette,M. P., and Greenwood, M. R. C. 1982. Effect of chronic paternal ethanol consumption on 19-day rat fetuses. *Fed Proc* 41:710.

Bland, C. E. 1960. Apert's syndrome (a type of acrocephalosyndactyly). *Ann Hum Genet* 24:151.

Bond, N. W., and DiGuisto, E. L. 1977. Prenatal alcohol consumption and open-field behavior in rats: Effects of age at time of testing. *Psychopharmacology (Berlin)* 52:311–12.

Borberg, A. 1951. Clinical and genetic investigations into tuberous sclerosis and Recklinghausen's neurofibromatosis. *Acta Psychiatr Neurol* 71:1.

Boveris, A., Fraga, C. G., Varsavski, A. I., and Koch, O. R. 1983. Increased chemiluminescence and superoxide production in the liver of chronically ethanol-treated rats. *Arch Biochem Biophys* 227:534–41.

Brady, K., Herrera, Y., and Zenick, H. 1975. Influence of parental lead exposure on subsequent learning ability of offspring. *Pharmacol Biochem Behav* 3:561–65.

Burton, R. 1977. *The Anatomy of Melancholy* (1621). New York: Vintage Books.

Cake, H., and Lenzer, I. 1985. On effects of paternal ethanol treatment on fetal outcome. *Psychol Rep* 57:51–57.

Cederbaum, A. I., Dicken, E., and Cohen, G. 1978. The effect of hydroxyl radical scavengers on microsomal oxidation of alcohols and on associated microsomal reactions. *Biochemistry* 17:3058–64.

Chauhan, P. S., Aravidakshan, M., Kumar, N. S., and Sundaram, K. 1980. Failure of ethanol to induce dominant lethal mutations in Wistar male rats. *Mutat Res* 79:263–75.

Cohen, A., ed. 1965. *The Minor Tractates of the Talmud*. London: Soncion Press.

Cohen, E. N., Brown, B. W., Bruce, D. L., Cascorbi, H., Corbett, T., Jones, T., and Whitcher, C. 1975. A survey of anaesthetic health hazards among dentists. *J Am Dent Assoc* 90:1291–96.

Cohen, E. N., Brown, B. W., Wu, M. L., Whitcher, C. E., Brodsky, J. B., Gift, H. C., Greenfield, W., Jones, T. W., and Driscoll, E. J. 1980. Occupational disease in dentistry and chronic exposure to trace anaesthetic gases. *J Am Dent Assoc* 101:21–31.

Cole, L. J., and Bachhaber, L. J. 1914. Effects of lead on germ cells of the male rabbit and as indicated by their progeny. *Proc Soc Exp Biol Med* 12:24–29.

Czajka, M. R., Tucci, S. M., and Kaye, G. I. 1980. Sister chromatid exchange frequency in mouse embryo chromosomes after in utero ethanol exposure. *Toxicol Lett* 6:257–61.

Dalterio, S., Steger, R. W., and Bartke, A. 1984. Maternal or paternal exposure to cannabinoids affects central neurotransmitter levels and reproductive function in male offspring. In *The Cannabinoids: Chemical Pharmacological, and Therapeutic Aspects*, New York: Academic Press. eds. S. Agurell, W. L. Dewey, and R. E. Willette 411–25.

Daniel, A., and Roane, D. 1987. Aneuploidy is not induced by ethanol during spermatogenesis in the Chinese hamster. *Cytogenet Cell Genet* 44:43–48.

Dicker, E., and Cederbaum, A. I. 1987. Hydroxyl radical generation by microsomes after chronic ethanol consumption. *Alcohol Clin Exp Res* 11: 309–14.

Erickson, J. D., and Cohen, M. M. 1974. A study of paternal age effects on the occurrence of fresh mutations of the Apert syndrome. *Ann Hum Genet* 38–89.

Erickson, J. D., Mulinare, J., McClain, P. W., Fitch, T. G., James, L. M., McClearn, A. B., and Adams, M. J. 1984a. Vietnam veterans' risks for fathering babies with birth defects. *JAMA* 252:903–12.

———. 1984b. Vietnam veterans risks for fathering babies with birth defects. U.S. Department of Health and Human Services, Public Health Service.

Fabia, J., and Thuy, T. 1974. Occupation of father at time of birth of children dying of malignant diseases. *Br J Prevent Med* 28:98–100.

Forman, H. J., and Boveris, A. 1982. Superoxide radical and hydrogen peroxide in mitochondria. In *Free Radicals in Biology*. Vol. 5, ed. W. A. Pryor, 65–89. New York: Academic Press.

Fridovich, I. 1983. Superoxide radical: An endogenous toxicant. *Annu Rev Pharmacol Toxicol* 23:239–57.

Fried, P. A., and Charlebois, A. T. 1979. Effects upon rat offspring following cannabis inhalation before and/or after mating. *Can J Psychol* 33:125–32.

Friedler, G. 1974. Morphine administration to male mice: Effects on subsequent progeny. *Fed Proc* 33:515.

Friedler, G., and Meadows, M. E. 1987. Effect of paternal ethanol on ethanol-induced hypothermia. *Fed Proc* 46:538.

Friedler, G., and Wheeling, H. S. 1979. Behavioral effects in offspring of male mice injected with opioids prior to mating. *Pharmacol Biochem Behav* 11:23–28.

Goodwin, D. W., Schulsinger, F., Hermansen, L., Guze, S. B., and Winokur, G. 1975. Alcoholism and the hyperactive child syndrome. *J Nerv Ment Dis* 160:349–53.

Graham, S., Levin, M., Lilienfeld, M., Schuman, L., Gibsen, R., Dowd, J., and Hempelmann, L. 1966. Preconception, intrauterine, and postnatal irradiation as related to leukemia. *NCI Monogr* 19:347–71.

Green, D. M., Fine, W. E., and Li, F. P. 1982. Offspring of patients treated for unilateral Wilms tumor. *Cancer* 49:2285–88.

Green, H. G. 1974. Infants of alcoholic mothers. *Am J Obstet Gynecol* 118:713–16.

Grisham, M. B., and McCord, J. M. 1986. Chemistry and cytotoxicity of reactive oxygen metabolites. In *Physiology of Oxygen Radicals*, ed. A. E. Taylor, S. Matalon, and P. Ward, 1–18. Baltimore: Williams & Williams.

Haggard, H. W., and Jellinek, E. M. 1942. *Alcohol Explored.* Garden City, N.Y.: Doubleday.

Hakulinen, T., Salonen, T., and Teppo, L. 1976. Cancer in the offspring of fathers in hydrocarbon-related occupations. *Br J Prevent Med* 30:138–40.

Hall, R. L., Hesselbrock, V. M., and Stabenau, J. R. 1983. Familial distribution of alcohol use: I. Assortive matings in the parents of alcoholics. *Behav Genet* 13:361–72.

Hemminki, K., Saloniemi, I., Salonen, T., Partanen, T., and Vainio, H. 1981. Childhood cancer and parental occupation in Finland. *J Epidemiol Community Health* 35:11–15.

Hicks, N., Zack, M., Caldwell, G. G., Fernbach, D. J., and Falletta, J. M. 1984. Childhood cancer and occupational radiation exposure in parents. *Cancer* 53:1637–43.

Hsu, L. L., and Adams, P. M. 1987. Cyclophosphamide: Effects of paternal exposure on the brain chemistry of the F_1 progeny. *J Toxicol Environ Health* 21:471–81.

Hugenholtz, A. P., and Bruce, W. R. 1983. Radiation induction of

mutations affecting sperm morphology in mice. *Mutat Res*
107:177–85.

Hunt, P. A. 1987. Ethanol-induced aneuploidy in male germ cells of the
mouse. *Cytogenet Cell Genet* 44:7–10.

Il'inskikh, N. N., Il'inskikh, I. N., Makarov, L. N., and Chernoskutora,
S. A. 1978. The effect of ethanol and its metabolite, acetaldehyde
on the chromosomal apparatus of rat and human cells. Translated
by National Clearing House for Alcohol Information, STIAR No.
56. *Tsitologiia* 20:421–25.

Infante, P., Wagoner, J., McMichael, A., Waxweiler, R., and Falk, H.
1976. Genetic risk of vinyl chloride. *Lancet* 1:734–35.

Jacob, T., and Bremer, D. A. 1986. Assortive mating among men and
women alcoholics. *J Stud Alcohol* 47:219–22.

Jenkinson, P. C., Anderson, D., and Gangolli, S. D. 1987. Increased
incidence of abnormal foetuses in the offspring of
cyclophosphamide-treated male mice. *Mutat Res* 188:57–62.

Joffe, J. M., Peterson, J. M., Smith, D. J., and Soyka, L. F. 1976.
Sublethal effects on offspring of male rats treated with methadone
before mating. *Res Commun Chem Pathol Pharmacol* 13:611–21.

Jones, K. L., and Smith, D. W. 1973. Recognition of the fetal alcohol
syndrome in early infancy. *Lancet* 2:999–1001.

Jones, K. L., Smith, D. W., Harvey, M. S. A., Hall, B. D., and Quan,
L. 1975. Older paternal age and fresh gene mutation: Data on
additional disorders. *J Pediatr* 86:84–88.

Kantor, A. F., Curnen, M. G., Meigs, J. W., and Flannery, J. T. 1979.
Occupations of fathers of patients with Wilms' tumors. *J Epidemiol
Community Health* 33:253–56.

Kappus, H. 1987. Oxidative stress in chemical toxicity. *Arch Toxicol*
60:144–49.

Klassen, R. W., and Persaud, T. V. N. 1979. Experimental studies on
the influence of male alcoholism on testicular function, pregnancy
and progeny. *Adv Stud Birth Defects* 2:239–56.

Klein, S. M., Cohen, G., Lieber, C. S., and Cederbaum, A. I. 1983.
Increased microsomal oxidation of hydroxyl radical scavengers and
ethanol after chronic consumption of ethanol. *Arch Biochem Biophys*
223:425–33.

Knill-Jones, R., Newman, B., and Spence, A. 1975. Anaesthetic
practice and pregnancy: Controlled survey of male anaesthetists in
the United Kingdom. *Lancet* 2:807–9.

Kocsis, J. J., Jollow, D. J., Witmer, C. M., Nelson, J. O., and Snyder,
R., eds. 1986. *Biological Reactive Intermediates*. New York: Plenum
Press.

Koike, M. 1985. Cytogenetic effects of maternal alcohol uptake on F_1 mouse fetuses. *Jpn J. Hyg* 40:575–84.

Krikun, G., and Cederbaum, A. I. 1986. Effect of chronic ethanol consumption on microsomal lipid peroxidation. *FEBS Lett* 208:292–96.

Krikun, G., Lieber, C. S., and Cederbaum, A. I. 1984. Increased microsomal oxidation of ethanol by cytochrome P-450 and hydroxyl radical-dependent pathways after chronic ethanol consumption. *Biochem Pharmacol* 33:3306–9.

Krzanowska, H. 1976. Inheritance of sperm head abnormality types in mice—the role of the Y chromosome. *Genet Res* 28:189–92.

Kwa, S., and Fine, L. J. 1980. The association between parental occupation and childhood malignancy. *J Occup Med* 22:792–94.

Latt, S. A. 1981. Sister chromatid exchange formation. *Annu Rev Genet* 15:11–56.

Leichter, J. 1986. Effects of paternal alcohol ingestion on fetal growth in rats. *Growth* 50:228–33.

Lester, R., and Van Thiel, D. H. 1977. Gonadal function in chronic alcoholic men. *Adv Exp Med Biol* 85A:399–414.

Levin, D. E., Hollstein, M., Christman, M. F., Schwiens, E. A., and Ames, B. N. 1982. New *Salmonella* tester strain with A. T. base pairs at the site of mutation detects oxidative mutagens. *Proc Natl Acad Sci USA* 79:7445–49.

Levine, S. A., and Kidd, P. M. 1985. *Antioxidant Adaptation*. San Leandro, Calif.: Allergy Research Group.

Li, F. P., Fine, W., Jaffe, N., Holmes, G. E., and Holmes, F. F. 1979. Offspring of patients treated for cancer in childhood. *J Natl Cancer Inst* 62:1193–97.

Li, F. P., and Jaffe, N. 1974. Progeny of childhood cancer survivors. *Lancet* 2:707–9.

Lieber, C. S., and DeCarli, L. M. 1970. Reduced NADP oxidase: Activity enhanced by ethanol consumption. *Science* 170:78–79.

Little, R. E., and Sing, C. F. 1987. Father's drinking and infant birthweight: Report of an association. *Teratology* 36:59–65.

Lutwak-Mann, C. 1964. Observations on progeny of thalidomide-treated male rabbits. *Br Med J* 1:1090–91.

McCord, J. M., and Fridovich, I. 1969. Superoxide dismutase: An enzymatic function for erythrocuprein. *J Biol Chem* 244:6049–55.

Mankes, R. F., LeFevre, R., Benitz, K. F., Rosenblum, I., Bates, H., Walker, A. I. T., and Abraham, R. 1982. Paternal effects of ethanol in the Long-Evans rat. *J Toxicol Environ Health* 10:871–78.

Martin, J. C., Martin, D. C., Sigman, G., and Radow, B. 1978.

Maternal ethanol consumption and hyperactivity in cross-fostered offspring. *Physiol Psychol* 6:362–65.

Matsunaga, E., Tonomura, A., Hidetsune, O., and Kikuchi, Y. 1978. Reexamination of paternal age effect in Down's syndrome. *Hum Genet* 40:259–68.

Meadows, M. E., Schmidt, J., and Friedler, G. 1987. Paternal ethanol alters side preference in mouse offspring. Paper presented to the International Society for Developmental Psychobiology, New Orleans. November 12, 1987.

Morrison, J. R., and Stewart, M. A. 1971. A family study of the hyperactive child syndrome. *Biol Psychiatry* 3:189–95.

Murdoch, J. L., Walker, B. A., Hall, J. G., Abbey H., Smith K. K., and McKusick, V. A. 1970. Achondroplasia—a genetic and statistical survey. *Ann Hum Genet* 33:227–44.

Murdoch, J. L., Walker, B. A., and McKusick, V. A. 1972. Paternal age effects on the occurrence of new mutations of the Marfan syndrome. *Ann Hum Genet* 35:331–36.

Nagy, F., Pendergrass, P. B., Bown, D. C., and Yeager, J. C. 1986. A comparative study of cytological physiological parameters of semen obtained from alcoholics and non-alcoholics. *Alcohol* 21:17–29.

Nelson, B. K., Brightwell, W. S., and Burg, J. R. 1985. Comparison of behavioral teratogenic effects of ethanol and *n*-propanol administered by inhalation to rats. *Neurobehav Toxicol Teratol* 7:779–83.

Nelson, C. J., Holson, J. F., Green, H. G., and Caylor, D. W. 1979. Retrospective study of the relationship between agricultural use of 2,4,5-T and cleft palate occurrence in Arkansas. *Teratology* 19:377–84.

Obe, G., and Ristow, H. 1977. Acetaldehyde but not ethanol induces sister chromatid exchanges in Chinese hamster cells in vitro. *Mutat Res* 56:211–14.

Peters, J. M., Preston, M. S., and Yu, M. C. 1981. Brain tumors in children and occupational exposure of parents. *Science* 213:235–37.

Pfeifer, W. D., Mackinnon, J. R., and Seiser, R. L. 1977. Adverse effects of paternal alcohol consumption on offspring in the rat. *Bull Psychonom Sci Soc* 10:246.

Polaska, K. L., Syner, F. N., and Zameveld, L. J. D. 1976. Biochemistry of human seminal plasma. In *Human Semen and Fertility Regulation in Men*, ed. E. S. Hafez, 133–43. St. Louis: C. V. Mosby.

Randall, C. L., Burlings, T. A., Lochry, E. A., and Sutker, P. B. 1982. The effect of paternal alcohol consumption on fetal development in mice. *Drug Alcohol Depend* 9:89–95.

Riley, E. P., Shapiro,N. R., and Lochry, E. A. 1979. Nose-poking and head-dipping behaviors in rats prenatally exposed to alcohol. *Pharmacol Biochem Behav* 11:513–19.

Ristow, H., and Obe, G. 1978. Acetaldehyde induces cross-links in DNA and causes sister-chromatid exchanges in human cells. *Mutat Res* 58:115–19.

Rustin, G. J. S., Booth, M., Dent, J., Salt, S., Rustin, F., and Bagshawe, K. D. 1984. Pregnancy after cytotoxic chemotherapy for gestational trophoblastic tumours. *Br Med J* 288:103–6.

Sangelsdorff, P., and Lutz, W. K. 1987. Sensitivity of DNA and nucleotides to oxidation by permanganate and hydrogen peroxide. *Arch Toxicol* 11:84–88.

Schane, F. A. X., Kane, A. B., Young, E. E., and Farber, J. L. 1979. Calcium dependence of toxic cell death: A final common pathway. *Science* 206:700–702.

Scheig, R. 1971. Effects of ethanol on lipid metabolism in adipose tissue. *Biochim Biophys Acta* 248:48–60.

Schwartz, D. C., and Cantor, C. R. 1984. Separation of yeast chromosome sized DNAs by pulsed field gradient gel electrophoresis. *J Cell* 37:67–75.

Secretary of Health and Human Services. 1987. *Alcohol and Health.* Washington, D. C.: U.S. Department of Health and Human Services.

Semczuk, M. 1978. Further investigations on the ultrastructure of spermatozoa in chronic alcoholics. *Mikrosk Anat Forsch* 92:494–508.

Senturia, Y. D., Peckham, C. S., and Peckham, M. J. 1985. Children fathered by men treated for testicular cancer. *Lancet* 2:766–69.

Shaw, S., and Jayatilleke, E. 1987. Acetaldehyde-mediated hepatic lipid peroxidation: Role of superoxide and ferritin. *Biochem Biophys Res Commun* 143:984–90.

Shaw, S., Jayatilleke, E., and Lieber, C. S. 1984. The effect of chronic alcohol feeding in lipid peroxidation in microsomes: Lack of a relationship to hydroxyl radical generation. *Biochem Biophys Res Commun* 118:233–38.

Shaw, S., Jayatilleke, E., Ross, W. A., Gordon, E. R., and Lieber, C. J. 1981. Ethanol-induced lipid peroxidation: Potentiation by long-term alcohol feeding and attenuation by methionine. *J Lab Clin Med* 98:417–24.

Sirtori, C. 1971. Effects of stress induced in male mice, as assessed in their offspring: Research in the framework of preconceptional preparation. In *Malformations, Tumors, and Mental Defects:*

Pathogenic Correlations, ed. H. Tuchmann-Duplessis, H. G. Fanconi, and G. Burgio. 54–70. Milan:Carlo Erba Foundation.

Slater, T. F. 1984. Free-radical mechanisms in tissue injury. *Biochem J* 222:2–15.

Smith, D. J., and Joffe, J. M. 1975. Increased neonatal mortality in offspring of male rats treated with methadone or morphine before mating. *Nature* 253:202–3.

Sonderegger, T., O'Shea, S., and Zimmermann, E. 1979. Progeny of male rats addicted neonatally to morphine. *Proc West Pharmacol Soc* 22:137–39.

Spitz, M. T., and Johnson, C. C. 1985. Neuroblastoma and paternal occupation. *Am J Epidemiol* 121:924–29.

Stene, J., and Stene, E. 1978. On data and methods in investigations on parental-age effects: Comments on a paper by J. D. Erickson. *Ann Hum Genet* 41:465–68.

Stene, J., Stene, E., Stengel-Rutkowski, S., and Murken, J. D. 1981. Paternal age and Down's syndrome data from prenatal diagnoses (DFG). *Hum Genet* 59:119–24.

Stevenson, A. C. 1957. Achondroplasia: An account of the condition in Northern Ireland. *Am J Hum Genet* 9:81–91.

Stowe, H. D., and Goyer, R. A. 1971. The reproductive ability and progeny of F lead-toxic. *Fertil Steril* 21:755–60.

Tanaka, H., Suzuki, N., and Armina, M. 1982. Experimental studies on the influence of male alcoholism on fetal development. *Brain Dev* 4:1–6.

Taylor, A. E., and Townsley, M. I. 1986. Assessment of oxygen radical tissue damage. In *Physiology of Oxygen Radicals*, ed. A. E. Taylor, S. Matolon, and P. Ward, 19–38. Baltimore: Williams & Williams.

Thurman, R. G. 1973. Induction of hepatic microsomal reduced nicotinamide adenine dinucleotide phosphate-dependent production of hydrogen peroxide by chronic prior treatment with ethanol. *Mol Pharmacol* 9:670–75.

Tomlin, P. J., 1979. Health problems of anaesthestists and their families in the West Midlands. *Br Med J* 1:779–84.

Trasler, J. M., Hales, B. F., and Robaire, B. 1985. Paternal cyclophosphamide treatment of rats causes fetal loss and malformation without affecting male fertility. *Nature* 316:144–46.

Watson, R. 1951. *Merry Gentlemen*. London: T. W. Laury.

Weller, C. 1915. The blastophthoric effect of chronic lead poisoning. *J Med Res* 33:271–93.

White, I. G., Darin-Bennett, A., and Poulos, A. 1976. Lipids of human semen. In *Human Semen and Fertility Regulation in Man*, ed. E. S. Hafez, 144–52. St. Louis: C. V. Mosby.

Wyrobek, A. J., Heddle, J. A., and Bruce, W. R. 1975. Chromosomal abnormalities and the morphology of mouse sperm heads. *Can J Genet Cytol* 17:675–81.

Zack, M., Cannon, S., Loyd, D., Heath, C. W., Falletta, J. M., Jones, B., Housworth, J., and Crowley, S. 1980. Cancer in children of parents exposed to hydrocarbon-related industries and occupations. *Am J Epidemiol* 111:329–36.

6

The Effects of Marijuana Use on Offspring

Susan L. Dalterio, Ph.D., and Peter A. Fried, Ph.D.

THE HISTORICAL BACKGROUND

As DESCRIBED in a lucid and engrossing manner by Abel (1980a), the relationship (real or perceived) between marijuana and aspects of reproduction is far from a twentieth century issue. In the vast folklore of Eastern European medicine dating back several centuries, marijuana was ascribed the property of being able to increase the vigor of contractions during labor and thereby hasten protracted labor. The report of the Indian Hemp Drug Commission (1893/1894), perhaps the earliest commissioned scientific report, included a discussion of marijuana as both a sexual stimulant and an inhibitor. Aphrodisiac properties of the drug were described in sixteenth century Arab literature, and these writings (including chapters such as "The Tale of the Hashish Eater" in the collection of *The Thousand and One Nights*) had quite an influence in Europe toward the end of the Napoleonic Wars. It was during this age of Romanticism that the Hashish Club of Paris came into existence, with its membership including some of the best-known literary and artistic personages of the times. The vivid writings of this club were widely read, and the intoxicating and sexual potential of the drug as perceived by these members became well known to the general population.

At a more contemporary level, there have been numerous reports associating marijuana use with increased sexual pleasure, but because of the complexity of the issue conclusions are difficult to draw. For example, the interactive relationship between the overall life-style (particularly values placed on sexual activity) and the effect of the drug is extremely difficult to separate (Abel 1980a, 1981).

161

Studies of Animal Reproduction

Placental Transfer

Cannabinoids cross the placental barrier and can be transferred via the milk in lactating females (Idanpäan-Heikkila 1969; Bloch et al. 1978). Studies in different animal species have determined that, depending on the route of administration, the majority of cannabinoid given to the mother stays in the maternal compartment, with significant storage in adipose tissue (Mantilla-Plata, Clewe, and Harbison 1975). There is a decreased concentration of cannabinoids in the placenta, with even lower levels in the fetus. However, maternal adipose tissue and the placenta may continue to release lipophilic cannabinoids to the fetus. In addition, cannabinoids accumulate in fetal tissue, including the brain (Dalterio 1980; Rosenkrantz 1984). In view of these findings it is of considerable importance to determine the short-term effects on pregnancy and the fetus, as well as the consequent long-term effects on the development of cannabinoid-exposed offspring. The emphasis in this chapter will be on the latter.

The Early Effects on the Fetus/Neonate

The majority of studies investigating the teratological potential of either marijuana or its purified constituents have focused on the number of implantations and resorptions, the litter size and sex ratio, and/or the evaluation of gross congenital defects (reviews by Fleischman et al. 1979 and by Rosenkrantz 1984). When administered by the inhalation route in rats, marijuana smoke produced no adverse effects on conception rate, maternal weight gain, or the total number of implants (Rosenkrantz 1984). In contrast, this same study noted a dose-related increase in the number of dams presenting evidence of early fetal resorptions. In addition, these studies indicated that oral Δ^9-tetrahydrocannabinol (THC) exposure produced a dose-related interruption of pregnancy in mice and rats. Total litter weight, mean fetal weight, and sex ratio seem to be unaltered by inhalation exposure to marijuana. These latter findings contrast with a report indicating a significant selective embrolethality in female rat fetuses exposed to THC in utero (Hutchings et al. 1987).

There seems to be a significant temporal relationship for embryocidal effects of THC, with maximal susceptibility in rodents occurring on days 7–9 of gestation (Mantilla-Plata, Clewe, and Harbison 1975;

Fleischman et al. 1979), although a clear dose/response relationship has not been established. This effect may also exhibit cannabinoid specificity, since Dalterio and Bartke (1981) observed an increase in fetal resorptions in female mice treated with Δ^9-tetrahydrocannabinol (THC) on days 12–16 of gestation, whereas the administration of cannabinol (CBN), a relatively nonpsychoactive component, had no effect.

Long-term Effects

REPRODUCTIVE FUNCTION

In mice, exposure to THC or CBN on the day before parturition and for the first six days postpartum had no apparent immediate effects on neonates. However, just before puberty THC- and CBN-exposed male offspring were significantly underweight compared to control mice. In addition, hormonal alterations were observed in association with the apparent pubertal delay. Specifically, levels of the pituitary gonadotropin, luteinizing hormone, were markedly elevated in males previously exposed to THC, whereas testicular weights were significantly reduced. In contrast, males exposed to CBN had significant decreases in both luteinizing hormone and testosterone levels in plasma (Dalterio 1980). In adulthood, testes size was still reduced, and pituitary gonadotropin release remained significantly elevated in THC-exposed mice. In contrast, in males exposed to CBN, reproductive indices were quite comparable to those in control mice. Therefore, it is possible that maternal CBN exposure may induce a maturational delay in reproductive development at puberty for which the animal eventually compensates. However, effects of THC on the male reproductive system persist into adulthood. Although their specific effects on any particular parameter are not identical, these results indicate that maternal exposure to either psychoactive or nonpsychoactive components of marijuana have an effect on the development of reproductive functions in mice.

FERTILITY

Male and female rats that were exposed to marijuana in utero and received injections of THC before mating exhibited reduced fertility, as well as a decrease in the size of their reproductive organs (Fried and Charlebois 1979). This study also reported that the F_1 generation of females that became pregnant experienced increased numbers of resorptions. Furthermore, their offspring were smaller at birth through 30 days of age. In additional studies, adult male mice perinatally exposed to THC, CBN, or cannabidiol produced smaller litter sizes than normal after mating with non-drug-exposed females (Dalterio and De-Rooij 1986).

NEUROLOGICAL DEVELOPMENT

Kawash, Yeung, and Berg (1980) reported a significant increase in brain weight at 37 days of age in rat offspring exposed prenatally to cannabis, despite the fact that body weights were reduced. In addition, DNA levels were significantly higher in these rats (Kawash, Yeung, and Berg 1980). This contrasts with the more recent findings of Hutchings et al. (1987) that brain levels of DNA and RNA were not affected by maternal exposure to either 15 or 50 mg of THC per kg throughout gestation, although brain protein concentration was significantly reduced in offspring of dams receiving the higher THC dose. Interestingly, in an earlier report, prenatal exposure to THC also significantly reduced brain RNA, DNA, and protein in rats (Luthra 1979).

Peripheral neuronal functions can also be affected by perinatal cannabinoid exposure, since a reduction in the sensitivity of the vas deferens to enkephalin and norepinephrine was observed in adult male mice perinatally exposed to THC (Dalterio et al. 1980). Animals receiving THC only as adults did not exhibit these changes in peripheral sensitivity; thus, it is apparent that perinatal exposure may represent a critical period for these cannabinoid effects.

BEHAVIOR

Maternal cannabinoid exposure produces dose-related alterations in the behavior of rat offspring. In one study a hypersensitivity response characterized by vertical jumping was evident after the administration of a single oral dose of THC to rats whose mothers had been treated with THC during gestation (Rosenkrantz 1984). This intriguing finding suggests that prenatal exposure influences the neural sensitivity of the animal to subsequent cannabinoid exposure. These findings are consistent with results of a study reported by Fried (1976), in which young rats previously exposed to marijuana in utero demonstrated an increased sensitivity to THC in terms of tolerance development. Furthermore, we recently observed that perinatal THC exposure significantly influenced the activity of hepatic cytochrome P-450 enzymes in adulthood

(Dalterio et al. 1986). Furthermore, these changes in enzyme activity were also associated with functional effects on the metabolism of the gonadal steroids in these animals. Thus, prenatal cannabinoid exposure affects subsequent sensitivity to cannabinoid reexposure and may also influence the response to other drugs.

Certain effects of perinatal marijuana exposure may represent developmental delay. High doses of THC were reported to delay reflex development in rodents (Borgen, Davis, and Pace 1973), whereas lower doses were without effect (Fried 1976; Charlebois and Fried 1980). Open-field behavior in neonatal rats was either decreased (Fried 1976) or increased (Borgen, Davis, and Pace 1973), depending on whether the marijuana exposure occurred throughout gestation or briefly during midgestation, respectively.

In other studies involving prenatal exposure to cannabis resin (Kawash, Yeung, and Berg 1980), pups from treated dams took significantly longer than controls to reach criterion in a maze learning task. These cannabis-exposed offspring also exhibited a reduction in open-field behavior. However, other studies have not reported similar effects on maze learning and passive avoidance responses in rodents after perinatal marijuana exposure (Charlebois and Fried 1980; Abel 1980b).

Male mice perinatally exposed to either THC or CBN exhibited alterations in sexual behavior as adults (Dalterio et al. 1980). In this study a significant proportion of THC-exposed adults failed to initiate copulatory behavior when paired with a sexually receptive female. In males that did mate, however, performance was comparable to that observed in normal mice. It is possible that an apparent inability of the testes in these THC-exposed males to be stimulated by pituitary gonadotropic hormones (Dalterio 1980) may have influenced behavioral responsiveness to the mating situation. It is well known that exposure of a male to a female or to the stimulation associated with mating evokes release of the gonadal hormone, testosterone (Kamel et al. 1977).

In contrast to the effects observed in THC-exposed males, animals exposed to CBN readily initiated mating behavior but ceased sexual activity before ejaculation (Dalterio et al. 1980). This unusual behavior may indicate that perinatal exposure to CBN results in a neural deficit involving central or peripheral sensory input from sexual stimulation. Prenatal cannabinoid exposure influences the expression of male copulatory behavior in mice. These actions may be mediated by endocrine effects in the case of THC, whereas those for CBN seem to involve alterations in neural sensitivity. Apparent cannabinoid specificity for these effects is further suggested by a report in which combined perinatal exposure to cannabichromine was capable of attentuating the long-term effects of THC on male reproductive functions and behavior in mice (Hatoum et al. 1981).

THE MECHANISMS OF ACTION

Maternal Factors

The precise mechanisms by which cannabinoids alter developmental processes remain to be determined. Certainly, potential indirect effects of cannabinoid exposure have been identified, including those potentially mediated by alterations in maternal nutrition, lactational performance, or maternal behaviors (reviews by Abel 1980b and Dalterio et al. 1986). However, in view of the well-documented ability of cannabinoids to influence endocrine functions after exposure in the adult, similar effects on the fetal endocrine system could potentially contribute to or mediate certain developmental actions of this drug.

Fetal Endocrine Factors

Cannabinoid exposure influences gonadal steroid production in laboratory animals and in humans (reviews by Bloch et al. 1978 and by Bloch 1983). It is well documented that the presence and timing of androgenic steroid exposure are critical for the establishment of male sexual dimorphism in mammals. Thus, alterations in the perinatal hormonal environment have been associated with changes in hypothalamic neuroendocrine regulation as well as in sexual behavior patterns (Gorski 1971; McEwen 1978). In addition, the morphological and functional development of reproductive structures is critically and permanently influenced by the fetal endocrine milieu (Jost 1972). Perinatal androgens also exert an organizational effect on the hepatic enzymes involved in drug and hormone metabolism (Chung, Raymond, and Fox 1975) and on immune system responsivity (Sitteri et al. 1980). Certainly, cannabinoid-related inhibition of fetal androgen production, even transiently, would be consistent with the alterations in hepatic, gonadal, neuroendocrine, and behavioral function observed in several studies (Dalterio et al. 1980, 1984a, 1984b, 1986).

Effects on Neurotransmitters

Effects of cannabinoid administration to adult animals on neurotransmitter activity have been quite inconsistent (Dewey 1986; Martin 1986). However, alterations in brain biogenic amine functions during development may be involved in the long-term developmental consequences resulting from perinatal cannabinoid exposure. Dalterio et al. observed changes in the concentrations of dopamine, norepinephrine, and serotonin in cannabinoid-exposed male mice (Dalterio et al. 1984a, 1984b). These effects appeared to be related to the timing of drug exposure and the particular cannabinoid administered. However, the relationship, if any, between specific changes in brain biogenic amine activity and those for endocrine parameters or sexual behavior were not obvious. In another report (Walters and Carr 1986), long-term alterations in neurotransmitter activity, including effects on receptor sensitivity, were observed in rats prenatally exposed to cannabinoids. It is, at present, difficult to demonstrate a relationship between such long-lasting effects on neurotransmitter functions and behavioral teratogenesis or other potential effects of perinatal cannabinoid exposure.

Calcium Membrane Transport

In recent studies the effects of THC exposure on calcium (Ca^{++}) membrane transport functions have been observed (Dalterio, Bernard, and Esquivel 1987a, 1987b). Prenatal exposure to THC influenced the subsequent activity of the Ca^{++} ATPase enzyme in testicular and pituitary plasma membranes (Dalterio, Bernard, and Esquivel 1987b). Calcium has a major second messenger role in the secretion-coupled release of neurotransmitters and hormones (Rasmussen and Waisman 1981). In recent studies we identified effects of THC treatment in adult mice on pituitary and testicular activity of Ca^{++} ATPase, a plasma membrane enzyme that serves as a major buffering mechanism regulating intracellular Ca^{++} concentrations (Dalterio, Bernard, and Esquivel 1987a). In addition, prenatal exposure to THC also produced long-term changes in the activity of Ca^{++} ATPase in these tissues (Dalterio, Bernard, and Esquivel 1987b). Certainly, cannabinoid actions on Ca^{++} membrane transport activity may mediate cannabinoid actions on neurotransmitter and endocrine functions.

CLINICAL STUDIES

The Incidence of Use during Pregnancy

In attempting to explore the relationship between marijuana use during pregnancy and persistent or long-term effects in human offspring, one is immediately struck by the paucity of objective information, which is surprising from two aspects. Marijuana is not a drug that has just arrived on the scene, nor is it a drug that is limited to a very select few women of reproductive age.

The extent of marijuana use by pregnant women has been examined by several investigators. In retrospective studies at the Boston City Hospital, postpartum interviews of inner city respondents reported usage of 10–14% (Hingson et al. 1982; Linn et al. 1983). At the Yale-New Haven Hospital it was estimated that 10% of the women delivering used marijuana during pregnancy (Hatch and Bracken 1986). This was a relatively low-risk population. Among another low-risk home-delivery population in California (Greenland et al. 1983) and in the Seattle, Washington, area (Barr et al. 1984) the rate was 16%.

In Ottawa, Canadian usage information was gathered from predominantly middle class women who volunteered to take part in a study (described in detail below) dealing with "life-style practices" (Fried, Innes, and Barnes 1984). When interviewed during pregnancy and asked about prepregnancy habits, the women reported that during the year before pregnancy 80% did not use any marijuana, 12% used irregularly, 3% smoked two to five joints per week, and 5% smoked six or more joints per week. Upon recognition of pregnancy, usage declined significantly. During each of the trimesters, however, the percentages remained relatively constant, with 6% reporting irregular use, 1% smoking two to five joints weekly, and 3% reporting six or more joints per week. It may be reflective of the lack of objective information about marijuana available to pregnant women that, compared to alcohol and cigarette use, heavy marijuana consumption was the least reduced during the course of pregnancy.

A year after delivery of the baby there were further differences between alcohol, cigarette, and marijuana consumption patterns. Women who were categorized as heavy social drinkers before pregnancy reduced their drinking during pregnancy and this reduction was still evident one year postpartum. Similarly, cigarette usage, which declined during pregnancy, continued to remain at the reduced level one year postpartum. However, heavy marijuana use, which was the least reduced during pregnancy, returned to prepregnancy levels a year after the baby's birth (Fried, Barnes, and Drake 1985).

The clinical focus of this chapter is the long-term or persistent effects of fetal exposure to marijuana. Data pertaining to postnatal effects beyond the neonatal period are limited to a report by Tennes et al. (1985) describing one-year-old children and a series of reports describing the findings from Fried's Ottawa sample. Because of our reliance on the latter work, the protocol and limitations of this study will be described in some detail.

The Ottawa Prenatal Prospective Study

When the Ottawa work was initiated in the late 1970s there were, other than two polydrug case reports, no human research studies pertaining to maternal cannabis use. The striking absence of objective information regarding the potential consequences of marijuana use by pregnant women, the results from the animal studies discussed earlier in this chapter, the extent of marijuana use by women of reproductive age, and the cooperation of the major teaching hospitals in the area all served as an impetus for the Ottawa Prospective Study. The project started in 1978. Commencing in 1979, data have been collected from approximately 700 pregnant women in the Ottawa, Canada, region. Mothers-to-be were informed of the study by their obstetricians or by notices in waiting rooms or prenatal clinics. In all cases the initial information did not mention marijuana; rather it discussed, in general terms, how life-style habits during pregnancy may influence the unborn child. Upon contacting the research facility, the prospective subject was given further details about the particular habits in which we were interested (i.e., alcohol, cigarette, and marijuana use). It was also emphasized that for comparison purposes we were also interested in women who did not use any of these substances during pregnancy. Upon volunteering to participate, each subject was interviewed once during each of the trimesters remaining in her pregnancy.

The volunteer method of participation was dictated primarily by ethical considerations and has both negative and positive consequences. The procedure certainly limits the generalizability of the epidemiological information collected because of the possible bias inherent in a volunteer sample. However, as reported elsewhere (Fried et al. 1980; Fried, Innes, and Barnes 1984), on a number of demographic factors (e.g., parity, income, age) the sample was similar to the overall characteristics of women living in Ottawa and giving birth in the local hospitals. On the positive side, the volunteer method of recruiting subjects has served to increase the reliability of the self-report of drug use (as elaborated below) and to increase the probability of a long-term commitment to the study. Aside from subjects who have moved away from the Ottawa region (32%), there has been a retention rate of over 95% during the past seven years.

During each of the interviews, conducted in the mother's home in virtually all cases, information was collected pertaining to socioeconomic status, the mother's health (both current and prior to pregnancy), the health of the father, the obstetrical history of previous pregnancies, a 24-hour dietary recall (including assessment of caffeine intake), and past and present drug use, with particular emphasis on marijuana, alcohol, and cigarette use. For the establishment of drug use, information was gathered both for the year preceding the pregnancy and for each trimester of the pregnancy. Alcohol and cigarette use were considered carefully, as it was anticipated that these drugs would be used extensively by the marijuana users. Thus, to facilitate the unraveling of potential confounding observations, detailed information about the use of drugs other than marijuana and their possible effects would be required.

As the range of marijuana use in the sample was considerable and the drug was not used by a similar number of subjects across the range, the marijuana data were treated categorically for descriptive and certain statistical purposes. There were the nonusers, the irregular users (one joint or less a week or exposure to the exhaled smoke of others), the moderate users (two to five joints per week), and the heavy users (more than six joints per week).

Many of the women who smoked marijuana regularly during pregnancy differed from the remainder of the sample on a number of factors that could be associated with adverse effects on the course of pregnancy and the development of the offspring. These potentially confounding factors included lower socioeconomic level, less formal education, and more cigarette smoking. Heavier alcohol consumption was also associated with heavy marijuana use, but not as strongly as was cigarette smoking. Although no difference in parity was noted between the heavy marijuana users and the nonusers, the heavy users were a significant

3.2 years younger. In terms of nutritional adequacy, as calculated by recommended dietary standards, there was no difference between the nonusers and those in the three categories of marijuana use.

The method of using self-report to assess such variables as nutrition and drug habits raises the critical issues of validity and reliability. Despite the potential, obvious shortcomings of self-reporting interviews, there is no practical alternative. In the Ottawa study, a number of procedures were implemented to enhance the probability of accurate data collection. First, to develop a comfortable rapport, the same female interviewer "followed" the mother-to-be during her entire pregnancy. Second, the questionnaire was administered once during each trimester and, during each of these interviews, the questions pertaining to drug use for each three-month period were repeated to measure test-retest reliability.

The Possible Interactive Effects of Additional Risk Factors

In several reports based on the Ottawa Prenatal Prospective Study, the course of pregnancy has been examined (Fried, Buckingham, and Vov Kulmiz 1983; Fried, Innes, and Barnes 1984). One aspect of these studies may have particular relevance for the interpretation of long-term effects of prenatal exposure to marijuana. In the Ottawa study no differences were observed between marijuana users and control subjects when considering such variables as miscarriage rates, type of presentation at birth, Apgar status, and the frequency of complications or major physical abnormalities at birth. No evidence of increased meconium staining among the newborns of the heavy marijuana users was noted. This latter observation contrasts with those in the first of two reports by Greenland and associates (Greenland et al. 1982, 1983). In the second of Greenland's reports no significant increase in meconium staining was noted. One of the primary differences between Greenland's two studies was the generally higher level of health and living standards among the sample who participated in the second study (Greenland et al. 1983). The women in the second report were more similar in terms of ethnicity, education, and general health to the Ottawa subjects than were the participants in Greenland's first study (Greenland et al. 1982).

The possible critical role that overall life-style may have in interacting with the teratogenic effects of marijuana has ramifications for interpreting some of the literature described below. A study using an animal model also bears directly on this issue.

Pregnant rats were exposed to marijuana smoke, placebo smoke (cannabis product with cannabinoids removed), or no smoke while the diet of the animals was manipulated (Charlebois and Fried 1980). In each of the three drug conditions the animals received one of three diets differing in protein content. One diet was relatively poor in protein, one was a standard laboratory rat chow, and the third was an enriched protein diet. The drug plus diet manipulations (3 × 3 design) were administered commencing 20 days before conception and were continued throughout gestation. There was a striking interaction between marijuana exposure and dietary manipulation. Outcomes such as stillbirths, litter destruction, and postnatal deaths were markedly potentiated by the combination of the low-protein diet and marijuana smoke. Conversely, some physiological and developmental milestones that were delayed in the rats receiving normal diet/marijuana smoke were attenuated in the high-protein/marijuana smoke condition. These results are certainly suggestive; as with all animal work, however, the extent of extrapolation is problematic. It is not unreasonable, however, to view these results (plus those of Greenland's described above) as suggesting that marijuana's potential teratogenic effects are more likely to manifest themselves in the human environment in which the overall life-style creates a high-risk situation before marijuana even enters the scene. Thus, in a relatively low-risk population (of which the Ottawa sample is a case in point), the fetus may be relatively less susceptible to some of marijuana's consequences.

Physical Congenital Anomalies

The argument of a drug by life-style interaction may have a direct bearing upon the relationship between physical anomalies and prenatal marijuana exposure. In the Ottawa study, no evidence of major physical anomalies was noted at birth. An examination was also undertaken to determine whether in utero cannabis exposure was associated with an increased risk of minor physical anomalies in children ranging in age from six months to four years (O'Connell and Fried 1984). The children of 25 marijuana-using women and the offspring of 25 matched controls were examined for the presence of over 40 types of minor physical anomalies. Neither the frequency of particular anomalies nor their total number was significantly different between the two groups of subjects. Although no specific pattern of anomalies was seen among the children born to the marijuana users, two anomalies associated with the visual system were noted among the offspring of heavy users of the drug. One anomaly was the presence of severe epicanthal folds (unusual amount of skin covering the nasal portion of the eye). The other anomaly found uniquely among three other children born to heavy marijuana users was true ocular hypertelorism (unusually wide separation of the eyes). It may be noteworthy that, in four-day-old neonates, visual behavior was also found to be altered in the offspring of marijuana users (Fried and Makin 1987). This latter result is described later in this chapter.

The lack of a clear relationship between minor physical anomalies and prenatal marijuana exposure is consistent with the findings of several other reports (Linn et al. 1983; Tennes et al. 1985; N. L. Day, personal communication, 1988). There are, however, two apparent exceptions. One is a large, mixed prospective and retrospective study (Hingson et al. 1982), and the other are two reports of five individual cases (Qazi et al. 1982, 1985).

The reports of congenital defects related to maternal cannabis use have described anomalies that are part of the diagnostic criteria of the fetal alcohol syndrome (FAS). In the large study (Hingson et al. 1982), it was reported that women who smoked marijuana during pregnancy were five times more likely than nonusers to have a baby with FAS features.

In the case reports, Qazi et al. (1982, 1985) suggested a link between prenatal cannabis exposure and FAS features because, in four of the five cases reported, mothers were regular users of marijuana but denied the use of alcohol or any other psychoactive drugs during pregnancy. The denial of alcohol consumption by 80% of these women seems questionable as virtually all reports in the literature have noted a moderately high correlation between regular marijuana use and alcohol consumption. Furthermore, in these case reports little demographic information or medical history was provided and no control (matching or otherwise) was undertaken to assess the role of potentially confounding variables.

The absence of a significant association between FAS features and prenatal exposure in the Ottawa study could be due to a number of factors. Among these are sample size, age of subjects, and, as discussed earlier, the "risk status" of the women in the sample. The relatively small size of the Ottawa sample may certainly have decreased the likelihood of finding a significant relationship among the variables examined. In the study of Hingson et al. (1982), the rate of occurrence of FAS features among the marijuana-exposed offspring was 2%. If that figure is representative and was applied to the Ottawa study, only one child would be expected to meet these criteria.

A second, potentially important differentiating feature between the Hingson study and that in Ottawa is that the former examined subjects during the first week after birth. The average age at examination of the infants in the Ottawa study was 29 months. There is evidence that some minor physical anomalies are transient, being observed only during the neonatal period (Smith 1974). Thus, the age of the infants at the time of examination may be of considerable significance. Some European research suggests that some anomalies indicative of alcohol exposure during fetal development normalize with age (Majewski 1981). Such observations could be interpreted as indicating that some of the FAS features represent a delay rather than a deficit in development.

As described previously, there may well be an interaction between maternal nutrition and the consequences of maternal use of marijuana. Using maternal weight gain as an indicator of nutrition during pregnancy, there was evidence that the Ottawa sample was better nourished than that in the Hingson study, with the mean weight gain during pregnancy being 16.02 kg in the former versus 13.64 kg in the latter study. Additional risk factors that were more prevalent in the Hingson report were lower socioeconomic status and more chronic illnesses. The presence or absence of such intervening risk variables may be a vital factor in determining the effects of marijuana on dysmorphology in the neonate.

Neurobehavioral Observations

Although this chapter focuses on the long-term effects of prenatal marijuana exposure, findings in newborns will be briefly mentioned as they may indicate the potential for more persistent long-term outcomes. The Ottawa study used a sample of 250 babies, of whom 47 were exposed to marijuana during fetal development. Canonical and regression analyses were used to explore the multivariate relationships between prenatal exposure to marijuana (and other drugs) and performance on the Brazelton Neonatal Assessment Scale. The infants were less than one week old when examined (Fried and Makin 1987). Prenatal exposure to marijuana was associated with increased tremors, frequently accompanied by exaggerated startles, both spontaneous and in response to minimal stimuli. This central nervous system excitation was not accompanied by other signs that are typically associated with neonatal drug withdrawal, such as hyperactivity or constant signs of distress. There was, however, a marginal trend toward increased irritability associated with marijuana exposure. Prenatal cannabis exposure was also related to poorer habituation to visual stimuli, although no effect on auditory habituation was observed. Habituation to repeated stimuli is thought to be an indicator of nervous system integrity. However, the level within the nervous system at which the possible dysfunction is occurring, as well as the reason for the apparent particular vulnerability of the visual system, remains to be determined.

It is intriguing that the literature on studies in animals also suggests that the visual system may be a target for the teratogenic effects of marijuana. For example, a study (Golub, Sassenrath, and Chapman 1981) examined the behavior of the offspring of rhesus monkeys exposed daily to psychoactive THC before and during pregnancy and throughout lactation. The category of behavior that distinguished the marijuana-exposed from control offspring was that the former failed to habituate to novel visual stimuli. In rodents, visual developmental milestones are also delayed in the offspring of marijuana-treated animals (Borgen, Davis, and Pace 1973; Fried 1976; Fried and Charlebois 1979).

The Ottawa study cited above (Fried and Makin 1987) primarily focused on the behavior of the newborns, with the unstated but underlying assumption that behavior reflected the neurological status of the infant. This implicit assumption was examined in a somewhat more direct fashion when the babies were slightly older (at 9 and 30 days) using the Prechtl neurological assessment (Fried et al. 1987). Data were collected on approximately 250 babies born to healthy, white, predominantly middle-class women. Of these infants, 32 were born to women who had used marijuana regularly during pregnancy. For this study, regular use was defined as smoking more than one joint per week. Discriminate function analysis was used to control for such potentially confounding variables as birth weight; socioeconomic status; nicotine, alcohol, and caffeine exposure; maternal weight gain and nutrition; and maternal age.

Marijuana use during pregnancy was associated with relatively similar observational effects in the neonate at 9 and 30 days of age. At both ages fine tremors, tremors associated with the Moro reflex, and startles were more pronounced, as were a number of motor reflexes in the marijuana-exposed offspring. At 9 days of age increased hand-to-mouth behavior in infants was associated with maternal marijuana use. Overall, these observations are consistent with but much milder in degree than those reported among infants born to opioid-addicted women and undergoing neonatal withdrawal. The increased tremors and startles among the offspring of marijuana users are consistent with observations made on newborns described previously (Fried and Makin 1987). At 9 and 30 days of age, however, no statistical associations were apparent between marijuana exposure levels and a number of eye variables examined in the Prechtl test, including pupil dilatation, doll's eye movements, nystagmus, and acoustic blink. However, compared to the rest of the sample, more marijuana-exposed babies demonstrated strabismus, as well as a lack of optical blink and habituation.

The Possible Delaying Effect on Nervous System Maturation

Data derived from the newborn as well as the 9- and 30-day-old infants suggest that marijuana exposure in utero may subtly depress the normal rate of development of the central nervous system. Functional manifestations of a reduction in the rate of maturation would probably be most evident in systems that depend upon the cooperative interaction of many components. Given the observations on the newborns and the suggestive nature of both the dysmorphology study and the Prechtl examination, the visual pathways were thought to represent an appropriate target for assessment of the course of nervous system development in the offspring of marijuana users. The working hypothesis was that the visual pathways are dependent upon the interaction of a large number of components, each with its own characteristic rate of maturation. This would be expected to result in a relatively greater degree of "normal" variability in immature than in mature visual systems. As more and more of these components reach maturation, the overall system variability would be expected to decrease.

To test this hypothesis we needed a measure that reflected functional maturation and could be administered to children with an acceptable degree of efficiency, accuracy, and objectivity. The transient pattern-evoked visual cortical potential was chosen, as both the amplitude and the latency of the major components of this evoked response exhibit systematic changes from birth to adulthood.

With the use of a reversing checkerboard pattern as a stimulus, children participating in the Ottawa study, averaging four years of age, were examined under monocular and binocular conditions (Tansley, Fried, and Mount 1986). Of this sample, 31 children had been exposed to marijuana during fetal development. For statistical purposes each marijuana-exposed child was "matched" to another child in terms of age and mother's use of alcohol and tobacco.

The evoked-potential wave forms obtained from the children were grossly similar to those from adults. Although the pattern and amplitude were similar among these groups of children, there was a trend for the marijuana-exposed offspring to have slightly longer latencies for the major wave form component of this visual evoked potential—a sign of immaturity in the system. More striking, however, was a significantly greater degree of variability in the marijuana-exposed children compared to age-matched control groups. Although far from conclusive, these data are consistent with the notion that exposure in utero to constituents of marijuana may act to slow the rate of maturation of visual components in the human nervous system.

Cognitive Functioning

In addition to the attempt to ascertain whether there is an association between maternal marijuana use and nervous system function in the offspring, the Ottawa Prenatal Prospective Study has also examined longer-term behavioral and cognitive functioning. At 12 and 24 months of age, the Bayley Scales of Infant Development were used as an assessment tool and, at the 24-month test session, the Reynell Developmental Language Scales and the Home Observation Measurement of the Environment (HOME) was also administered (Fried and Watkinson 1988). The Bayley test consists of three scales that include assessments of mental development and motor development and an infant behavior record that evaluates the infant's attitude, interests, and temperament. The investigators examined 217 infants at 12 months of age and 153 at 24 months. Multiple regression analysis was used to assess the association between outcome measures and prenatal marijuana exposure while adjusting for potential confounding factors.

The variable of exposure to marijuana in utero did not significantly contribute to either the mental or motor components of the Bayley test or the Reynell language test. A surprising and at this time inexplicable observation was a positive relationship between maternal marijuana use and a cluster of items in the infants' behavioral records that reflect a cognitive factor (Matheny, Dolan, and Wilson 1974), for example, attention span, goal directedness, object orientation, and reactivity. Maternal marijuana use was not related to a visual composite score derived from the infant behavioral record. Items that entered into this score included responsiveness to objects, manipulation of objects, and sights-looking.

FUTURE RESEARCH

Studies in Animals

It is imperative that the issue of repeated or intermittent maternal exposure, as well as the consequences of potential tolerance development, be evaluated in the context of long-term effects of cannabinoids on development. In addition, the entire life-span of cannabinoid-exposed offspring should be assessed, including the ability to adapt to environmental stresses, susceptibility to disease, and aging processes.

Clinical Studies

The lack of clear, negative effects of prenatal marijuana exposure at 12 and 24 months of age contrasts to the neonatal observations, perhaps suggesting that drug effects are transitory. On the other hand, it may be that the effects of marijuana exposure in utero are quite subtle and that facets of cognitive behavior affected by marijuana exposure may become apparent only as the child becomes older. Preliminary analysis of data on three- and four- year-old children tentatively supports the importance of assessing complex cognitive abilities in the older child, which cannot be assessed at a very early age. The cognitive effects of prenatal marijuana exposure may manifest themselves only when complex demands are placed on nervous system functions. Subtle deviations and nonoptimal performance, not visible at an earlier age, may then become apparent. In a pragmatic sense, the onset of school attendance represents such an example of additional demands on the child. Thus, critical questions still remain to be addressed pertaining to the potential long-term behavioral teratogenicity of marijuana in the human.

REFERENCES

Abel, E. 1980a. *Marijuana: The First Twelve Thousand Years*. New York: Plenum Press.

———. 1980b. Prenatal exposure to cannabis: A critical review of effects on growth, development and behavior. *Behav Neurol Biol* 29:137–56.

———. 1981. Marijuana and sex: A critical review. *Drug Alcohol Depend* 8:1–22.

Barr, H. M., Streissguth, A. P., Martin, D. C., and Hermes, C. S. 1984. Infant size at 8 months of age: Relationship to maternal use of alcohol, nicotine and caffeine during pregnancy. *Pediatrics* 74:336–41.

Bloch, E. 1983. Effects of marijuana and cannabinoids on reproduction, endocrine function, development and chromosomes. In *Cannabis and Health Hazards*, ed. K. O. Fehr and H. Kalant, 355–432. Toronto: Addiction Research Foundation.

Bloch, E., Thysen, B., Morrill, G. A., Gardner, E., and Fujimoto, G. 1978. Effects of cannabinoids on reproduction and development. *Vitam Horm* 36:203–58.

Borgen, L. A., Davis, W. M., and Pace, H. B. 1973. Effects of prenatal THC on the development of the rat offspring. *Pharmacol Biochem Behav* 1:203–6.

Charlebois, A. T., and Fried, P. A. 1980. The interactive effects of nutrition and cannabis upon rat perinatal development. *Dev Psychobiol* 13:591–605.

Chung, L. W. K., Raymond, G., and Fox, S. 1975. Role of neonatal androgen in the development of hepatic microsomal drug-metabolizing enzymes. *J Pharmacol Exp Ther* 193:621–30.

Dalterio, S. L. 1980. Perinatal or adult exposure to cannabinoids alters male reproductive functions in mice. *Pharmacol Biochem Behav* 12:143–53.

Dalterio, S., Bartke, A., and Mayfield, D. 1981. Fetal testosterone in mice: Effect of gestational age and cannabinoid exposure. *J Endocrinol* 91:509–14.

Dalterio, S. L., Bernard, S. A., and Esquivel, C. R. 1987a. Acute Δ^9-tetrahydrocannabinol exposure alters Ca^{++} ATPase activity in neuroendocrine and gonadal tissues in mice. *Eur J Pharmacol* 137:91–100.

———. 1987b. Perinatal cannabinoid exposure: Effects on Ca^{++} ATPase activity in mice. In: *Functional Teratogenesis*, ed. T. Fujii and P. M. Adams, 101–8. Tokyo: Teikyo University Press.

Dalterio, S., Blum, K., Dellalo, L., Sweeney, C., Briggs, A., and Bartke, A. 1980. Perinatal exposure to Δ^9-THC in mice: Altered enkephalin and norepinephrine sensitivity in vas deferens. *Subst Alcohol Actions/Misuse* 1:467–71.

Dalterio, S. L. and DeRooij, D. G. 1986. Maternal cannabinoid exposure: Effects on spermatogenesis in male offspring. *Int J Androl* 9:250–58.

Dalterio, S., Steger, R., Mayfield, D., and Bartke, A. 1984a. Early cannabinoid exposure influences neuroendocrine and reproductive functions in male mice: I. Prenatal exposure. *Pharmacol Biochem Behav* 20:107–14.

———. 1984b. Early cannabinoid exposure influences neuroendocrine and reproductive functions in mice: II. Postnatal exposure. *Pharmacol Biochem Behav* 20:115–24.

Dalterio, S., Thomford, P. J., Michael, S. D., DeAngelo, L., and Mayfield, D. 1986. Perinatal cannabinoid exposure: Effects on hepatic cytochrome P-450 and plasma protein levels in male mice. *Teratology* 33:195–201.

Dewey, W. L. 1986. Cannabinoid pharmacology. *Pharmacol Rev* 38:151–78.

Fleischman, R. W., Hayden, D. W., Naqui, R. H., Rosenkrantz, H., and Braude, M. C. 1979. The embryonic effects of cannabinoids in rats and mice. *J Environ Pathol Toxicol* 4:471–82.

Fried, P. A. 1976. Short and long-term effects of prenatal cannabis inhalation upon rat offspring. *Psychopharmacology* 50:185–290.

Fried, P. A., Barnes, M. V., and Drake, E. R. 1985. Soft drug use after pregnancy compared to use before and during pregnancy. *Am J Obstet Gynecol* 151:787–92.

Fried, P. A., Buckingham, M., and Vov Kulmiz, P. 1983. Marijuana use during pregnancy and perinatal risk factors. *Am J Obstet Gynecol* 144:922–24.

Fried, P. A., and Charlebois, A. T. 1979. Cannabis administered during pregnancy: First- and second-generation effects. *Physiol Psychol* 7:307–10.

Fried, P. A., Innes, K. S., and Barnes, M. V. 1984. Soft drug use prior to and during pregnancy: A comparison of samples over a four-year period. *Drug Alcohol Depend* 13:161–76.

Fried, P. A., and Makin, J. E. 1987. Neonatal behavioral correlates of prenatal exposure to marijuana, cigarettes and alcohol in a low risk population. *Neurotoxicol Teratol* 9:1–7.

Fried, P. A., and Watkinson, B. 1988. 12- and 24-month neurobehavioral follow-up of children prenatally exposed to marijuana, cigarettes and alcohol. *Neurotoxicol Teratol* 4:305–13.

Fried, P. A., Watkinson, B., Dillon, R. F., and Dulberg, C. S. 1987. Neonatal neurological status in a low-risk population after prenatal exposure to cigarettes, marijuana and alcohol. *J Dev Behav Pediatr* 8:318–26.

Fried, P. A., Watkinson, B., Grant, A. and Knights, R. M. 1980. Changing patterns of soft drug use prior to and during pregnancy: A prospective study. *Drug Alcohol Depend* 6:323–43.

Fried, P. A., Watkinson, B., and Willan, A. 1984. Marijuana use during pregnancy and decreased length of gestation. *Am J Obstet Gynecol* 150:23–27.

Golub, M. S., Sassenrath, E. N., and Chapman, C. F. 1981. Regulation of visual attention in offspring of female monkeys treated chronically with delta-9-tetrahydrocannabinol. *Dev Psychobiol* 14:507–12.

Gorski, R. A. 1971. Gonadal hormones and the perinatal development of neuroendocrine function. In *Frontiers in Neuroendocrinology*, ed. L. Martini and W. F. Ganong, 237–90. London: Oxford University Press.

Greenland, S., Staisch, K., Brown, N., and Gross, S. 1982. The effects of marijuana use during pregnancy: I. A preliminary epidemiological study. *Am J Obstet Gynecol* 143:408–13.

———. 1983. Effects of marijuana on human pregnancy, labor and delivery. *Neurobehav Toxicol Teratol* 4:447–50.

Hatch, E. E., and Bracken, M. R. 1986. Effect of marijuana use in pregnancy on fetal growth. *Am J Epidemiol* 124:986–93.

Hatoum, N. S., Davis, W. M., ElSohly, M. A., and Turner, C. E. 1981. Perinatal exposure to cannabichromine and Δ^9-tetrahydrocannabinol: Separate and combined effects on viability of pups and on male reproductive system at maturity. *Toxicol Lett* 8:141–46.

Hingson, R., Alpert, J., Day, N., Dooling, E., Kayne, H., Morelock, S., Oppenheimer, E., and Zuckerman, B. 1982. Effects of maternal drinking and marijuana use on fetal growth and development. *Pediatrics* 70:539–46.

Hutchings, D. E., Morgan, B., Brake, S. C., Shi, T., and Lasalle, E. 1987. Delta-9-tetrahydrocannabinol during pregnancy in the rat: I. Differential effects of maternal nutrition, embryotoxicity and growth in the offspring. *Neurotoxicol Teratol* 9:39–43.

Idanpään-Heikkila, J. 1969. Placental transfer of tritiated delta-1-tetrahydrocannabinol. *N Engl J Med* 281:330 (abstr).

Indian Hemp Drug Commission. 1893/1894. *Marijuana*. Reprinted in 1969. Silver Spring, Md.: Thomas Jefferson.

Jakubovic, A., Tait, R. M., and McGeer, P. L. 1974. Excretion of THC and its metabolites in ewe's milk. *Toxicol Appl Pharmacol* 28:38–43.

Jost, A. 1972. A new look at the mechanisms controlling sex differentiation in mammals. *John Hopkins Med J* 130:38–53.

Kamel, F., Wright, W. W., Mock, E. S., and Frankel, A. I. 1977. The influence of mating and related stimuli on plasma levels of luteinizing hormone, prolactin and testosterone in the male rat. *Endocrinology* 101:421–29.

Kawash, G. F., Yeung, D. L., and Berg, S. D. 1980. Effects of administration of cannabis resin during pregnancy on emotionality and learning in rats' offspring. *Percept Mot Skills* 50:359–65.

Linn, S., Schoebaum, S. C., Monson, R. R., Rosner, R., Stubblefield, P. C., and Ryan, K. J. 1983. The association of marijuana use with outcome of pregnancy. *Am J Public Health* 73:1161–64.

Luthra, Y. K. 1979. Brain biochemical alterations in neonates of dams treated orally with delta-9-tetrahydrocannabinol during gestation and lactation. In *Marijuana: Biological Effects*, ed. G. G. Nahas and W. D. M. Paton, 531–37. New York: Pergamon Press.

Majewski, F. 1981. Alcohol embryopathy: Some facts and speculations about pathogenesis. *Neurobehav Toxicol Teratol* 3:129–44.

Mantilla-Plata, B., Clewe, G. L., and Harbison, R. D. 1975. Δ^9-Tetrahydrocannabinol-induced changes in prenatal growth and development of mice. *Toxicol Appl Pharmacol* 33:333–40.

Martin, B. R. 1986. Cellular effects of cannabinoids. *Pharmacol Rev* 38:45–74.

Matheny, A. P., Dolan, A. B., and Wilson, R. S. 1974. Bayley's infant behavior record: Relations between behaviors and mental test scores. *Dev Psychobiol* 10:696–702.

McEwen, B. S. 1978. Sexual maturation and differentiation: The role of gonadal steroids. *Prog Brain Res* 48:291–308.

O'Connell, C. M., and Fried, P. A. 1984. An investigation on prenatal cannabis exposure and minor physical anomalies in a low-risk population. *Neurobehav Toxicol Teratol* 6:345–50.

Qazi, Q. H., Mariano, E., Bellar, E., Milman, D., and Crumbleholme, W. 1982. Is marijuana smoking fetotoxic? *Pediatr Res* 16:272A.

———. 1985. Abnormalities associated with prenatal marijuana exposure. *Dev Pharmacol Ther* 8:141–48.

Rasmussen, H., and Waisman, D. M. 1981. The messenger function of calcium in endocrine systems. In *Biochemical Actions of Hormones*, ed. G. Litwara. New York: Academic Press.

Rosenkrantz, H. 1984. Effects of cannabinoids on fetal development of rodents. In *Marijuana '84*, ed. G. G. Nahas and W. D. M. Paton. Oxford, England: IRL Press.

Sitteri, P. K., Jones, L. A., Roubinian, J., and Talal, N. 1980. Sex steroids and the immune system: I. Sex differences in autoimmune disease in NZB/N2W hybrid mice. *J Steroid Biochem* 15:425–32.

Smith, D. W. 1974. *Recognizable Patterns of Human Malformations*. Philadelphia: W. B. Saunders.

Tansley, B. W., Fried, P. A., and Mount, H. T. J. 1986. Visual processing in children exposed prenatally to marijuana and nicotine. *Can J Public Health* 77:72–78.

Tennes, K., Avitable, N., Blackard, C., Boyles, C., Hassoun, B., Holmes, L., and Kreye, M. 1985. Marijuana: Prenatal and postnatal exposure in the human. In *Current Research on the Consequences of Maternal Drug Abuse. NIDA Res Monogr* 59.

Walters, D. E., and Carr, L. A. 1986. Changes in brain catecholamine mechanisms following perinatal exposure to marijuana. *Pharmacol Biochem Behav* 25:763–68.

7

Cocaine Use during Pregnancy: Neurobehavioral Changes in the Offspring

Diana Dow-Edwards, Ph.D., Ira J. Chasnoff, M.D., and Dan R. Griffith, Ph.D.

COCAINE USE by pregnant women has become a major issue of concern for health workers in the United States. However, there is little information about the exact effects of cocaine upon pregnancy and the developing fetus. Our preliminary study of 23 cocaine-using women and their offspring gave an initial indication that cocaine would have significant effects on pregnancy outcome (Chasnoff et al. 1985). These initial impressions have been borne out in subsequent studies.

CLINICAL STUDIES

In an ongoing research project at Northwestern University Medical School from April 1986 to June 1987, 70 infants were born to cocaine-using women enrolled in the Perinatal Center for Chemical Dependence. Each of these women used cocaine intranasally, intravenously, or by freebasing during the first trimester of pregnancy, and 60% of the women continued to use cocaine throughout the pregnancy. Urine samples obtained on a regular basis were screened for the use of licit and illicit drugs (opiates, amphetamines, barbiturates, marijuana, benzodiazepines, propoxyphene, cocaine, phencyclidine, tobacco, and alcohol).

For evaluation of outcome of the cocaine-exposed infants, a drug-free comparison group (n = 70) was selected from the population of the Prentice Ambulatory Care Clinic representing pregnant women of a similar racial and socioeconomic distribution. These women had no history or evidence of licit or illicit drug use and were selected for the control group on the basis of social, demographic, and environmental

Table 7-1. Maternal Characteristics

Characteristic	Cocaine-treated	Drug-free
Age (years	26.7	27.1
Gravidity	3.5	2.7
Cigarettes (no./day)	12.7	9.2
Alcohol (ml/week)	16.7 (7 women)	—
Marijuana (joints/month)	7.8 (15 women)	—
Weight gain (pounds)	27.1	28.6
Education (years)	11.4	11.0

Note: *t* test, not significant; each group contained 70 subjects. Values are means.

backgrounds; they also were comparable for cigarette use during pregnancy (table 7.1).

Obstetric management of pregnancy was similar for the two groups of women and has been described in previous publications (Chasnoff, Hatcher, and Burns 1982; Chasnoff 1985). The reproductive histories of all women were reviewed, and labor and delivery data were recorded at the time of delivery. All neonates were examined at birth. When the infants delivered at term (38–42 weeks gestation) were 12 to 72 hours old, the Neonatal Behavioral Assessment Scale (Brazelton 1984) was administered by trained examiners who were blinded to the infants' prenatal history. Appropriate statistical measures for parametric and nonparametric data were utilized to analyze differences between the cocaine-exposed and drug-free groups.

Evaluation of outcome revealed that, as in other substance-abusing populations, the cocaine-addicted women had a high incidence of infectious disease complications, especially hepatitis (24%) and venereal disease (10.5%). There was an increase in complications of labor and delivery in cocaine-using women as compared to drug-free women (table 7.2).

All of the infants were of singleton birth, and there was a similar distribution of infants according to sex in each group. A similar number of infants in each group had Apgar scores of less than 7 at one and five minutes. Meconium staining occurred in the cocaine-exposed group with greater frequency as compared to the control group of infants.

Table 7.2 Complications of Labor and Delivery

	Cocaine-treated		Drug-free	
Complication	*n*	%	*n*	%
Premature labor	17	24	2	3
Precipitous labor	7	10	2	3
Abruptio placentae	12	17	1	1
Fetal monitor abnormality	7	10	4	5

Note: χ^2 analysis, $p < .05$ for all results.

Table 7-3. Neonatal Growth Parameters

Parameter	Cocaine-treated ($n = 61$)	Drug-free ($n = 68$)
Weight (g)	3094	3473
Length (cm)	48.9	51.1
Head circumference (cm)	33.1	34.8

Note: t test, $p < .02$. Values are means. All infants were born at ≥ 38 weeks gestation.

There was an increased incidence of premature labor among the cocaine-complicated pregnancies, and mean gestational age was reduced for the cocaine group of infants. There were significant differences in birth weights, lengths, and head circumferences between infants in the two groups (table 7.3) who were delivered at term (≥ 38 weeks gestation).

Perinatal complications are shown in table 7.4. The most significant are the reduced mean gestational age and the high rate of small-for-gestational age neonates in the cocaine group. No infant in the cocaine group required pharmacological therapy for symptoms of abstinence. Eight cocaine-exposed infants had malformations of the genitourinary tract (Chasnoff, Chisum, and Kaplan 1988): two with "prune belly syndrome," one with female pseudohermaphroditism, two with first degree

Table 7-4. Perinatal Morbidity

Parameter	Cocaine-treated ($n = 70$)	Drug-free ($n = 70$)
Gestation age in weeks $(\bar{x})$[a]	37.1	39.3
Small for gestational age[b]	13 (19%)	2 (3%)
Ileal atresia	3 (4%)	—
Cerebral infarction	2 (3%)	—

[a] t test, $p < .05$.
[b] χ^2, $p < .05$.

hypospadias and undescended testes, and three with hydroureter/hydronephrosis. Two infants in the cocaine-exposed group suffered a perinatal cerebral infarction during the 48 to 72 hours before delivery, which was related to their mother's cocaine use (Chasnoff et al. 1986), and three cocaine-exposed infants presented with ileal atresia at 24 hours of age. Cluster analysis (Lester, Als, and Brazelton 1978) of the Neonatal Behavioral Assessment Scale revealed that cocaine-exposed newborn infants exhibited poor motor, orientation, and state regulation behaviors, which had improved significantly by one month of age. In the cases of orientation and state regulation, however, abilities were still significantly poorer than the same abilities in drug-free newborns (Griffith et al. 1988).

The drug-free group of women in the present study had an incidence of complications of labor and delivery similar to that of the general population. However, the cocaine-using women had a higher rate of complications of labor and delivery than the control women. Cocaine acts peripherally to inhibit nerve conduction. It also prevents norepinephrine reuptake at the nerve terminals, producing increased norepinephrine levels with subsequent vasoconstriction and tachycardia and a concomitant abrupt rise in blood pressure (Ritchie and Greene 1980). Placental vasoconstriction also occurs (Sherman and Gautieri 1972), decreasing blood flow to the fetus. An increase in uterine contractility has also been reported in human beings (Lederman et al. 1978). The increased incidence of preterm labor and abruptio placentae is consistent with these pharmacological actions of cocaine.

Maternal problems at delivery are reflected in the high rate of fetal distress noted in the cocaine-exposed infants, as manifested by fetal monitor abnormalities and fetal meconium staining. The perinatal cerebral infarction noted in two infants is a severe example of the morbidity associated with intrauterine exposure to cocaine (Chasnoff et al. 1986) and is similar to intracerebral insults reported in adults who use cocaine. The occurrence of genitourinary malformations in the cocaine-exposed infants is consistent with studies in animals, which found an increased incidence of cryptorchidism and hydronephrosis in mice (Mahalik, Gautieri, and Mann 1980); however, larger numbers of cocaine-exposed infants must be studied before conclusions regarding the association of congenital malformation with cocaine use can be reached. The impaired intrauterine growth noted in the infants exposed to cocaine is consistent with the vasoconstrictive action of cocaine.

Infant responses to the Neonatal Behavioral Assessment Scale indicated that newborn cocaine-exposed infants as a group experienced deficiencies in their ability to move adaptively through the various states of arousal in response to the demands of testing and in their ability to attend to and actively engage auditory and/or visual stimuli. The majority of the cocaine-exposed infants had very few self-protective mechanisms for avoiding overstimulation and required considerable assistance from caretakers to maintain control of their hyperexcitable nervous systems.

During testing with the Neonatal Behavioral Assessment Scale, the cocaine-exposed newborns often made abrupt changes in state which were inappropriate for the level of stimulation being presented. Varying patterns of state control were observed, but the one characteristic that these patterns shared in common was the infants' use of sleeping and crying to shut themselves off from external stimulation.

This tendency to shut out rather than interact with external stimuli seemed to have its greatest effect on the interactive capabilities of the cocaine-exposed newborn. Drug-free newborns could typically achieve repeated episodes of alert responsiveness to external stimuli with varying degrees of help from the examiner, but many of the cocaine-exposed newborns never reached an alert state during the examination. The majority of those infants who did achieve alertness required a high degree of examiner-induced controls designed to reduce the intensity of extraneous stimuli and to allow the infants to focus on one specific stimulus. Even though the examiner might tightly swaddle the infants, hold their hands, give them pacifiers, and rock them gently in a vertical position, most of the newborn cocaine-exposed infants were capable of only fleeting attention to a given stimulus before displaying signs of distress, including color changes, rapid respiration, disorganized motor activity, and frantic gaze aversion. With careful use of examiner's controls and "time-out" periods for the infant at the first signs of stress, some of the infants were able to regain enough organization to respond in like manner to another stimulus. Each infant, however, seemed to have a threshold for overstimulation which could not be exceeded without the infant terminating the examination by moving into a completely unavailable state of sleeping or frantic crying.

Recent research has indicated that, by one month of age, the present sample of cocaine-exposed infants had made significant improvements with regard to their state control and interactive capabilities (Griffith et al. 1988). They still, however, performed significantly more poorly than drug-free newborns in their management of states of arousal and their ability to maintain alert, responsive periods without becoming overloaded. The worst of the one-month-old cocaine-exposed infants continued to vacillate between sleeping and crying in response to the demands of the examination. Most of them, however, were capable of achieving at least brief periods of alert responsiveness if given a good deal of caretaker assistance. Swaddling and pacifiers were still essential for many of these infants to be able to attend to stimulation without losing control and moving into a state of unavailability through crying. With these controls and repeated time-outs, most of the one-month-old cocaine-exposed infants were able to complete the examination but were obviously exhausted by the effort this required.

The abnormal characteristics found in the newborn cocaine-exposed infants go beyond their performance on state-control and orientation-interaction dimensions to the quality of their psychomotor abilities. Many of these infants display a number of abnormal reflexes and the imbalance in muscle tone which are usually displayed as hypertonicity. These difficulties have been shown to persist through at least four months of age (Schneider and Chasnoff 1987). More recent studies confirmed the high rates of prematurity and growth retardation in cocaine-exposed infants (Chasnoff et al. 1989; Zuckerman et al. 1989). One study also demonstrated, however, that, if the cocaine-using women entered treatment and became drug-free by the end of the first trimester, the risk for poor obstetric outcome was significantly reduced. Even infants exposed to cocaine only during the first trimester still demonstrated impaired neurobehavioral outcome (Chasnoff et al. 1989). It was hypothesized that early gestational exposure of the devloping fetal catecholamine system to cocaine leads to neurobehavioral deficiencies evident at birth.

STUDIES IN ANIMALS

Teratological Studies

Just as interest in the clinical effects of cocaine use during pregnancy has increased, interest in basic research on the developmental toxicity of cocaine has also expanded recently. There were, however, basic science publications on the teratology of cocaine as early as 1980. Mice given a single subcutaneous dose of cocaine at 60 mg/kg between gestation days 6 and 12 and examined on gestation day 18 (one day before delivery) demonstrated soft tissue and skeletal abnormalities, increased resorption, and altered sex ratio (Mahalik, Gautieri, and Mann 1980). However, these single doses had no effect on maternal weight gain or mean fetal weights. Fantel and MacPhail (1982) did find that repeated intraperitoneal cocaine doses of 60 mg/kg between days 7 and 16 of gestation in the mouse significantly reduced fetal weights. In general, the fetuses appeared to be normal. This same dose given daily to pregnant rats (between days 8 and 12 of gestation) also caused a decrease in maternal and fetal weights, an increase in the number of resorptions, and the presence of edema in 13 fetuses of nine litters examined. Higher doses (75 mg/kg) were lethal, and lower doses (50 mg/kg) only increased the resorption rate slightly. Since these authors used ether to anesthetize the animals before the daily injection, the results of this study needed to be verified. A fairly complete dose/ response curve for subcutaneous administration of cocaine during pregnancy has now been established for the rat. A cocaine dose of 40–90 mg/kg induced decreases in maternal food and water consumption and maternal weight gain in a dose/response manner (Church, Dintcheff, and Gessner 1988). Fetal weights were, however, affected only at the highest dose. This relative sparing of the fetuses is perhaps due to the increased fetal death observed at all doses of the drug, perhaps resulting in a greater share of the maternal nutrients being provided to the survivors. Fetal edema, abruptio placentae, and cephalic hemorrhage were also identified in the fetuses. Together, these animal data indicate that low birth weight, abruptio placentae, cephalic hemorrhage, and other effects also identified in the clinical population are effects of cocaine exposure per se and not merely the result of polydrug interactions, which are common and difficult to control in the human population.

Neurobehavioral Studies

Scientists were quick to recognize that cocaine might potentially have its greatest developmental effects on the nervous system. In adults, cocaine is known to be a powerful central nervous system stimulant with lasting neurobehavioral effects after even a single dose of the drug. The first to identify behavioral alterations in young rats exposed to cocaine in utero were Spear et al. (1987). They found that 40 mg of cocaine per kg given between gestational days 8 and 20 has no effect on the development of certain reflexes; rather, the treated pups showed decreased learning and memory in one test using appetitive conditioning. Cocaine also was associated with a transient decrease in wall climbing and an increase in locomotor activity after mild foot shock during the preweaning period. This dose had minimal effects on the physical development of the fetus as a whole and had no effect on the number and weight of live offspring or on the length of gestation. Apparently, prenatal cocaine exposure at a dose too small to induce obvious malformations does induce abnormal behavioral development, which persists at least until the time of weaning. These and more recent studies investigating the responses of exposed pups to dopamine agonists and antagonists (Spear, Kirstein, and Frambes 1989) resulted in the working hypothesis that prenatal cocaine exposure may induce a down-regulation of central dopamine pathways.

The first published report showing a neurobehavioral effect of prenatal cocaine exposure was that by Hutchings, Fico, and Dow-Edwards (1989). We examined two doses (30 and 60 mg/kg per os), utilized both nontreated and pair-fed control groups, and fostered the pups at birth to another group of untreated dams to eliminate the possible residual effects of the cocaine or pair-feeding treatments on the postnatal development of the pups. Cocaine at 30 and 60 mg/kg per os given between days 8 and 22 of gestation had minimal effects on fetal development, but maternal weight gain was significantly reduced at both doses. Interestingly, when activity levels of the litters were determined every 3

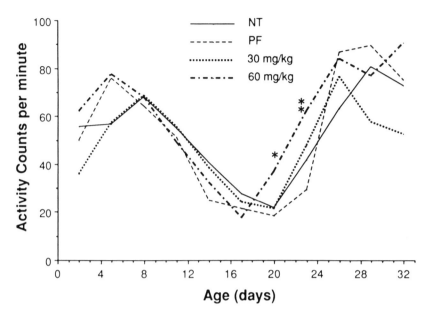

Figure 7.1. Mean activity counts per minute for 8 not treated (NT), 8 pair-fed (PF), and 18 cocaine-exposed (7 to 30 mg/kg and 11 to 60 mg/kg) litters from postnatal days 2–32. *p < .001, univariate F test, significantly different from all other groups; **p < .006, univariate F test, significantly different from pair-fed groups.
Source: Hutchings, Fico, and Dow-Edwards 1989.

days for the first 32 days of life, all groups showed a peak activity level at 5 days and a decrease at 15–17 days (fig. 7.1). On postnatal days 20 and 23, those litters receiving 60 mg/kg prenatally showed statistically significant *increases* in activity, which were no longer apparent at 26 days of age. Since this normal increase in activity occurs at a time when several forebrain regions associated with motor control are undergoing synaptogenesis (Hartley and Seeman 1983), it is possible that prenatal cocaine exposure may alter the normal developmental sequence in these important central neuronal pathways.

Several other groups have now also identified long-term neurobehavioral changes induced by prenatal cocaine exposure. Foss and Riley (1988) reported that prenatal cocaine was associated with an enhanced reflex-startle response in male rats when measured at 90 days of age. Interestingly, female rats did not show a similar effect. Raum et al.

(1990) reported that prenatal cocaine alters male sexually dimorphic behavior when rats are examined at 60 days of age. Cocaine exposure also resulted in an increase in luteotrophic hormone levels and a decrease in sperm count by 40% at 80 days of age.

To assess the function of specific central neuronal pathways, we (Dow-Edwards, Freed, and Fico 1990) used the deoxyglucose method to measure brain functional activity (Sokoloff et al. 1977) in adult rats selected from litters receiving either 60 mg of cocaine per kg or pair-feeding during gestation days 8–22. This method is based on the quantification of the incorporation of an analog of glucose during a specified period in the brain of awake, freely moving animals. Since the analog is radiolabeled, placing sections of the brain with the analog incorporated in vivo against x-ray film produces a map of the metabolism of glucose in each region throughout the entire neuraxis simultaneously. There were no differences in most of the physiological parameters measured (mean arterial blood pressure, body weight and temperature, etc.), but there was a significant increase in hematocrit in the exposed adult males. Persistent decreases in functional activity were observed in several brain areas, including the primary motor and somatosensory cortices, and in components of the limbic system, including the hippocampus, amygdala, and septum (table 7.5). The hypothalamus showed the greatest concentration of decreases in glucose utilization, with five of nine structures showing statistically significant decreases compared to controls. Other laboratories have reported that a similar period of cocaine exposure at a lower dose than we utilized results in the development of males with alterations in sexually dimorphic behaviors and increased levels of leuteotropic hormone (Raum et al. 1990). If the rat is an appropriate model for human development, we should be concerned that children exposed to cocaine prenatally may show abnormal sexual development from puberty into adulthood.

The possible mechanisms whereby cocaine induces these neurobehavioral alterations have also been the subject of much interest. Woods, Plessinger, and Clark (1987) reported that cocaine lowers fetal oxygen tension and raises heart rate and blood pressure in a dose-dependent manner when administered intravenously to a preterm ewe. Chronic hypoxia, which might also be induced in the rat model by daily cocaine administration, would certainly be expected to have significant effects on brain development, just as it does on whole-body development. Many studies also show that cocaine is associated with a decrease in

Table 7.5 Glucose Utilization in Selected Structures from Adult Male Rats Treated Prenatally with 60 mg Cocaine per kg

Structure	Activity (μmol/100 g/min)		
	Control (n = 7)	Treated (n = 6)	% Change
Cortex			
Visual	109.4 ± 5.8	98.9 ± 4.1	− 10
Auditory	140.7 ± 6.6	131.3 ± 3.5	− 7
Parietal	93.0 ± 3.0	87.5 ± 3.8	− 6
Forelimb/motor	96.3 ± 3.4	87.6 ± 2.0*	− 9
Forelimb/sensory	94.9 ± 3.9	82.6 ± 3.1*	− 13
Piriform	118.9 ± 4.4	106.6 ± 3.4	− 8
Cingulate	105.8 ± 6.6	90.7 ± 3.2	− 14
Motor Structures			
Red n.	77.6 ± 3.7	73.6 ± 1.9	− 5
Substantia nigra			
Pars reticulata	58.7 ± 2.9	53.3 ± 1.8	− 9
Pars compacta	71.5 ± 2.0	65.1 ± 1.6*	− 9
Zona incerta	89.9 ± 3.1	80.3 ± 3.0*	− 11
Globus pallidus	55.7 ± 2.4	51.4 ± 1.3	− 8
Caudate n.	95.8 ± 3.1	87.6 ± 2.0*	− 9
Sensory Structures			
Superior olive	135.1 ± 6.3	130.6 ± 5.2	− 3
Vent. caud. n. lat. lemniscus	114.6 ± 5.7	115.5 ± 2.8	+ 1
Inferior colliculus	154.3 ± 7.3	148.7 ± 4.2	− 4
Medial geniculate	127.6 ± 4.7	121.7 ± 2.6	− 5
Superior colliculus	93.4 ± 3.2	82.3 ± 2.2*	− 12
Lateral geniculate	95.1 ± 3.1	90.1 ± 3.0	− 5
External plexiform layer	102.4 ± 5.7	93.5 ± 3.6	− 9
Ventral thalamus	91.5 ± 2.4	89.8 ± 1.6	− 2
Vestibular n.	107.9 ± 5.3	108.5 ± 4.0	+ 1

Table 7.5 (*Continued*)

Structure	Activity (μmol/100 g/min)		
	Control ($n = 7$)	Treated ($n = 6$)	% Change
Limbic Structures			
Median raphe	97.3 ± 4.6	89.0 ± 2.7	−9
Interpeduncular n.	112.4 ± 4.9	113.5 ± 3.8	+1
Habenula			
Medial	56.7 ± 1.1	52.0 ± 2.5	−8
Lateral	106.5 ± 2.7	99.3 ± 4.0	−7
Mediodorsal thalamus	123.7 ± 5.8	110.4 ± 4.3	−11
Amygdala			
Anterior	86.0 ± 3.8	77.4 ± 2.8	−10
Central	39.0 ± 0.8	34.5 ± 1.4*	−12
Cortical	85.1 ± 2.9	79.2 ± 5.4	−7
Hippocampus			
Molecular/CA1	86.0 ± 2.2	73.2 ± 2.7*	−18
Dentate gyrus	52.6 ± 1.7	49.6 ± 2.3	−6
Ventral tegmentum A10	70.7 ± 3.8	62.0 ± 1.6	−12
Lateral septal n.	58.1 ± 1.8	48.6 ± 2.1*	−16
Accumbens	70.4 ± 3.6	60.2 ± 2.2*	−17
VDBV	83.2 ± 2.8	75.1 ± 2.2*	−10
Hypothalamic Structures			
Mammillary body	128.2 ± 6.6	122.1 ± 4.8	−5
Median eminence	42.1 ± 1.6	37.1 ± 2.7	−12
Arcuate n.	43.8 ± 1.6	36.0 ± 2.2*	−18
Ventromedial n.	58.8 ± 7.2	40.8 ± 2.0*	−31
Dorsomedial n.	59.1 ± 1.8	51.4 ± 2.2*	−13
Paraventricular n.	52.6 ± 1.4	45.5 ± 1.3*	−14
Lateral	66.4 ± 2.6	59.3 ± 2.5	−11
Suprachiasmatic n.	68.8 ± 3.2	61.9 ± 2.4	−10
Medial preoptic area	44.5 ± 1.1	38.2 ± 2.1*	−14

Source: Dow-Edwards, Freed, and Fico 1990.
Note: Activity values are means ± SE.
* Significantly different from control by Student's *t* test, $p < .05$.

maternal weight gain (Hutchings, Fico, and Dow-Edwards 1989; Church, Dintcheff, and Gessner 1988), which might be expected to result in poor nutritional status. Prenatal undernutrition is associated with intrauterine growth retardation (an effect of cocaine identified clinically) and abnormal brain development (Dodge, Prensky, and Feigen 1975). Cocaine is also known to have potent effects on the neuroendocrine systems (particularly prolactin), which would also be expected to produce a variety of developmental abnormalities, including those reported by Raum et al. (1990). Therefore, the established effects of cocaine in adult animals, as well as those recently identified in pregnant animals, could certainly contribute to many of the growth and neurobehavioral effects of the drug which have appeared in recent studies on the rat, as well as those identified clinically.

Studies of Cocaine Administered Directly to the Developing Organism

The rat brain, unlike the human brain, undergoes a significant amount of development during the early postnatal period. For example, the eyes are open and able to perceive light soon after birth in the human, but eye opening does not occur until about day 15 in the rat. Whereas much of the brain undergoes synaptogenesis during the third trimester in humans, this process occurs during the first three weeks of postnatal life in the rat (Levitt and Moore 1979; Hartley and Seeman 1983; Fillion and Bauguen 1984; Moon-Edley and Herkenham 1984; Murrin, Gibbens, and Ferrer 1985). It is these processes of axonal and dendritic expansion and synaptogenesis which are most sensitive to environmental influences (Dobbing 1968). In the adult cocaine acts at the synapse by inhibiting the reuptake of dopamine, norepinephrine, and serotonin (Komiskey et al. 1977; Fuxe, Hamberger, and Malmfors 1967); thus, one might predict that the presence of cocaine during the processes of synapse formation would have significant effects on the development of these important neurotransmitter systems.

Manipulation of transmitter substances with agonists or antagonists during critical periods of development results in long-term alterations in the function of the specific brain regions and associated pathways (Loizou 1972; Coyle and Henry 1973; Rosengarten and Friedhoff 1979; Friedhoff and Miller 1983). Reuptake of catecholamines, the inhibition of which is the presumed action of cocaine in the synapses of adult brain, is functioning during the early postnatal period (Coyle and Axelrod 1972; Coyle and Campochiaro 1976; Deskin et al. 1981); therefore, the receptors for cocaine may be functioning and pharmacologically affected by neonatal cocaine treatment, as in the adult. Our approach has been to administer the drug during the early postnatal period, when the forebrain regions are undergoing synaptogenesis, and to examine brain functional activity, specific neurochemical indices, and behavior in the 60–70-day-old animals.

In the first study, we administered 50 mg of cocaine hydrochloride per kg to one half of the pups in a litter and the vehicle (water) to the other half during the first 10 days of life (Dow-Edwards, Freed, and Milhorat 1988). All litters were culled to eight, and the pups were weighed daily. The development of certain reflex behaviors such as day of walking, etc., was assessed on a small sample of pups throughout this early period and found not to be affected. Body weights of the pups both before and after weaning (day 21) were also not affected. At 60 days of age, brain glucose metabolism was determined using the deoxyglucose method (Sokoloff et al. 1977), as previously described (Vingan, Dow-Edwards, and Riley 1986). The female rats were all examined during diestrus to minimize differences in brain metabolism which occur with the different days of the estrus cycle (Nehlig et al. 1985). Using the fully quantified method, we found that 40% of the limbic structures examined were metabolically stimulated in the treated adult females compared to the controls (table 7.6). The motor and sensory systems were less significantly affected, although most of the regions examined in the female rats had mean glucose utilization rates above those of the controls. This is in sharp contrast to the findings with the male rats (table 7.7). Here, neonatal cocaine treatment had little effect on brain glucose metabolism. Only 1 of 40 structures examined was statistically significantly affected. This structure, the auditory cortex, was depressed in the treated males.

We repeated these studies in animals treated between postnatal days 11 and 20, and the results resemble those seen after 1–10 days of exposure but encompass different brain regions. The female treated rats showed large increases in glucose metabolism in many brain regions, including the many cortical regions, the subcortical motor areas, and the hippocampus. The male treated rats showed increases in activity in the auditory system and decreases in the structures in the medial forebrain bundle. From these data it is evident that cocaine has specific

Table 7-6. Brain Metabolism in Cocaine-treated Female Rats (Days 1–10)

Structure	Activity (μmol/100 g/min)		% Change
	Control (n = 6)	Cocaine-treated (n = 6)	
Motor Structures			
Motor cx	69 ± 4	79 ± 3	+ 14
Caudate n.	78 + 4	89 ± 2*	+ 14
Globus pallidus	45 ± 2	47 ± 1	+ 4
Thalamus			
Ventral n.	67 ± 3	80 ± 2*	+ 19
Substantia nigra	44 ± 2	48 ± 1	+ 9
Red n.	59 ± 3	68 ± 2*	+ 15
Pontine nuclei	46 ± 2	51 ± 1*	+ 11
Cerebellar cx	38 ± 4	41 ± 1	+ 8
Corpus callosum	36 ± 2	38 ± 2	+ 6
Mesolimbic forebrain			
Accumbens	74 ± 1	84 ± 5	+ 14
Bed n. stria terminalis	34 ± 1	36 ± 1	+ 6
Horizontal limb of diagonal band	77 ± 3	89 ± 3*	+ 16
Septum			
Medial	64 ± 2	70 ± 4	+ 9
Lateral	47 ± 1	48 ± 1	+ 2
Limbic cx			
Cingulate cx	86 ± 2	102 ± 4*	+ 19
Piriform cx	84 ± 5	91 ± 4	+ 8
Insular cx	112 ± 6	125 ± 6	+ 12
Hippocampus			
CA1	61 ± 3	70 ± 2*	+ 15
Dentate gyrus	43 ± 3	47 + 1	+ 9
Amygdala			
Lateral n.	64 ± 2	70 ± 1*	+ 9
Cortical n.	44 ± 1	48 ± 2	+ 9
Habenula			
Medial n.	58 ± 3	67 ± 3	+ 16
Lateral n.	97 ± 2	109 ± 5*	+ 12

Table 7-6. (*Continued*)

Structure	Activity (μmol/100 g/min)		
	Control (*n* = 6)	Cocaine-treated (*n* = 6)	% Change
Thalamus			
mediodorsal n.	88 ± 4	106 ± 6*	+20
Ventral tegmental area	51 ± 2	59 ± 1*	+16
Interpeduncular n.	83 ± 5	100 ± 5*	+20
Medial raphe n.	82 ± 3	99 ± 7*	+21
Central gray	51 ± 3	57 ± 1	+12
Sensory Structures			
Sensory cx			
Head	74 ± 4	83 ± 2	+12
Vibrissa	76 ± 4	83 ± 4	+9
Association (parietal) cx	69 ± 3	76 ± 3	+10
Primary olfactory cx	94 ± 4	106 ± 3*	+13
Occipital cx	77 ± 4	86 ± 4	+12
Lateral geniculate n.	69 ± 3	78 ± 2*	+13
Superior colliculus	63 ± 3	73 ± 5	+16
Auditory cx	113 ± 11	130 ± 6	+15
Medial geniculate n.	103 ± 8	123 ± 4*	+19
Inferior colliculus	129 ± 11	143 ± 5	+11

Source: Dow-Edwards, Freed, and Milhorat 1988.
Note: Activity values are means ± SE.
* Significant difference from control value; $p \leq .05$ by *t* test.

effects on brain functional development which depend, first, on the time when the drug is administered and, second, on the gender of the animal. (See chapter 2 for additional information on gender-specific effects.)

Other workers in the field have described similar sex-related differences in response to cocaine (Glick, Hinds, and Shapiro 1983; Glick and Hinds 1984; Post 1981). However, prenatal cocaine exposure seems to have greater effects on males (Foss and Riley 1988; Raum et al. 1990). Therefore, more work must be completed before possible sex differences in the developmental toxicity of cocaine are established. In

Table 7.7. Brain Metabolism in Cocaine-treated Male Rats (Days 1–10)

	Activity (μmol/100 g/min)		
	Control (n = 5)	Cocaine-treated (n = 6)	% Change
Motor Structures			
Motor cx	83 ± 3	82 ± 3	−1
Caudate n.	89 ± 2	93 ± 4	+4
Globus pallidus	52 ± 1	52 ± 2	0
Thalamus			
ventral n.	86 ± 2	85 ± 2	−1
Substantia nigra	49 ± 1	50 ± 2	+2
Red n.	70 ± 3	67 ± 2	−4
Pontine nuclei	55 ± 3	54 ± 4	−2
Cerebellar cx	42 ± 4	41 ± 2	−2
Corpus callosum	33 ± 3	37 ± 2	+12
Mesolimbic Forebrain			
Accumbens	85 ± 4	85 ± 4	0
Bed n. stria terminalis	41 ± 1	41 ± 1	0
Horizontal limb of diagonal band	96 ± 6	93 ± 4	−3
Septum			
Medial	82 ± 2	77 ± 3	−6
Lateral	51 ± 3	49 ± 2	−4
Limbic cx			
Cingulate	114 ± 6	109 ± 6	−4
Piriform	103 ± 6	98 ± 4	−5
Insular cx	137 ± 7	130 ± 5	−5
Hippocampus			
Ca1	73 ± 4	70 ± 3	−4
Dentate gyrus	49 ± 3	47 ± 1	−4
Amygdala			
Lateral n.	78 ± 1	75 ± 2	−4
Cortical n.	56 ± 3	57 ± 2	+2
Habenula			
Medial n.	66 ± 4	66 ± 2	0
Lateral n.	113 ± 4	108 ± 3	−5

Table 7.7. Brain Metabolism in Cocaine-treated Male Rats (Day 1–10)

	Activity (μmol/100 g/min)		
	Control (*n* = 5)	Cocaine-treated (*n* = 6)	% Change
Thalamus			
Mediodorsal n.	111 ± 7	116 ± 5	+4
Ventral tegmental area	58 ± 2	57 ± 2	−2
Interpeduncular n.	101 ± 4	95 ± 4	−6
Medial raphe n.	108 ± 6	97 ± 2	−10
Central gray	67 ± 5	60 ± 2	−10
Sensory Structures			
Sensory cx			
Head	85 ± 4	86 ± 2	+1
Vibrissa	86 ± 3	87 ± 3	+1
Association (parietal) cx	80 ± 3	83 ± 3	+4
Primary olfactory cx	117 ± 7	116 ± 5	−1
Occipital cx	97 ± 9	91 ± 5	−6
Lateral geniculate n.	81 ± 2	83 ± 3	+3
Superior colliculus	79 ± 5	76 ± 3	−4
Auditory cx	148 ± 7	126 ± 5*	−15
Medial geniculate n.	124 ± 3	125 ± 3	+10
Inferior colliculus	153 ± 8	152 ± 1	−1

Source: Dow-Edwards, Freed, and Milhorat 1988.
Note: Activity values are means ± SE.
* Significant difference from control value; $p \leq .05$ by *t* test.

addition, the metabolic changes identified in the female treated rats are unlikely to be the result of an altered physiological status of the animals because mean arterial blood pressure, arterial blood gases, hematocrit, and plasma glucose were all within the range of the control values in treated male and female rats. The increase in metabolism in the affected areas could be the result of increased neuronal firing, a greater concentration (density) of cells or neuropil, or perhaps an increase in a specific or general metabolic process in the neurons or glia in those regions.

Since the dopaminergic regions showed the greatest concentration of structures affected by early cocaine exposure, we measured the concentrations of dopamine receptors using ligands with high specificity for the D_1 subtype (^{3}H-SCH23390) and for the D_2 subtype (^{3}H-sulpiride). These analyses are still ongoing. It seems, however, that early (days 1–10) cocaine treatment results in a decrease in the concentration of D_1 receptors in the caudate nucleus, whereas later treatment (days 11–20) results in an increase in D_1 receptor binding. Thus, it seems that cocaine exposure during the time of dopaminergic synaptogenesis results in alterations in the dopaminergic system depending upon the time of drug administration.

Further evidence for the period-specific effects of cocaine can be seen in the behavioral response to an amphetamine challenge. We found that adult females exposed during the early postnatal period exhibit more locomotion activity as measured in the Omnitech activity chamber compared to controls that received the vehicle postnatally (Hughes et al. 1991). Late exposure produced the opposite effect; the cocaine-exposed females showed a decrease in response to low doses of amphetamine. This decrease in amphetamine response is consistent with a relative increase in serotonergic function compared to dopaminergic function. We are continuing our study of the effects of postnatal drug administration by examining the acute response of developing brain to cocaine.

In conclusion, we have presented evidence that exposure to cocaine during critical periods of development in the rat can induce lasting changes in several neurobehavioral measures. Therefore, although low to moderate exposure to cocaine during pregnancy does not seem to induce obvious structural abnormalities in the rat, our data as well as the data of others suggest that cocaine use may place exposed children at risk for the development of serious neurobehavioral abnormalities, which may persist into adulthood.

SUMMARY

The correlation between the findings of human and animal studies as to the effects of cocaine on the developing organism is striking. The neurobehavioral deficiencies exhibited by the offspring in both clinical and animal populations are consistent and serve as a warning of the long-term risks for infant growth and development. Further studies will help to define and delineate these risk factors and serve as the basis for intervention programs as prenatally exposed children reach school age.

REFERENCES

Brazelton, T. B. 1984. *Neonatal Behavioral Assessment Scale*. Philadelphia: Spastics International.

Chasnoff, I. J. 1985. Effects of maternal narcotic vs. non-narcotic addiction on neonatal neurobehavior and infant development. In *Consequences of Maternal Drug Abuse*, ed. T. M. Pinkert, 84–95. Washington, D.C.: National Institute on Drug Abuse.

Chasnoff, I. J., Burns, W. J., Scholl, S. H., and Burns, K. A. 1985. Cocaine use in pregnancy. *N Eng J Med* 313:666–69.

Chasnoff, I. J., Bussey, M. E., Savich, R., and Stack, C. M. 1986. Perinatal cerebral infarction and maternal cocaine use. *J Pediatr* 108:456–59.

Chasnoff, I. J., Chisum, G. M., and Kaplan, W. E. 1988. Maternal cocaine use and genitourinary tract malformations. *Teratology* 37:201–4.

Chasnoff, I. J., Griffith, D. R., MacGregor, S. N., Kirkes, K., and Burns, K. 1989. Temporal patterns of cocaine use in pregnancy. *JAMA* 261:1741–44.

Chasnoff, I. J., Hatcher, R., and Burns, W. J. 1982. Polydrug- and methadone-addicted newborns: A continuum of impairment? *Pediatrics* 70:210–13.

Church, M. W., Dintcheff, B. A., and Gessner, P. K. 1988. Dose-dependent consequences of cocaine on pregnancy outcome in the Long-Evans rat. *Neurotoxicol Teratol* 10:51–58.

Coyle, J. T., and Axelrod, J. 1972. Dopamine-B-hydroxylase in the rat brain: Developmental characteristics. *J Neurochem* 19:449–59.

Coyle, J. T., and Campochiaro, P. 1976. Ontogenesis of dopaminergic-cholinergic interactions in the rat striatum: A neurochemical study. *J Neurochem* 27:673–78.

Coyle, J. T., and Henry, D. 1973. Catecholamines in fetal and newborn rat brain. *J Neurochem* 21:61–67.

Deskin, R., Seidler, F. J., Whitmore, W. L., and Slotkin, T. A. 1981. Development of a-noradrenergic and dopaminergic receptor systems depends on maturation of their presynaptic nerve terminals in the rat brain. *J Neurochem* 36:1683–90.

Dobbing, J. 1968. Vulnerable periods in developing brain. In *Applied Neurochemistry*, ed. A. Davison and J. Dobbing, 287–316. Philadelphia: Davis.

Dodge, P. R., Prensky, A. L., and Feigen, R. D. 1975. *Nutrition and the Developing Nervous System*. St. Louis: C. V. Mosby.

Dow-Edwards, D. L., Freed, L. A., and Fico, T. A. 1990. Structural and functional effects of prenatal cocaine exposure in adult rat brain. *Dev Brain Res* 57:263–68.

Dow-Edwards, D. L., Freed, L. A., and Milhorat, T. H. 1988. Stimulation of brain metabolism by perinatal cocaine exposure. *Brain Res* 42:137–41.

Fantel, A. G., and MacPhail, T. 1982. The teratogenicity of cocaine. *Teratology* 26:17–19.

Fillion, G., and Bauguen, C. 1984. Postnatal development of ^{3}H-5-HT binding in the presence of GTP in rat brain cortex. *Dev Pharmacol Ther* 7(suppl):1–5.

Foss, J. A., and Riley, E. P. 1988. Behavioral evaluation of animals exposed prenatally to cocaine. *Teratology* 37:517 (abstr).

Friedhoff, A. J., and Miller, J. C. 1983. Prenatal psychotropic drug exposure and the development of central dopaminergic and cholinergic neurotransmitter systems. *Monogr Neural Sci* 9:91–98.

Fuxe, K., Hamberger, B., and Malmfors, T. 1967. The effect of drugs on accumulations of monoamines in tubero-infundibular dopamine neurons. *Eur J Pharmacol* 1:334–41.

Glick, S. D., and Hinds, P. A. 1984. Sex differences in sensitization to cocaine-induced rotation. *Eur J Pharmacol* 99:119–23.

Glick, S. D., Hinds, P. A., and Shapiro, R. M. 1983. Cocaine-induced rotation: Sex-dependent differences between left- and right-sided rats. *Science* 221:775–77.

Griffith, D. R., Chasnoff, I. J., Dirkes, K., and Burns, K. 1988. Neurobehavioral development of cocaine-exposed infants in the first month of life. *Pediatr Res* 23:55 (abstr).

Hartley, E. J., and Seeman, P. 1983. Development of receptors for dopamine and noradrenaline in rat brain. *Eur J Pharmacol* 91:391–97.

Hughes, H. E., Pringle, G., Scribani, L., and Dow-Edwards, D. L. 1991. Cocaine treatment in neonatal rats affects adult behavioral response to amphetamine. *Neurotoxicol Teratol* 13:335–39.

Hutchings, D. E., Fico, T. A., and Dow-Edwards, D. L. 1989. Prenatal cocaine: Maternal toxicity, fetal effects and motor activity in rat offspring. *Neurobehav Toxicol Teratol* 11:65–69.

Komiskey, H. L., Miller, D. D., LaPidus, J. B., and Patil, P. N. 1977. The isomers of cocaine and tropacocaine: Effect on [^{3}H] catecholamine uptake by rat brain synaptosomes. *Life Sci* 21:1117–22.

Lederman, R. P., Lederman, E., Work, B. A., Jr., and McCann, D. S. 1978. The relationship of maternal anxiety, plasma catecholamines, and plasma cortisol to progress in labor. *Am J Obstet Gynecol* 132:495–500.

Lester, B. N., Als, H., and Brazelton, T. B. 1978. Scoring criteria for seven clusters of the Brazelton scale. Boston: Children's Hospital Medical Center.

Levitt, P., and Moore, R. V. 1979. Development of the noradrenergic innervation of neocortex. *Brain Res* 162:243–59.

Loizou, A. L. 1972. The postnatal ontogeny of monoamine-containing neurons in the CNS of albino rats. *Brain Res* 40:395–418.

Mahalik, M. P., Gautieri, R. F., and Mann, D. E. 1980. Teratogenic potential of cocaine hydrochloride in CF-1 mice. *J Pharm Sci* 69:703–9.

Moon-Edley, S., and Herkenham, M. 1984. Comparative development of striatal opiate receptors and dopamine revealed by autoradiography and histofluorescence. *Brain Res* 305:27–42.

Murrin, L. C., Gibbens, D. L., and Ferrer, J. R. 1985. Ontogeny of dopamine serotonin and spirodecanone receptors in rat forebrain—an autoradiographic study. *Dev Brain Res* 23:91–109.

Nehlig, A., Porrino, L., Crane, A., and Sokoloff, L. 1985. Local cerebral glucose utilization in normal female rats: Variations during the estrus cycle and comparison with males. *J Cereb Blood Flow Metab* 5:393–400.

Post, R. M. 1981. Central stimulants: Clinical and experimental evidence on tolerance and sensitization. In *Research Advances in Alcohol and Drug Problems*, ed. Y. Israel, F. Glaser, H. Kalant, R. E. Dopham, W. Schmidt, and R. Smart, 1–65. New York: Plenum Press.

Raum, W. J., McGiven, R. F., Peterson, M. A., Shryne, J. H., and Gorski, R. A. 1990. Prenatal inhibition of hypothalamic sex steroid uptake by cocaine: Effects on neurobehavioral sexual differentiation in male rats. *Dev Brain Res* 53:230–36.

Ritchie, J. M., and Greene, N. M. 1980. Local anesthesia. In *The Pharmacological Basis of Therapeutics*. 6th ed., ed. A. G. Gilman, L. S. Goodman, and A. Gilman, New York: Macmillan.

Rosengarten, H., and Friedhoff, A. J. 1979. Enduring changes in dopamine receptor cells of pups from drug administration to pregnant and nursing rats. *Science* 203:1133–35.

Ross, S. B., and Kent, A. L. 1961. Inhibition of the uptake of tritiated 5-HT in brain tissue. *Eur J Pharmacol* 7:270–77.

Schneider, J. W., and Chasnoff, I. J. 1987. Cocaine abuse during pregnancy: Its effects on infant motor development—a clinical perspective. *Top Acute Care Trauma Rehab* 2:59–69.

Sherman, W. T., and Gautieri, R. F. 1972. Effects of certain drugs on perfused human placenta: X. Norepinephrine release by bradykinin. *J Pharm Sci* 61:878–83.

Sokoloff, L., Revich, M., Kennedy, C., Des Rosiers, M. H., Patlak, C. S., Pettigrew, K. D., Sakurada, O., and Shinohara, M. 1977. The [^{14}C] deoxyglucose method for measurement of local cerebral glucose utilization: Theory, procedure and normal values in the conscious and anesthetized albino rat. *J Neurochem* 28:897–16.

Spear, L. P., Kirstein, C., Bell, J., Greenbaum, R., O'Shea, J., Yoottanasumpum, V., Hoffmann, H., and Spear, N. E. 1987. Effects of prenatal cocaine on behavior during the early postnatal period in rats. *Teratology* 35:8B (abstr).

Spear, L. P., Kirstein, C., and Frambes, N. A. 1989. Cocaine effects on developing central nervous system: Behavioral, psychopharmacological, and neurochemical studies. *Ann NY Acad Sci* 562:290–307.

Vingan, R. D., Dow-Edwards, D. L., and Riley, E. P. 1986. Effects of prenatal exposure to ethanol on local cerebral glucose utilization. *Alcohol Clin Exp Res* 10:22–26.

Woods, J. R., Plessinger, M. A., and Clark, K. E. 1987. Effect of cocaine on uterine blood flow and fetal oxygenation. *JAMA* 257:957–61.

Zuckerman, B., Frank, D. A., Hingson, R., Amaro, H., Levenson, S., Kayne, H., Parker, S., Vinci, R., Aboagye, K., Fried, L., Cabral, H., Timperi, R., and Bauchner, H. 1989. Effects of maternal marijuana and cocaine use on fetal growth. *N Eng J Med* 320:762–68.

8

The Perinatal Opioid Syndrome: Laboratory Findings and Clinical Implications

---

Ian S. Zagon, Ph.D., and Patricia J. McLaughlin, D.Ed.

THE CONSUMPTION of opium for medicinal, religious, social and personal reasons dates back 6,000 years (Blum 1969; Terry and Pellens 1970; Musto 1973). A decidedly important aspect of opium consumption is the passive dependence of the fetus, neonate, and infant when this drug is consumed by a pregnant or nursing woman. It is unclear how long this relationship between opium and dependence of the fetus/offspring has been known, although Hippocrates mentioned opium in connection with "uterine suffocation" (see Martin 1893). Clinical reports about unusual behavior of the fetus/neonate were evidenced by publications as early as the 1870s.

"Chronic opium intoxication" described infants with excessive nervousness, rapid breathing, and convulsive movements soon after birth, with death occurring within the first week of life (Terry and Pellens 1970). Review of the early literature proves quite revealing with regard to the effects of opioids on the fetus and neonate. (*Opioids* will be the term used to signify naturally occurring compounds—both exogenous and endogenous—and synthetic drugs with morphine-like properties.) Bureau, in 1895, reported that morphine could pass through the human placenta. A number of other workers recognized that drug addiction by the mother could have considerable effect on the fetus (Sainsbury 1909) and that enough opium could pass into the breast milk to alleviate withdrawal (Laase 1919; Langstein 1930; Petty 1912) or even to render the normal infant dependent through breast-feeding on an opium-consuming woman (Lichenstein 1915).

By the beginning of the twentieth century, the use of morphine, heroin, or paregoric to prevent withdrawal of the neonate was in clinical practice (Menninger-Lerchenthal 1934). As far back as 1888 (Earle), concern that fetal opioid exposure could be associated with a number of abnormalities in childhood and even adulthood was discussed. Early information about the prevalence of the perinatal opioid syndrome often presented conflicting portraits. Perlstein (1947) and Petty (1913) found this situation to be "rare." However, in 1926 Graham-Mulhall (1981) recorded over 800 pregnant women consuming opioids during a one-year period in New York during the early 1900s. The opioid of choice serving as the abusive substance over the past 100 years has undergone a change. Early in the literature, opium and morphine seemed to be the major opioids abused, with a change to heroin signaled in the report of Goodfriend, Shey, and Klein (1956). Subsequent to Dole and Nyswander's (1965) advocation of methadone as a substitute for heroin, numerous reports document methadone-dependent offspring.

Given recent estimates that the birth rate of heroin- and methadone-addicted mothers is roughly 3,000/year in New York City alone (Carr 1975) and assuming that New York City has one third to one half of the total number of chronic heroin and methadone users in the United States (Carr 1975), one could extrapolate 6,000 to 9,000 births per year to opium-consuming women. Placed within the context of roughly 3.3 million births every year in the United States, at least 1 in 1,000 births involves a mother using heroin or methadone. The incidence for the perinatal opioid syndrome rivals estimates for many well-known and highly publicized problems of early life, including the fetal alcohol syndrome, Down's syndrome, and neural tube defects, and it far exceeds the incidence of cancer in children aged 1 to 15 years. Thus, over the last 30–40 years, well over a quarter of a million infants, children, and young adults have been maternally exposed to opium; the number of offspring paternally exposed to opium has not been estimated but certainly enters the picture as well. This would indicate that at least 1 in every 1,000 people in the United States has been subjected to opioids in early life. These estimates are only from numbers known about maternal opioid addiction, not from paternal addiction (as mentioned), nor does it include the births by opioid-addicted parents who are not documented.

In this book, the clinical findings as to the fetus, neonate, and infant offspring born of mothers consuming opioid substances are reviewed in chapter 10 concerning methadone and chapter 9 with respect to heroin and morphine. As in most areas of human research, data collection and interpretation may be associated with numerous difficulties. In the study of perinatal opioid exposure and human development, the potential for problems is magnified. In actuality, two individuals—the mother and her offspring—are involved, and both must be considered in evaluating all of the repercussions associated with maternal opioid abuse. Confounding issues such as polydrug abuse, demographics, socioeconomic states, length of hospitalization, poor prenatal or postnatal care, neonatal withdrawal, breast-feeding, mother-infant/child interactions, paternal influences, sample selection, type of tests utilized for investigation, structuring of appropriate comparison/control groups, "dropout" rate of patients in the study, and statistical analysis must be—and often are—recognized (e.g., Householder et al. 1982; Strauss et al. 1979; Wilson, Desmond, and Wait 1981; Aylward 1982).

LABORATORY FINDINGS

In view of the potential difficulties involved in studying the human consumption of opioid substances and the effect of this consumption on the fetus/neonate/infant/child/adult and the need for further information as to whether opioid compounds are adverse agents in the developmental process, laboratory investigations are warranted. Laboratory models permit us to address such questions with a variety of methods that include maternal models of opioid consumption and studies on postnatally developing animals, regenerating tissues, tissues and cells in culture, and other in vitro preparations. Thus, the laboratory has allowed investigators to be more unrestricted in research design to address the important question of whether opioids influence biological development. If they do, one then asks what are the mechanisms involved and what are some possible strategies for intervention and treatment. A number of reviews (e.g., Zagon 1983, 1985; Zagon and McLaughlin 1984a) and bibliographies (Zagon et al. 1982; Zagon, McLaughlin, and Zagon 1984; Zagon, Zagon, and McLaughlin 1989) have been published, and the reader is referred to this earlier literature.

The methods and confounding influences used in studies of perinatal opioid abuse were recently reviewed (Zagon and McLaughlin 1990a) and will not be described herein. However, routes of administration, drug dosages, and schedules of treatment should be mentioned as some of the more important variables. Maternal exposure to opioids seems to have little effect on the estrous cycle, fertility, length of gestation, and parturition (Zagon and McLaughlin 1977a, 1977b, 1977c), although difficulties with conception and a protraction of the gestational period (Buchenauer, Turnbow, and Peters 1974), as well as positional malformations of the fetus (Chandler et al. 1975), have been reported. Fujinaga and Mazze (1988), implanting osmotic minipumps containing morphine into pregnant rats, found a significantly lower pregnancy rate in animals receiving 35 or 70 mg/kg/day but not in animals treated with 10 mg/kg/day. A reduction in maternal body weight during pregnancy is a common finding in terms of the effects of maternal opioid consumption (McGinty and Ford 1980; White, Zagon, and McLaughlin 1978; Seidler, Whitmore, and Slotkin 1982; Zagon and McLaughlin 1977a), but these weight deficits do not seem to reflect poor nutritional status (Ford and Rhines 1979; White, Zagon, and McLaughlin 1978). Maternal exposure to morphine or methadone, in general, does not have a detrimental influence on litter size, although some decreases in litter size with higher doses of methadone have been reported (Middaugh and Simpson 1980). Teratogenicity seems to be associated with high drug dosages administered acutely or over a short time period (Geber and Schramm 1975; Jurand 1973, 1980, 1985), but not with drugs administered chronically (e.g., Fujinaga and Mazze 1988). An increase in stillborns with high drug dosages was observed by Freeman (1980) and Sobrian (1977), but other investigations revealed little problem in this area (Davis and Lin 1972; Fujinaga and Mazze 1988).

The effect of transplacental exposure to opioids on postnatal viability seems to be determined by drug dosage and by whether the neonates continue to receive opioids postnatally (e.g., breast milk, direct injection). Neonates that do not continue to receive opioids after birth often may be hypersensitive to stimuli and may exhibit tremors at birth, with substantial neonatal mortality during the first few days of life (e.g., Davis and Lin 1972; Zagon and McLaughlin 1977d; Freeman 1980; Fujinaga and Mazze 1988).

Evaluation of the developmental pattern in offspring exposed to opioids can be determined in many laboratory animals, since the timetables of behavioral and physical maturation are well documented. Delays in physical characteristics (e.g., eye opening), spontaneous motor function (e.g., walking), and reflexes (e.g., visual orientation) all have been recorded. Interestingly, animals exposed only prenatally to opioids (i.e., permitted to go through withdrawal at birth and not receiving drug postnatally) exhibit the greatest number of delays in attaining behavioral capabilities and physical characteristics. Those animals receiving drug prenatally and postnatally (a situation more comparable to that in humans when opioids are administered to prevent or diminish withdrawal) are often closest to the normal timetable of maturation.

The behavior of rats during the period shortly after weaning (post-natal days 21 to 44) is often characterized by a reduction in activity and a decreased emotionality in opioid-exposed animals as compared to control offspring (Freeman 1980; Grove, Etkin, and Rosencrans 1979; Zagon, McLaughlin, and Thompson 1979a). An abnormally high incidence of wet-dog shake and head-shake behaviors, often resembling drug withdrawal, was recorded in opioid-subjected rats (Zagon and McLaughlin 1981b). In contrast to the reduced activity levels in opioid-treated animals at weaning, young adults (postnatal days 45 to 89) generally were hyperactive and more emotional (Davis and Lin 1972; Grove, Etkin, and Rosencrans 1979; Zagon, McLaughlin, and Thompson 1979a). Methadone-exposed pups often exhibited head-shake and wet-dog shake behaviors, indicating a protracted phase of withdrawal. Peters (1978) also accumulated preliminary evidence of learning disabilities in methadone- and morphine-exposed rats at this age.

Adult rats perinatally exposed to opioids often exhibit a lasting impairment in the ability to acquire fear (Sonderegger and Zimmerman 1976), a reduction in social dominance (Thompson and Zagon 1982), problems in learning (Middaugh and Simpson 1980; Zagon, McLaughlin, and Thompson 1979b), and a facilitation toward self-administrative behavior (Rech, Lomuscio, and Algeri 1980). Hovious and Peters (1985) reported an increased self-administration of morphine in adult rats subjected to methadone during gestation and lactation, suggesting an increased susceptibility to some opioids after perinatal opioid exposure.

A number of studies have explored anatomical, physiological, and biochemical correlates to opioid exposure in early life. Somatic growth retardation (e.g., McLaughlin and Zagon 1980; McLaughlin, Zagon, and White 1978; Slotkin, Lau, and Bartolome 1976; Slotkin, Seidler, and Whitmore 1980), smaller brain dimensions (Zagon and McLaughlin 1977b, 1978), and deficits in organ weights (McLaughlin and Zagon 1980; McLaughlin, Zagon, and White 1978) were noted. Physiological dysfunction with regard to thermoregulation (Thompson and Zagon 1981; Thompson, Zagon, and McLaughlin 1979), nociceptive thresholds (Zagon and McLaughlin 1980, 1981a, 1982b), and aberrant response to opioids and nonopioid drugs (Zagon and McLaughlin 1981a, 1984b) were also reported. Offspring exposed to opioids, especially those exposed to drugs only prenatally, often exhibit deficits in brain cell number, as well as alterations in brain RNA and protein concentrations and content (Zagon and McLaughlin 1978). Changes in polyamine metabolism (Slotkin, Lau, and Bartolome 1976; Slotkin et al. 1979) and in the ontogeny of catecholaminergic systems, as well as a retardation in the synaptic development of 5-hydroxytryptamine, dopamine, and epinephrine neurons in the nervous system, were recorded (McGinty and Ford 1980; Rech, Lomuscio, and Algeri 1980; Slotkin et al. 1982). Morphological investigations demonstrated that the timetable of neurogenesis is dependent on the schedule of drug exposure (Zagon and McLaughlin 1982b) and that prenatal exposure to opioids is related to reductions in cortical thickness and in the number of cells in the neocortex during the first two weeks of rat development, in addition to neuronal density changes in the hippocampus up to postnatal day 28 (Ford and Rhines 1979). It does not seem that either maternal undernutrition or inadequate nutrition of the offspring is the etiological basis for opioid-related problems (e.g., Ford and Rhines 1979; Zagon and McLaughlin 1982a; McLaughlin and Zagon 1980; Seidler, Whitmore, and Slotkin 1982; White, Zagon, and McLaughlin 1978; Raye, Dubin, and Blechner 1977; Smith, Hui, and Crofford 1977). Moreover, hypoxia due to opioid consumption does not seem to be responsible for the sequelae recorded (White and Zagon 1979), although this may be related to acute or short-term studies, since a hypoxic response can be noted after initial injections. Obviously, protocols calling for the drug to be administered for a period before pregnancy, thereby allowing adjustment to the respiratory depressive reactions of opioids, essentially remove this confounding variable. Other studies using paradigms of acute administration or those in which tolerance to respiratory depression has not been established may well be at risk of introducing hypoxia-related effects.

The mechanism(s) underlying opioid action on the fetus and neonate and its long-term implications in disturbing the well-being of children and young adults are of interest. Opioids seem to accumulate selectively in the brains and nervous tissues of fetal rats (Peters, Turnbow, and Buchenauer 1972) and preweaning rats (Shah and Donald 1979), presumably because of an increased permeability of the blood-brain barrier in developing organisms. Opioids exert a stereospecific effect on the growth of animals (Smith, Hui, and Crofford 1977; Crofford and Smith 1973), which suggests that opioid action is quite specific and involves opioid receptors. The effects of opioids can be blocked by the concomitant administration of opioid antagonists such as naloxone (Crofford and Smith 1973; Hui, Krikun, and Smith 1978; Meriney, Gray, and Pilar 1985), indicating again that opioid action resides at the level of the opioid receptor. Also, opioid receptors have been found in body and brain tissues of developing organisms (e.g., Gibson and Vernadakis 1982; Clendeninn, Petraitis, and Simon 1976), often appearing only or at the greatest concentration during the developmental period. Morphine administered to one-day-old rats inhibits [³H]thymidine incorporation into brain DNA in a naloxone-reversible manner, suggesting that exogenous opioids can depress cell proliferation (Kornblum, Loughlin, and Leslie 1987). Tempel et al. (1988) reported that chronic administration of morphine to pre- and postnatal rats produces a marked decrease in brain μ-opioid receptor density without a change in receptor affinity; no change in δ- or κ-receptors was observed. Interestingly, Tempel et al. observed a tolerance to the analgesic reactions of morphine in these animals, suggesting that exposure to some types of opioids may have notable functional influences with respect to receptor regulation. Alterations in receptor profiles by perinatal opioid exposure were also found by Vernadakis and Gibson (1985). These investigators reported that α-*l*-acetylmethadol (LAAM), a long-acting opioid that was considered a substitute for methadone, altered both the binding affinity and the binding capacity of [³H]etorphine binding, in both in vivo and in vitro preparations.

Tissue culture studies verified the stereospecific and naloxone-reversible effects of opioid agonists on cell growth and also revealed that tolerance can develop to these influences (e.g., Zagon and McLaughlin 1984c). Additionally, cells that are physically dependent on opioid agonists and are removed from drugs go through a withdrawal. A principle sign of cellular withdrawal is a diminution in mitotic activity. Vernadakis et al. (1982), using tissue cultures of neuronal and glial cells, reported that ornithine decarboxylase (ODC), thought to play a role in neural growth, was altered in methadone-subjected cultures. Sakellaridis, Mangoura, and Vernadakis (1986) showed that brain cell cultures derived from chick embryos may react in a neurotoxic fashion to morphine, but not to methadone. However, methadone may influence some cholinergic functions, since a decrease in choline acetyltransferase activity was noted in opioid-treated cultures. Finally, Choi and Visekul (1988) reported a selective attenuation of N-methyl-D-aspartate neurotoxicity of cortical neurons in opioid-subjected cultures.

CONCLUSIONS AND FUTURE DIRECTIONS

The laboratory information gained in experiments with opioids such as morphine, methadone, and heroin with regard to the clinical picture is worthy of discussion. A number of striking parallels between clinical and laboratory observations exist. These include passive dependence of the fetus on opioids, occurrence of the neonatal abstinence syndrome, high rate of morbidity and mortality of the neonate when not given supportive therapy for withdrawal, delays in sensorimotor development, retardation in somatic growth, smaller head circumferences in humans/smaller brain sizes in laboratory animals, delays in walking, problems in visual and/or auditory systems, neuropathology, diminished alertness, poor attention spans in early phases of development, hyperactivity in later phases of development, learning disabilities, and social maladjustments. However, in neither clinical nor laboratory studies are there pathognomonic features, characteristics that distinguish opioid effects from the manifestations exerted by other detrimental agents and/or conditions. Of course, the same end result does not imply the same means. Smaller head size may be due to a number of distinct situations such as cell death or diminishment of cell proliferation, with the final outcome showing a similarity.

The results of laboratory studies indicate that opioid agonists serve to inhibit growth at the level of the opioid receptor. It can be envisioned that maternal opioid consumption subjects the fetus and infant by way of the placenta and breast milk, respectively, to these substances and that these agonists alter developmental events until tolerance is established. The magnitude of these effects depends on such things as drug dosage and the length of time needed to establish tolerance in the developing organism. Withdrawal from opioid agonist exposure at birth or even during fetal life would force developing cells that have become tolerant to the opioid agonist to readjust to the absence of drug. This withdrawal reaction could result in delayed growth, and the extent of these delays would correlate with the magnitude of withdrawal. Obviously, opioid agonists given during withdrawal would serve to eliminate or minimize the withdrawal reaction and to circumvent the need of the tissues and cells to readjust to a new environment. This hypothesis fits very well with laboratory findings that prenatal exposure followed by postnatal withdrawal is often the most detrimental to developmental processes, whereas prenatal exposure along with the administration of opioids during the postnatal period usually causes the least damage. It is understandable that elimination or a substantial reduction of the opioid withdrawal syndrome probably attenuates many detrimental influences. Therefore, it is hardly any wonder that difficulties might exist in establishing firm evidence separating the effects of perinatal opioid exposure from those of other potentially damaging influences.

Finally, recent information suggests that endogenous opioids, just like their exogenous counterparts, also serve to inhibit growth and do so in a stereospecific and naloxone-reversible fashion (e.g., Zagon and McLaughlin 1983a, 1983b, 1984a, 1984b, 1984c, 1986a, 1986b, 1987, 1990a, 1990b, 1991; Zagon, Gibo, and McLaughlin 1990, 1991; Hauser, McLaughlin, and Zagon 1987, 1989; Hess and Zagon 1988; Isayama, McLaughlin, and Zagon 1991). With paradigms that involve opioid antagonists to block opioids from access to receptors for only a short time or permanently, or the utilization of endogenous opioids given directly to the organism or cell culture, endogenous opioid systems normally seem to regulate growth. A total blockade of endogenous opioid-opioid receptor interaction during the first three weeks of postnatal life in the rat, a time of remarkable growth, results in an acceleration in development. In particular, animals given opioid antagonists to block receptors completely for the entire period exhibit a greater number of neurons and glia engaged in postnatal proliferation, an increase in dendritic elaboration and synaptogenesis, and acceleration in the acquisition of physical and behavioral characteristics. These studies suggested that endogenous opioids must serve as inhibitory growth factors and that endogenous opioid systems must be quite active during this time. Continuing research revealed that the control of cell proliferation seems to be the target for opioid action; endogenous opioids depress DNA synthesis in proliferating neural cells destined to become neurons and glia. Extensive study showed that the pentapeptide, met[5]-enkephalin, is one of the most potent peptides in the regulation of cell proliferation. Concentrations as low as 100 µg of met[5]-enkephalin per kg result in a marked reduction in DNA synthesis of replicating brain cells; administration of naloxone blocked the effects of met[5]-enkephalin. Opioids selective for other receptors such as mu, delta, kappa, epsilon, and sigma did not alter DNA synthesis. These findings also indicate that proenkephalin A, the parent of met[5]-enkephalin, must be the family of opioid peptides involved in growth. With the use of radiolabeled met[5]-

enkephalin and homogenates of developing cerebellum, recent studies demonstrated specific and saturable binding with high affinity. The binding affinity (K_d) of radiolabeled met[5]-enkephalin to developing cerebellar homogenates was 2.2 nM, and the binding capacity (B_{max}) was 22.3 fmol/mg protein. Competitive inhibition profiles of met[5]-enkephalin to cerebellar preparations were different from those of other opioid ligands, and the location of met[5]-enkephalin binding was nuclear rather than cytoplasmic/membranous (where other opioid binding sites are located). This receptor has been termed zeta (ζ), in reference to its association with the proliferation of life (Greek *zoe*). It seems that the developing human brain also contains the ζ receptor (Zagon, Gibo, and McLaughlin 1990).

Precisely how the exogenous opioids such as heroin and methadone interact with endogenous opioid control of growth is only beginning to be explored. Because endogenous opioids serve a number of other roles (e.g., neurotransmission) in the organism, a variety of other alterations also might be displayed. For example, the normal ontogeny of certain neurotransmitters might be delayed or diminished because of the reaction to exogenously administered opioids. In essence, exogenous opioids would be mistaken in the regulatory pathways, leading to alterations in the biological profile of the organism. The role of endogenous opioids as normal, trophic factors in growth is extremely exciting and is being actively pursued. In combination with studies on opioid abuse during the perinatal period, these studies may well lead to new insights into the mechanisms of the detrimental influence of opioids.

REFERENCES

Aylward, G. P. 1982. Methadone outcome studies: Is it more than the methadone? *J Pediatr* 101:214–15.

Blum, R. H. 1969. A history of opium. In *Society and Drugs: I. Social and Cultural Observations*, ed. R. H. Blum et al., 45–58. San Francisco: Jossey-Bass.

Buchenauer, C., Turnbow, M., and Peters, M. A. 1974. Effect of chronic methadone administration on pregnant rats and their offspring. *J Pharmacol Exp Ther* 189:66–71.

Bureau, A. 1895. Accouchement d'une morphinomane: Prévue chimique du passage de la morphine à travers le placenta. Réflexions. *Bull Mem Soc Obstet Gynecol* 356–362.

Carr, J. N. 1975. Drug patterns among drug-addicted mothers:

Incidence, variance in use, and effects on children. *Pediatr Ann* 4:408–17.

Chandler, J. M., Robie, P., Schoolar, J., and Desmond, M. M. 1975. The effects of methadone on maternal-fetal interactions in the rat. *J Pharmacol Exp Ther* 192:549–54.

Choi, D. W., and Viseskul, V. 1988. Opioids and non-opioid enantiomers selectively attenuate N-methyl-D-aspartate neurotoxicity on cortical neurons. *Eur J Pharmacol* 155:27–35.

Clendeninn, N. J., Petraitis, M., and Simon, E. J. 1976. Ontological development of opiate receptors in rodent brain. *Brain Res* 118:157–60.

Crofford, M., and Smith, A. A. 1973. Growth retardation in young mice treated with *dl*-methadone. *Science* 181:947–49.

Davis, W. M., and Lin, C. H. 1972. Prenatal morphine effects on survival and behavior of rat offspring. *Res Commun Chem Pathol Pharmacol* 3:205–14.

Dole, V. P., and Nyswander, M. A. 1965. Medical treatment for diacetyl-morphine (heroin) addiction. *JAMA* 193:646–50.

Earle, F. B. 1888. Maternal opium habit and infant mortality. *M Standard (Chicago)* 3:2.

Ford, D., and Rhines, R. 1979. Prenatal exposure to methadone HCl in relationship to body and brain growth in the rat. *Acta Neurol Scand* 59:248–62.

Freeman, P. R. 1980. Methadone exposure in utero: Effects on open-field activity in weanling rats. *Int J Neurosci* 11:295–300.

Fujinaga, M., and Mazze, R. I. 1988. Teratogenic and postnatal developmental studies of morphine in Sprague-Dawley rats. *Teratology* 38:401–10.

Geber, W. F., and Schramm, L. C. 1975. Congenital malformations of the central nervous system produced by narcotic analgesics in the hamster. *Am J Obstet Gynecol* 123:705–13.

Gibson, D. A., and Vernadakis, A. 1982. [^{3}H]Etorphine binding in early chick embryos: Brain and body tissue. *Brain Res* 4:23–29.

Goodfriend, M. J., Shey, I. A., and Klein, M. D. 1956. The effects of maternal narcotic addiction on the newborn. *Am J Obstet Gynecol* 71:29–36.

Graham-Mulhall, S. 1981. *Opium the Demon Flower* (1926). New York: Arno Press.

Grove, L. V., Etkin, M. K., and Rosencrans, J. A. 1979. Behavioral effects of fetal and neonatal exposure to methadone in the rat. *Neurobehav Toxicol* 1:87–95.

Hauser, K. F., McLaughlin, P. J., and Zagon, I. S. 1987. Endogenous opioids regulate dendritic growth and spine formation in developing rat brain. *Brain Res* 416:157–61.

――――. 1989. Endogenous opioid systems and the regulation of dendritic growth and spine formation. *J Comp Neurol* 281:13–22.

Hess, G. D., and Zagon, I. S. 1988. Endogenous opioid systems and neural development: Ultrastructural studies in the cerebellar cortex of infant and weanling rats. *Brain Res Bull* 20:473–78.

Householder, J., Hatcher, R., Burns, W., and Chasnoff, I. 1982. Infants born to narcotic-addicted mothers. *Psychol Bull* 92:453–68.

Hovious, J. R., and Peters, M. A. 1985. Opiate self-administration in adult offspring of methadone-treated female rats. *Pharmacol Biochem Behav* 22:949–53.

Hui, F. W., Krikun, E., and Smith, A. A. 1978. Inhibition by *d,l*-methadone of RNA and protein synthesis in neonatal mice: Antagonism by naloxone or naltrexone. *Eur J Pharmacol* 49:87–93.

Isayama, T., McLaughlin, P. J., and Zagon, I. S. 1991. Endogenous opioids regulate cell proliferation in the retina of developing rat. *Brain Res* 544:79–85.

Jurand, A. 1973. Teratogenic activity of methadone hydrochloride in mouse and chick embryos. *J Embryol Exp Morphol* 30:449–58.

――――. 1980. Malformations of the central nervous system induced by neurotropic drugs in mouse embryos. *Dev Growth Diff* 22:61–78.

――――. 1985. The interference of naloxone hydrochloride in the teratogenic activity of opiates. *Teratology* 31:235–40.

Kornblum, H. I., Loughlin, S. E., and Leslie, F. M. 1987. Effects of morphine on DNA synthesis in neonatal rat brain. *Dev Brain Res* 31:45–52.

Laase, C. F. J. 1919. Narcotic drug addiction in the newborn: Report of a case. *Am J Med* 25:283–86.

Langstein, L. 1930. Uber das schicksal von morphiumsuchtigen frauen gebornener sauglinge. *Med Klin* 26:500–501.

Lichenstein, P. M. 1915. Infant drug addiction. *NY Med J* 15:905.

Martin, E. 1893. *L'opium, ses abus, mangeurs et fumeurs d'opium morphinomanes*. Paris.

McGinty, J. F., and Ford, D. H. 1980. Effects of prenatal methadone on rat brain catecholamines. *Dev Neurosci* 3:224–34.

McLaughlin, P. J., and Zagon, I. S. 1980. Body and organ development of young rats maternally exposed to methadone. *Biol Neonate* 38:185–96.

McLaughlin, P. J., Zagon, I. S., and White, W. J. 1978. Perinatal methadone exposure in rats: Effects on body and organ development. *Biol Neonate* 34:48–54.

Menninger-Lerchenthal, E. 1934. Die morphinkrankheit der neugeboren morphinstinscher mutter. *Monatsschr Kinderheilkd* 60:182–83.

Meriney, S. D., Gray, D. B., and Pilar, G. 1985. Morphine-induced delay of normal cell death in the avian ciliary ganglion. *Science* 228:1451–53.

Middaugh, L. D., and Simpson, L. W. 1980. Prenatal maternal methadone effects on pregnant C57BL/6 mice and their offspring. *Neurobehav Toxicol* 2:307–13.

Musto, D. F. 1973. *The American Disease.* New Haven: Yale University Press.

Perlstein, M. A. 1947. Congenital morphinism: A rare cause of convulsions in the newborn. *JAMA* 135:633.

Peters, M. A. 1978. A comparative study on the behavioral response of offspring of female rats chronically treated with methadone and morphine. *Proc West Pharmacol Soc* 21:411–18.

Peters, M. A., Turnbow, M., and Buchenauer, D. 1972. The distribution of methadone in the nonpregnant, pregnant, and fetal rat after acute methadone treatment. *J Pharmacol Exp Ther* 181:273–78.

Petty, G. E. 1912. Congenital morphinism with report of cases: General treatment of morphinism. *Memphis M Monthly* 32:37–63.

———. 1913. *Narcotic Drug Diseases and Allied Ailments.* Memphis, Tenn.: J. A. Davis.

Raye, J. R., Dubin, J. W., and Blechner, J. N. 1977. Fetal growth retardation following maternal morphine administration: Nutrition or drug effects. *Biol Neonate* 32:222–28.

Rech, R. H., Lomuscio, G., and Algeri, S. 1980. Methadone exposure in utero: Effects on brain biogenic amines and behavior. *Neurobehav Toxicol* 2:75–78.

Sainsbury, H. 1909. *Drugs and the Drug Habit.* London: Methuen Co.

Sakellaridis, N., Mangoura, D., and Vernadakis, A. 1986. Effects of opiates on the growth of neuron-enriched cultures from chick embryonic brain. *Int J Dev Neurosci* 4:293–302.

Seidler, F. J., Whitmore, W. L., and Slotkin, T. A. 1982. Delays in growth and biochemical development of rat brain caused by maternal methadone administration: Are the alterations in synaptogenesis and cellular maturation independent of reduced maternal food intake? *Dev Neurosci* 5:13–18.

Shah, N. S., and Donald, A. G. 1979. Pharmacological effects and metabolic fate of levo-methadone during post-natal development in rat. *J Pharmacol Exp Ther* 208:491–97.

Slotkin, T. A., Lau, C., and Bartolome, M. 1976. Effects of neonatal or maternal methadone administration on ornithine decarboxylase activity in brain and heart of developing rats. *J Pharmacol Exp Ther* 199: 141–48.

Slotkin, T. A., Seidler, F. J., and Whitmore, W. L. 1980. Effects of maternal methadone administration on ornithine decarboxylase in brain and heart of the offspring: Relationships of enzyme activity to dose and to growth impairment in the rat. *Life Sci* 26:861–67.

Slotkin, T. A., Weigle, S. J., Whitmore, W. L., and Seidler, F. J. 1982. Maternal methadone administration: Deficient in development of alpha-noradrenergic responses in developing rat brain as assessed by norepinephrine stimulation of ^{33}Pi incorporation into phospholipids in vivo. *Biochem Pharmacol* 31:1899–1902.

Slotkin, T. A., Whitmore, W. L., Salvaggio, M., and Seidler, F. J. 1979. Perinatal methadone addiction affects brain synaptic development of biogenic amine systems in the rat. *Life Sci* 24:1223–30.

Smith, A. A., Hui, F. W., and Crofford, M. J. 1977. Inhibition of growth in young mice treated with *d,l*-methadone. *Eur J Pharmacol* 43:307–14.

Sobrian, S. K. 1977. Prenatal morphine administration alters behavioral development in the rat. *Pharmacol Biochem Behav* 7:285–88.

Sonderegger, T., and Zimmerman, E. 1976. Persistent effects of neonatal addiction in the rat. In *Tissue Responses to Addictive Drugs*, ed. D. H. Ford and D. H. Clouet, 589–609. New York: Spectrum Publications.

Strauss, M. E., Lessen-Firestone, J. K., Chavez, C. J., and Stryker, J. C. 1979. Children of methadone-treated women at five years of age. *Pharmacol Biochem Behav* 2(suppl):3–6.

Tempel, A., Habas, J. E., Paredes, W., and Barr, G. A. 1988. Morphine-induced down-regulation of μ-opioid receptors in neonatal rat brain. *Dev Brain Res* 41:129–33.

Terry, C. E., and Pellens, M. 1970. *The Opium Problem* (1928), 312–48. Montclair, N.J.: Patterson Smith.

Thompson, C. I., and Zagon, I. S. 1981. Long-term thermoregulatory changes following perinatal methadone exposure in rats. *Pharmacol Biochem Behav* 14:653–59.

———. 1982. Decreased dominance in adult rats perinatally exposed to methadone. Paper presented to the Eastern Psychological Association, Baltimore, Md.

Thompson, C. I., Zagon, I. S., and McLaughlin, P. J. 1979. Impaired thermal regulation in juvenile rats following perinatal methadone exposure. *Pharmacol Biochem Behav* 10:551–56.

Vernadakis, A., Estin, C., Gibson, D. A., and Amott, S. 1982. Effects of methadone on ornithine decarboxylase and cyclic nucleotide phosphohydrolase in neuronal and glial cultures. *J Neurosci Res* 7:111–17.

Vernadakis, A., and Gibson, A. 1985. Neurotoxicity of opiates during brain development: In vivo and in vitro studies. In *Prevention of Physical and Mental Congenital Defects: Part C. Basic Medical Science Education and Future Strategies. Prog Clin Biol Res* 163:245–53.

White, W. J., and Zagon, I. S. 1979. Acute and chronic methadone exposure in adult rats: Studies on arterial blood gas concentrations and pH. *J Pharmacol Exp Ther* 209:451–55.

White, W. J., Zagon, I. S., and McLaughlin, P. J. 1978. Effects of chronic methadone treatment on maternal body weight and food and water consumption in rats. *Pharmacology* 17:227–32.

Wilson, G. S., Desmond, M. M., and Wait, R. B. 1981. Follow-up of methadone-treated and untreated narcotic-dependent women and their infants: Health, developmental, and social implications. *J Pediatr* 98:716–22.

Zagon, I. S. 1983. Behavioral effects of prenatal exposure to opiates. In *Drugs and Hormones in Brain Development*, ed. M. Schlumpf and W. Lichstensteiger. *Monogr Neural Sci* 9:159–68.

———. 1985. Opioids and development: New lessons from old problems. *NIDA Res Monogr* 60:58–77.

Zagon, I. S., Gibo, D. M., and McLaughlin, P. J. 1990. Adult and developing human cerebella exhibit different profiles of opioid binding sites. *Brain Res* 523:62–68.

———. 1991. Zeta (ζ), a growth-related opioid receptor in the developing rat cerebellum: Identification and characterization. *Brain Res.* 551:28–35.

Zagon, I. S., and McLaughlin, P. J. 1977a. The effect of chronic maternal methadone exposure on perinatal development. *Biol Neonate* 31:271–82.

———. 1977b. The effects of different schedules of methadone treatment on rat brain development. *Exp Neurol* 56:538–52.

———. 1977c. The effect of chronic morphine administration on pregnant rats and their offspring. *Pharmacology* 15:302–10.

———. 1977d. Morphine and brain growth retardation in the rat. *Pharmacology* 15:276–82.

———. 1978. Perinatal methadone exposure and brain development: A biochemical study. *J Neurochem* 31:49–54.

———. 1980. Protracted analgesia in young and adult rats maternally exposed to methadone. *Experientia* 36:3299–3330.

————. 1981a. Enhanced sensitivity to methadone in adult rats perinatally exposed to methadone. *Life Sci* 29:1137–42.

————. 1981b. Withdrawal-like symptoms in young and adult rats maternally exposed to methadone. *Pharmacol Biochem Behav* 15:887–94.

————. 1982a. Comparative effects of postnatal undernutrition and methadone exposure on protein and nucleic acid contents of the brain and cerebellum in rats. *Dev Neurosci* 5:385–93.

————. 1982b. Neuronal cell deficits following maternal exposure to methadone in rats. *Experientia* 38:1214–16.

————. 1983a. Increased brain size and cellular content in infant rats treated with an opiate antagonist. *Science* 221:1179–80.

————. 1983b. Naltrexone modulated growth in infant rats. *Life Sci* 33:2449–54.

————. 1984a. The neurobehavioral sequelae of perinatal opioid addiction: An overview. In *Neurobehavioral Teratology*, ed. J. Yanai, 197–234. Amsterdam: Elsevier/North Holland.

————. 1984b. Prenatal exposure of rats to methadone alters sensitivity to drugs in adulthood. *Neurobehav Toxicol Teratol* 6:319–24.

————. 1984c. Opiates alter tumor cell growth and differentiation in vitro. *NIDA Res Monogr* 49:344–51.

————. 1986a. Opioid antagonist (naltrexone) modulation of cerebellar development. *J Neurosci* 6:1424–32.

————. 1986b. Opioid-antagonist-induced modulation of cerebral and hippocampal development: Historical and morphometric studies. *Dev Brain Res* 28:233–46.

————. 1987. Endogenous opioid systems regulate cell proliferation in the developing rat brain. *Brain Res* 412:68–72.

————. 1990a. Drugs of abuse and the fetus and neonate: Considerations in the testing and evaluation of animals. In *Modern Methods in Pharmacology: Testing and Evaluation of Drugs of Abuse*, ed. M. Adler, and A. Cowan, 241–54. New York: A. R. Liss.

————. 1990b. Ultrastructural localization of enkephalin-like immunoreactivity in developing rat cerebellum. *Neuroscience* 34:479–89.

————. 1991. Identification of opioid peptides related to cell proliferation in the developing nervous system. *Brain Res* 542:318–23.

Zagon, I. S., McLaughlin, P. J., and Thompson, C. I. 1979a. Development of motor activity in young rats following perinatal methadone exposure. *Pharmacol Biochem Behav* 10:743–49.

————. 1979b. Learning ability in adult female rats perinatally exposed to methadone. *Pharmacol Biochem Behav* 10:889–94.

Zagon, I. S., McLaughlin, P. J., Weaver, D. J., and Zagon, E. 1982. Opiates, endorphins, and the developing organism: A comprehensive bibliography. *Neurosci Biobehav Rev* 6:439–79.

Zagon, I. S., McLaughlin, P. J., and Zagon, E. 1984. Opiates, endorphins, and the developing organism: A comprehensive bibliography, 1982–1983. *Neurosci Biobehav Rev* 8:387–403.

Zagon, I. S., Zagon, E., and McLaughlin, P. J. 1989. Opioids and the developing organism: A comprehensive bibliography, 1984–1988. *Neurosci Biobehav Rev*, 13:207–235.

9

Heroin Use during Pregnancy: Clinical Studies of Long-term Effects

Geraldine S. Wilson, M.D.

IN THE preceding chapter, Zagon and McLaughlin chronicled the history of the gradual expansion of knowledge concerning the use of opioids during pregnancy and reviewed mechanisms by which opioids might affect the developing fetus. Issues complicating the pregnancy of an opiate-dependent woman are reviewed in chapter 10. General areas of concern include increased obstetrical and perinatal morbidity, compromised fetal growth, and neonatal narcotic withdrawal (abstinence syndrome). Clinical reports of the effects of opioids on the developing fetus in the late 1950s and early 1960s emphasized the recognition and management of the newborn narcotic withdrawal syndrome (Goodfriend, Shey, and Klein 1956; Hill and Desmond 1963). In the late 1960s and early 1970s, knowledge of the newborn abstinence syndrome was broadened through neurophysiological studies (Behrendt and Green 1972; Glass, Rajegowda, and Floyd 1972; Schulman 1969). Despite a rich literature dealing with the fetal and neonatal effects of addiction, it was not until the early 1970s that observations were extended beyond the newborn period (Desmond and Wilson 1975; Wilson, Desmond, and Verniaud 1973). They suggested a continuation of neurobehavioral disruption in exposed infants. Subsequently, in the laboratory, investigators reported differences in learning and behavior of gestationally opiate-exposed rats (Zagon et al. 1982). Both clinical and laboratory data suggested the need for long-term studies of opiate-exposed infants to explore the possibility that heroin might have behavioral teratogenic effects.

As described by Kaltenbach and Finnegan (1984), follow-up studies have flourished since the popularization of methadone maintenance during pregnancy. Women's participation in treatment programs has facilitated sustained investigator contact with the mother-child dyad during both pregnancy and the postpartum period. Few studies have included children of untreated addicts, however, and the longitudinal study of heroin-exposed children has been limited indeed.

Preliminary studies suggested the hypothesis that heroin-exposed children would show a specific constellation of behavioral findings which occur with low frequency in the normal population and that the behaviors would be independent of later environmental experiences. The clinical investigations reviewed in this chapter address this hypothesis.

METHODOLOGICAL ISSUES

Clinical studies of the long-term effects of chronic exposure to narcotics during the period of fetal development are fraught with methodological problems (Aylward 1982). Associations between maternal opiate dependence and such effects as intrauterine growth retardation, the neonatal abstinence syndrome, and neurobehavioral sequelae have been established, but the underlying pathophysiology has remained elusive because of the sheer multitude of additional factors impinging upon the pregnancy of the addicted mother, the developing fetus, the infant during the perinatal period, and the developing toddler and child (Householder et al. 1982; Lawson and Wilson 1980).

Heroin addicts by definition frustrate the investigator who is committed to research design. The sine qua non of participation in a longitudinal study is long-term commitment, an unrealistic expectation of a drug-dependent personality. Furthermore, the documentation of drug use during pregnancy by serial urine screening or other toxicological measures is hindered by the absence or irregularity of prenatal care in untreated narcotic-dependent women. An accurate history of drug use is limited by the unreliability and distortion of long-term memory as well as by the impurity of drugs and lack of dosage standards. Sociodemographic data that may have a bearing on the child's neurodevelopmental function (i.e., history of educational attainment, occupation, or neurodevelopmental disability in the extended family) are often unavailable, since contact with the natural mother may be limited and her ability to cooperate may be impaired by the stress of perinatal events. The relevant paternal history is often unknown even to the mother.

The "background noise" introduced by these potentially confounding variables affecting the pregnancy and the fetus is compounded by perinatal morbidity and increases exponentially with the child's advancing age and the increasing influence of environmental factors. For those end points that cannot be measured until preschool or school age (i.e., attentional deficit disorder or language learning disability), the number and variety of intervening confounding variables may overwhelm prenatal events. To demonstrate behavioral teratogenesis, the observed effect must be of limited occurrence in the "normal" population, must be of adequate clinical scope to be identifiable, and must follow a recognizable pattern.

DESCRIPTIVE STUDIES

In our first published study, we reviewed the course of 30 infants who were born to women dependent on heroin during gestation, evaluated at birth, and followed through ages 3–34 months (Wilson, Desmond, and Verniaud 1973). Sixty percent of these babies required pharmacological treatment for moderate to severe withdrawal symptoms. An exacerbation of behavioral symptoms (restlessness, agitation, tremors, hyperphagia, brief sleep periods) after hospital discharge, designated "subacute withdrawal" (Desmond and Wilson 1975), persisted until 4 to 6 months of age. On follow-up the most notable difference between drug-exposed and other high-risk babies continued to be behavioral. Half of the 13 children examined at 1 year or older demonstrated high activity levels, sleep disturbances, tantrums, and low frustration tolerance. Developmental function as measured by the Gesell Developmental Schedules was within the normal range, although adaptive functioning tended to be low during the first 4 or 5 months. Neurological abnormality was seen in 5 patients.

Olofsson et al. (1983) reported the outcome at one to ten years of 72 children exposed in utero to a variety of drugs (heroin, methadone, or tranquilizers). They reported impaired psychomotor development in 21% of the sample and behavioral abnormalities (lack of concentration, hyperactivity, aggressiveness, and lack of social inhibition) in 50%. Behavioral findings were based on interviews with parents and with school and health-care personnel.

CROSS-SECTIONAL STUDY OF PRESCHOOL CHILDREN AND CONTROLS

The first comparison study of neurodevelopmental and behavioral function in 22 heroin-exposed children was cross-sectional and included three control groups evaluated at ages ranging from three to six years (Wilson et al. 1979). Comparison groups included children at environmental risk (i.e., raised by drug-dependent parent but not exposed in utero), children with other non-drug-related perinatal risk factors, and children of similar sociodemographic background without specific risk factors. Foster or adoptive families raised one half of the heroin-exposed infants from infancy, but evaluation of the primary caregiver revealed no intergroup differences in parental education and occupation, rating of the home environment, or parental attitudes.

Heroin-exposed children were rated by parents as having more adjustment problems than controls, differing on the following variables: impulsiveness, uncontrollable temper, self-confidence, aggressiveness, and peer relations. Examiners subjectively rated the heroin-exposed group as more active than controls, but ratings of cooperation and attention were comparable across all four groups. Objective measures of activity level in structured test situations did not differentiate among the groups.

Neurologically, heroin-exposed children differed only on a test of motor coordination. On neuropsychological testing, heroin-exposed children performed less well than the combined controls on tasks involving perception, organization, and short-term memory. Group means on standardized tests fell within the normal range for all four groups.

STUDIES OF CHILDREN RAISED BY ADDICTED PARENTS

Several studies reported disturbed function in children of heroin addicts regardless of gestational exposure to drugs. In 1973 Nichtern reviewed the experience of a New York foster-care agency with 95 children whose parent or parents were heroin dependent; children exposed to heroin in utero were not differentiated from those born to drug-free mothers and addicted fathers (Nichtern 1973). He reported a history of early problems with physiological patterning, behavioral concerns, developmental lags, and learning problems. As a psychiatrist, he was impressed with the subjects' difficulties in organizing and integrating impulses, as well as their impaired capacity for human relatedness. Sowder and Burt (1980) focused on 34 children three to seven years old raised by addicted parent(s); 44% reported that their children were exposed to heroin and/or other drugs gestationally. In comparison to neighborhood controls from drug-free households, children of addicts performed significantly less well on the Bender-Gestalt Test of Visual Motor Function and on two measures used to assess cognition (Stanford-Binet Vocabulary Sub-test and Draw-a-Person IQ Test). Groups did not differ in performance on the Peabody Picture Vocabulary Test. On the basis of cumulative performance on the four tests administered, 42% of the children of addicts and 20% of the comparison group were considered at high risk for early school problems and poor socioemotional development. When the children of addicts were dichotomized into "at-risk" and "average/superior" groups, the at-risk group tended to be of lower birth weight, to have a history of maternal drug exposure during pregnancy, and to have unemployed families with low income. However, the differences were not statistically significant in this small sample.

Herjanic et al. (1979) studied 32 children aged 6–17 years raised in the household of their heroin-addicted father and 37 comparison children. By history, children were not exposed to opiates in utero. Forty-four percent of the children of addicts were slow in mental development on the basis of screening tests and school performance, as compared to 10% of controls. Reports of behavioral concerns at home or school were comparable during the early elementary years, but by age 12 conduct disorders and behavioral problems at school were much more common in children of addicts. Both of these studies (Herjanic et al. 1979; Sowder and Burt 1980) suggested that the family dysfunction and environmental factors related to addiction may adversely influence children's cognitive and emotional function.

CONTROLLED LONGITUDINAL STUDY OF PRESCHOOL CHILDREN

The most comprehensive longitudinal study of heroin-exposed children was designed to compare their health, neurodevelopmental course, and behavior to that of infants born to methadone-treated women and to drug-free controls. A complete description of subjects, procedure, and findings during the first year of life has been published (Wilson, Desmond, and Wait 1981).

The study enrolled women known to be dependent upon heroin or methadone upon entry into Houston's public maternity hospital for prenatal care. Comprehensive obstetrical care was provided, and heroin-dependent women were encouraged to enroll in methadone treatment programs.

The group of drug-dependent women who continued to abuse heroin primarily are designated the "untreated heroin group." Women were categorized as methadone maintained if they received methadone treatment for at least two consecutive months during pregnancy; methadone maintenance did not preclude the use of other drugs. The comparison drug-free group was selected from the public maternity service, matching for age, race, marital status, and socioeconomic status. We attempted to match for another important variable, gestational timing at the beginning of prenatal care, but too few drug-free women without prenatal care agreed to participate in the study. Maternal measures included duration of prenatal care, maternal weight gain during pregnancy, prenatal risk score, and a narcotic score derived from reported use of methadone, heroin, and other psychoactive drugs during each trimester of pregnancy.

The longitudinal study included medical and neurodevelopmental assessments of infants and interviews of parents for social and behavioral information at 6 weeks and at 3-month intervals during the first year, at 18 months, at 2 years, and annually thereafter in a pediatric out-patient unit. To enhance compliance, a research team composed of a developmental pediatrician, a nurse, and a social worker coordinated all aspects of medical care and provided social services (Wilson, Desmond, and Wait 1981).

This study was undertaken with the expectation that methadone maintenance during pregnancy would eliminate many of the undesirable variables associated with the life-style of the untreated heroin addict. By comparing the infants and children of treated and untreated heroin-dependent women, we hoped to separate the effects of narcotic exposure from those of confounding variables such as poor nutrition, untreated infection, and continuing illegal activities.

We did, indeed, find differences between the methadone-maintained and untreated addict groups. A significantly greater number of white and married women in the methadone-treated group (versus single black untreated women) suggests that there may have been a selection bias in the subgroup of addicts who chose to enter methadone treatment (Wilson, Desmond, and Wait 1981). We were unable to document our impression that methadone-treated women came from better-educated and more stable families than untreated addicts because our limited contact with women without prenatal care (usually untreated addicts) precluded the in-depth interviews needed to obtain data about family background.

Benefits associated with methadone maintenance included more regular prenatal care and greater involvement in the child's care after hospital discharge. Methadone-maintained women showed no advantage in terms of nutritional status, obstetrical risk factors, or preterm delivery. Ninety-two percent reported polydrug use. Alcohol use and smoking were more prevalent among the methadone-treated than the untreated addicts.

Methadone maintenance was not associated with a reduction of newborn morbidity; the incidence of undergrowth for gestational age, infection, and abstinence syndrome was similar for treated and untreated groups, with a more prolonged withdrawal in infants of methadone-treated women (Wilson, Desmond, and Wait 1981).

Subjects

Ninety-three of the original sample (73%) were evaluated between the ages of three and six years. Subjects included 26 heroin-exposed, 26 methadone-treated, and 41 comparison children. One child had died (methadone group), 18 subjects had moved from the area, and 15 subjects could not be located. Those lost to study did not differ from the group studied on the following measures: socioeconomic status, race, sex, gestational age, birth measurements, need for pharmacological treatment of withdrawal symptoms, neurological status, or developmental performance at age nine months. Compliant children were more apt to be living with substitute parents at nine months than were those lost to study (30% versus 7%, $p < .01$).

Methods

Data for this report are based upon the evaluation of each subject at three to six years of age (mean, 4.2 ± 0.8 years) by a pediatrician and a psychologist unaware of the subject's background or drug classification. Evaluation included physical and neurological examination, using the procedure of Touwen and Prechtl for assessment of neuromaturational function in preschool children (Touwen and Prechtl 1970).

The McCarthy Scales of Children's Abilities (1972) were administered by the psychologist.

Behavior was rated by the psychologist and the pediatrician independently, using an adaptation of the Behavior Record of the Bayley Scales of Infant Development (Bayley 1969). Ratings of activity level and attention were combined, with higher scores indicating high activity level and inattention.

Families were interviewed by the social worker to obtain information regarding the child's current environment, the occupation and education of the parent or the parent substitute, and the extent of day care and preschool experience. In addition, the stability of the child's family structure was rated on a nine-point scale including such items as the consistency of parental figures, the reliability of family income, and involvement in criminal activities. The Caldwell Home Inventory (HOME) (Caldwell 1978), reporting characteristics of parenting and the home environment, was completed by the team social worker.

Data Analysis

For continuous variables the comparability of the three groups was tested initially by one-way analysis of variance. A multiple-comparison approach (Bonferroni modification of the t test) was then used to compare two groups at a time. Chi-square analysis was utilized to analyze categorical variables. For those variables with more than two categories (i.e., race), an overall χ^2 was followed by further $2 \times 2 \chi^2$ if the initial χ^2 indicated significance.

Correlation analyses were used initially to determine relationships of outcome measures to variables possibly affecting developmental and neurobehavioral outcome. These variables included race, maternal nutritional status, prenatal care score, pregnancy and intrapartum risk scores, smoking, narcotic score, education and occupation of the natural parents, Apgar scores, the infant's sex, birth measurements, duration of withdrawal treatment, education of the primary caretaker, HOME score, adequacy of the child's diet, day care or preschool attendance, and stability of the family, as well as measures of developmental, neurological, and behavioral outcome. Variables found to be associated with outcome ($r > .25$) were included in a multiple regression analysis to assess their relative effect on outcome. Separate analyses were performed for each outcome variable. For dichotomous outcome variables, multiple logistic regression analysis was utilized (Dixon 1981).

Results

Socioenvironmental Findings

At preschool evaluation, 80% of the heroin-exposed children, 38% of the methadone-exposed group, and 5% of the comparison group were not living with their biological parent(s). Ten children (eight heroin exposed, two methadone exposed) were in adoptive or court-appointed foster homes; the remainder lived with extended family or friends, although the natural mother retained legal custody.

The educational and occupational classification of the head of the household (parent or parent substitute) was similar for all three groups. The HOME score did not differentiate between groups (methadone, 34.8 ± 8.2; heroin, 34.1 ± 8.2; comparison, 32.6 ± 7.9). The range of HOME scores was similar for children living with natural parents (15–44) and for those living with extended family or friends (20–44) but tended to be higher for those in adoptive homes (27–44). Family stability did not differ significantly among groups (methadone, 6.4 ± 2.2; heroin, 7.2 ± 1.8; comparison, 7.3 ± 1.4). The adoptive homes were uniformly stable (range, 7–9), but stability scores for both natural and extended families were highly variable, ranging from 2 to 9. Day care was utilized by 27% of the methadone group, 32% of the heroin group, and 15% of controls. Special preschool educational services had been recommended for five methadone-treated subjects (19%), ten heroin-exposed subjects (38%), and six controls (15%).

Neurological Findings

Twelve methadone-treated subjects (46%), 11 heroin-exposed subjects (42%), and 18 controls (44%) had one or more abnormalities on neurological examination (table 9.1). Of the subjects in each group, 30–40% had motor incoordination, defined as immature motor patterns, weakness in gross or fine motor coordination, or weak visual-motor skills. Motor incoordination related directly to the severity of neonatal withdrawal ($r = .28$) and to the maternal nutritional state during pregnancy ($r = .26$). Multiple logistic regression confirmed this significant association between motor incoordination and the severity of newborn

Table 9-1. Neurobehavioral Findings in Preschool Children of Drug-dependent Women and Controls

Finding	Children of Untreated Heroin-dependent Women (n = 26)		Children of Methadone-treated Women (n = 26)		Comparison Group (n = 41)	
	No.	%	No.	%	No.	%
Neurological finding						
Motor incoordination	8	(31)	11	(42)	13	(32)
Articulation disorder	4	(15)	4	(15)	2	(5)
Tremor/dysmetria	3	(12)	1	(4)	2	(5)
Hydrocephalus, CP, MR[a]	1	(4)	0		0	
Strabismus	0		1	(4)	0	
Hearing impairment	0		0		1	(4)
Activity-attention						
ADHD[b]	2	(8)	6	(23)	6	(15)
Rating: mean ± SD	1.16	± 1.03	1.27	± 1.31	0.85	± 1.35

[a] CP, cerebral palsy; MR, mental retardation.
[b] ADHD, attention deficit hyperactivity disorder.

withdrawal ($p < .05$). Calculation of an odds ratio indicated that, after adjustment for possible confounding variables, the likelihood of motor incoordination was 2.9 times greater in children who were treated for newborn narcotic withdrawal than it was in those who either were asymptomatic or had mild withdrawal symptoms and required no medication.

Behavioral Findings

Behavioral patterns observed during evaluation did not differentiate between drug-exposed children and the comparison group. Fearfulness and an inability to establish rapport were seen in four compari-

Table 9.2. Developmental Performance in Preschool Children of
Drug-dependent Women and Controls

McCarthy Scale	Children of Untreated Heroin-dependent Women ($n = 26$)	Children of Methadone-treated Women ($n = 26$)	Comparison Group ($n = 41$)
General cognitive index	85.3 ± 15.7	90.4 ± 13.0	89.4 ± 10.8
Verbal	44.2 ± 9.5	44.0 ± 7.9	44.3 ± 8.6
Perceptual-performance	39.0 ± 10.3	42.6 ± 9.4	42.6 ± 8.5
Quantitative	44.3 ± 8.8	46.2 ± 8.9	44.3 ± 9.2
Memory	45.5 ± 11.7	44.5 ± 7.4	45.2 ± 7.9
Motor	40.5 ± 8.1	41.6 ± 10.0	42.1 ± 7.2

Note: Values are means ± SD.

son children and one of the heroin-exposed group. Oppositional or
negative behavior was reported in two controls and in one methadone-
exposed child. Disturbances in attention and activity level were judged
to be clinically significant in six controls, six methadone-exposed subjects, and two heroin-exposed children. Mean values on a five-point
scale of activity-attention did not differ significantly among groups
(table 9.1). However, on correlational analysis, the rating of activity-
attention correlated with the maternal narcotic score at a level of $r =$
.25. Multiple regression analysis also indicated that only the maternal
narcotic score related significantly to the activity-attention rating (coef-
ficient = .073, SD = 0.036, $p <$ .05).

Intellectual Potential

Lifschitz et al. (1985) analyzed the relationship of the intellectual
function of these same 93 preschool subjects to maternal drug use, to
perinatal factors including the character of neonatal abstinence symptoms, and to environmental factors. Intellectual potential, as measured
by the McCarthy general cognitive index (GCI), was comparable for
all groups (table 9.2). Five heroin-exposed children and one control
performed in the mildly retarded range, with GCI scores ranging from

56 to 68. A heroin-exposed child with hydrocephalus and severe neurological impairment was profoundly retarded.

Analysis failed to demonstrate a relationship between GCI and maternal narcotic score, birth size, or severity of neonatal abstinence. Factors predictive of intelligence included obstetric prenatal risk score, the amount of prenatal care, and the quality of the home environment.

Group means were also compared for the five McCarthy scales assessing verbal, perceptual-performance, quantitative, memory, and motor skills. No significant differences were found, and mean scores fell within the normal range (table 9.2).

Somatic Growth

Lifschitz et al. (1983) also studied the relationship of birth size and postnatal growth to maternal drug use and other factors. For this study they included the 71 subjects from the longitudinal study (22 heroin-exposed, 21 methadone-treated, and 28 comparison) who were examined at the age of three years. In analyzing maternal factors, Lifschitz et al. found that methadone-treated women showed no advantage over untreated addicts in terms of weight gain during pregnancy or in the rating of nutritional status (weight/height ratio).

Both heroin- and methadone-exposed infants were significantly smaller than comparison babies at birth despite similar gestational periods. Group differences were eliminated, however, by adjustment for sex, race, prenatal care, weight gain during pregnancy, prenatal risk score, maternal education, and smoking. By age three years, mean weight, height, and head circumference were comparable for all three groups. Three-year measurements, while unrelated to maternal drug use or perinatal morbidity, were predicted by birth length, midparental height, and cigarette smoking.

DISCUSSION

Although the short-term toxicity of chronic heroin exposure during gestation is clearly manifest by the neonatal abstinence syndrome, it has been difficult to link long-term negative effects directly to heroin use. Even such biological effects as the intrauterine growth retardation reported in infants of narcotic-dependent women (Zelson, Rubio, and Wasserman 1971; Wilson, Desmond, and Verniaud 1973) may not be directly attributable to narcotic use (Lifschitz et al. 1983); rather, these effects may be secondary to related factors. Although the literature in early studies suggested a cluster of neurobehavioral findings and learning patterns in the children of heroin-dependent women, their profile was not unique when compared to a matched demographic "life-style" control that was drug-free. In the controlled longitudinal study, heroin-exposed children failed to show the expected pattern of disability (i.e., impairment of attention, hyperactivity, and weak perceptual and organizational skills). Although the mean cognitive potential of heroin-exposed children did not differ significantly from that of controls, their high rate (19%) of mental retardation is important clinically and evokes a desire to study a larger sample size. The extent of maternal drug use and newborn withdrawal syndrome did not directly affect cognitive performance, but prenatal factors associated with drug use and the child's home environment significantly influence the level of cognition.

Although the frequency of neurological abnormalities and of attentional deficit disorder was not increased in drug-exposed children, it was only in this neurobehavioral arena that effects were related directly to maternal drug use. Motor incoordination was directly associated with the severity of neonatal withdrawal. The rating of activity and attention was related to the maternal narcotic score, but not to environmental measures. These findings suggest that drug use may have subtle effects on nervous system function which are not obscured by time or experience.

From these studies we conclude that heroin use during pregnancy is not associated with major developmental disability or a specific behavioral syndrome. The studies of children raised by addicted parents reinforce the impression that biological and environmental factors affect their behavior and cognitive performance (Herjanic et al. 1979; Sowder and Burt 1980; Nichtern 1973). Only in the neurophysiological area did a dose/effect relationship link maternal drug use to subtle impairment of motor coordination and high (but clinically insignificant) activity-inattention scores.

Because long-term detrimental effects of heroin use during pregnancy seem to be related to factors associated with the life-style of the drug-dependent woman, comprehensive treatment of the pregnant addict should be given high priority. Major objectives of treatment should include elimination of polydrug use, provision of consistent obstetrical care, and psychosocial support and parenting education. The major benefit of treatment may be the mother's ability to assume responsibility for her child's care. Intervention directed toward improving the environment of the infant and child may be as important as improving the environment in utero.

In summary, the data indicate that fetal exposure to narcotics and pursuant newborn nervous system dysfunction may have a direct but subtle effect on neurobehavioral function beyond the period of infancy. The study did not reveal a consistent pattern of major neurobehavioral dysfunction, but minor deficits in behavior and motor performance could be directly attributed to maternal drug use. However, the relatively high rate of minor neuromotor abnormalities, low intellectual potential, and marginal attentional abilities among all subjects suggests that the comparison group as well as the drug-exposed children are at risk for poor academic performance.

REFERENCES

Aylward, G. P. 1982. Methadone outcome studies: Is it more than the methadone? *J Pediatr* 101:214–15.

Bayley Scales of Infant Development. 1969. New York: The Psychological Corp.

Behrendt, H., and Green, M. 1972. Nature of the sweating deficit of prematurely born neonates: Observations of babies with the heroin withdrawal syndrome. *N Engl J Med* 286:1376–79.

Caldwell, M. M. 1978. *Manual for the Home Observation for Measurement of the Environment*. Little Rock: University of Arkansas.

Desmond, M. M., and Wilson, G. S. 1975. Neonatal abstinence syndrome: Recognition and diagnosis. *Addict Dis* 2(1):113–21.

Dixon, W. J., ed. 1981. *BMPD Statistical Software*, 330–45. Berkeley and Los Angeles: University of California Press.

Glass, L., Rajegowda, B. K., and Floyd, M. V. 1972. Effect of heroin withdrawal on respiratory rate and acid-base status in the newborn. *N Engl J Med* 286:746–48.

Goodfriend, M. J., Shey, I. A., and Klein, M. D. 1956. The effect of maternal narcotic addiction on the newborn. *Am J Obstet Gynecol* 71:29–36.

Herjanic, B. M., Barredo, V. H., Herjanic M., and Tomelleri, C. J. 1979. Children of heroin addicts. *Int J Addict* 14:919–31.

Hill, R. M., and Desmond, M. M. 1963. Management of the narcotic withdrawal syndrome in the neonate. *Pediatr Clin North Am* 10:67–85.

Householder, J., Hatcher, R., Burns, W., and Chasnoff, I. 1982. Infants born to narcotic-addicted mothers. *Psychol Bull* 92:453–68.

Kaltenbach, K., and Finnegan, L. 1984. Developmental outcome of children born to methadone-maintained women: A review of longitudinal studies. *Neurobehav Toxicol Teratol* 6:271–75.

Lawson, M. S., and Wilson, G. S. 1980. Parenting among women addicted to narcotics. *Child Welfare* 59:67–79.

Lifschitz, M. H., Wilson, G. S., Smith, E. O., and Desmond, M. M. 1983. Fetal and postnatal growth of children born to narcotic-dependent women. *J Pediatr* 102:686–91.

———. 1985. Factors affecting head growth and intellectual function in children of drug addicts. *Pediatrics* 75:269–74.

McCarthy Scales of Children's Abilities. 1972. New York: The Psychological Corp.

Nichtern, S. 1973. The children of drug users. *J Am Acad Child Psychiatry* 12:24–31.

Olofsson, M., Buckley, W., Anderson, G. E., and Friis-Hansen, B. 1983. Investigation of 89 children borne by drug-dependent mothers. *Acta Paediatr Scand* 72:407–10.

Schulman, C. A. 1969. Alterations of the sleep cycle in heroin-addicted and "suspect" newborns. *Neuropediatrie* 1:89–100.

Sowder, B. J., and Burt, M. M. 1980. *Children of Heroin Addicts*, ed. J. A. Inciardi. New York: Praeger Publishers.

Touwen, B., and Prechtl, H. 1970. *The Neurological Examination of the Child with Minor Nervous Dysfunction.* Philadelphia: J. B. Lippincott.

Wilson, G. S., Desmond, M. M. and Verniaud, W. M. 1973. Early development of infants of heroin-addicted mothers. *Am J Dis Child* 126:457–62.

Wilson, G. S., Desmond, M. M., and Wait, R. B. 1981. Follow-up of methadone-treated and untreated narcotic-dependent women and their infants: Health, developmental and social implications. *J Pediatr* 98:716–22.

Wilson, G. S., McCreary, R., Kean, J., and Baxter, J. C. 1979. The development of preschool children of heroin-addicted mothers: A controlled study. *Pediatrics* 63:135–41.

Zagon, I. S., McLaughlin, P. J., Weaver, D. J., and Zagon, E. 1982. Opiates, endorphins and the developing organism: A comprehensive bibliography. *Neurosci Biobehav Rev* 6:439–79.

Zelson, C., Rubio, E., and Wasserman, E. 1971. Neonatal narcotic addiction: Ten-year observation. *Pediatrics* 48:178–89.

10

Methadone Maintenance during Pregnancy: Implications for Perinatal and Developmental Outcome

Karol Kaltenbach, Ph.D., and Loretta P. Finnegan, M.D.

THE USE OF methadone maintenance as a treatment for heroin addiction has generated a number of questions regarding its use with pregnant narcotic-dependent women. Since the early 1970s (Blinick, Jerez, and Wallach 1973), methadone maintenance has been recommended for narcotic dependence in pregnancy. The use of methadone as a maintenance therapy for the pregnant woman stabilizes her addictive behavior and, by preventing erratic maternal drug levels, protects the fetus from repeated episodes of withdrawal. As methadone maintenance requires participation in a treatment program, the probability of receiving prenatal care is also enhanced; with such care morbidity and mortality are reduced. However, there has been concern about the perinatal and developmental outcome of infants exposed to methadone in utero. When considering the efficacy of methadone maintenance during pregnancy, one must take a number of factors into account.

MEDICAL AND OBSTETRICAL FACTORS AMONG PREGNANT NARCOTIC-DEPENDENT WOMEN

In general, all pregnant women who are substance abusers, regardless of the particular age and abuse, are considered to be in a higher than normal risk category because of the complications of illicit drug use. The three most common indicators of pregnancy are (1) a history of amenorrhea, (2) a positive pregnancy test, and (3) palpation of the gravid uterus. Unfortunately, in the narcotic-addicted woman, none of these indicators is reliable. Amenorrhea is common. In addition, the early signs or symptoms of pregnancy such as fatigue, headaches, nau-

Table 10.1. Obstetrical Complications in Drug-dependent Women

Spontaneous abortion	Placental insufficiency
Intrauterine death	Intrauterine growth retardation
Abruptio placentae	Premature rupture of membranes
Amnionitis	Premature labor
Chorioamnionitis	Postpartum hemorrhage
Septic thrombophlebitis	Preeclampsia

sea and vomiting, hot sweats, and pelvic cramps may be interpreted as withdrawal symptoms by both physician and patient. Not infrequently, the onset of these symptoms compels the drug-dependent woman to use additional drugs that not only are ineffective in alleviating her symptoms, but also expose the fetus to increased secondary, changing serum levels of narcotics and other drugs. Chronic parenteral drug abuse during pregnancy has a variety of concomitant obstetrical and medical complications due to the method of drug administration, potential withdrawal from reduced availability of drugs, and lack of prenatal care for identification and treatment of problems. Infections account for a high percentage of related medical complications, and they may have profoundly harmful effects on the pregnant addict and her unborn child, particularly if they remain untreated throughout gestation. Especially frequent are types A, B, and non-A, non-B hepatitis, bacterial endocarditis, septicemia, cellulitus, and venereal disease (Blinick, Wallach, and Jerez 1969; Cherubin 1971; Cherubin, Kane, et al. 1972; Cherubin and Millian 1968; Cherubin, Rosenthal, et al. 1972; Cherubin et al. 1976; Cushman and Grieco 1973; Naeye et al. 1973).

Obstetrical complications associated with heroin addiction are those usually seen in any woman lacking prenatal care (table 10.1). A frequent result is the birth of a low-weight infant who has an array of problems due to prematurity and whose withdrawal symptoms are therefore difficult to manage. In some cases, death of a pregnant woman and her fetus may occur from these untreated complications.

The obstetrical complications in women maintained on methadone are similar to those of heroin users but without the persistent danger of infection from contaminated needles. This is of paramount importance, specifically in regard to the perinatal transmission of the human immunodeficiency virus (HIV). According to estimates by the National Association of Children's Hospitals and related institutions, about 3,000 infants are infected with the HIV each year. Over 80% of children who contract the acquired immunodeficiency syndrome (AIDS) are born to drug-abusing mothers or mothers who have a sexual partner involved in drug abuse. Comprehensive methadone treatment programs for pregnant intravenous drug-dependent women are essential to reduce or eliminate the perinatal transmission of HIV infection.

Methadone maintenance, in and of itself, is not necessarily sufficient to reduce perinatal complications but must be offered in conjunction with prenatal care reinforced by psychosocial counseling. Within the framework of a comprehensive program, complications can be identified and treated, thereby reducing maternal and infant morbidity and mortality. Maternal nutrition is usually improved, and the woman is more receptive to prenatal care and social and psychological rehabilitation. Connaughton, Reeser, and Finnegan (1977) found that morbidity in infants born to drug-dependent women was directly related to the amount of prenatal care and to the type of maternal narcotic dependence. Nearly 75% of infants born to 63 heroin addicts who had no prenatal care suffered neonatal morbidity. Similarly, 82% of infants born to 78 methadone-dependent women with inadequate care suffered neonatal morbidity. The incidence of neonatal morbidity was decreased to 69.9% for infants born to methadone-dependent women receiving adequate prenatal care.

More importantly, infants born to women who use methadone have somewhat higher birth weights than do children born to women using heroin (Connaughton et al. 1975; Kandall et al. 1976; Zelson 1973). Kandall et al. (1976) reported a significant relationship between the first trimester maternal methadone dose and birth weight. This study indicated that methadone may promote fetal growth in a dose-related fashion even after maternal heroin use, whereas heroin itself causes fetal growth retardation that may persist beyond the period of addition. Stimmel et al. (1982) analyzed the birth records of 239 infants born to narcotic-dependent women (1) on supervised methadone maintenance, (2) on unsupervised methadone maintenance, (3) on street heroin, or (4) who were multiple drug users. Although the presence of withdrawal symptoms did not differ with respect to the type of drug abused, perinatal outcome was significantly improved in those infants born to women on supervised methadone maintenance, as compared to all other groups.

METHADONE MAINTENANCE DURING PREGNANCY

The pharmacology of methadone in the pregnant woman has been well evaluated. Methadone is widely distributed throughout the body after oral ingestion, with extensive nonspecific tissue binding creating reservoirs that release unchanged methadone back into the blood, thus contributing to its long duration of action (Dole and Kreek 1973). Peak plasma levels occur 2–6 hours after the ingestion of a maintenance dose of methadone, with less than 6% of the ingested dose in the total blood volume at this time (Inturrisi and Verebely 1972; Kreek 1973; Sullivan and Blake 1972). Lower sustained plasma concentrations are present during the remainder of the 24-hour period. Methadone is metabolized primarily by the liver and is excreted in the urine and feces as both unchanged methadone and a variety of metabolities. Studies of methadone distribution in pregnant women show marked intra- and interindividual variations, with a plasma level somewhat lower after a given dose during pregnancy than following delivery. This decrease in available methadone in a pregnant woman can be accounted for by an increased fluid space, a large tissue reservoir for storing methadone, and drug metabolism by both the placenta and the fetus (Kreek et al. 1974). Methadone-maintained women frequently need elevations of their oral dose to maintain the same plasma level and remain withdrawal-free (Finnegan and Wapner 1987). If detoxification is considered, it is not advised before 14 weeks gestation because of the potential risk of inducing abortion and should not be performed after the 32nd week of pregnancy because of possible withdrawal-induced fetal stress. The multiple medical and pharmacological complications that result from parenteral heroin abuse must be considered before one recommends detoxification from methadone during pregnancy. Moreover, there is a greater potential for relapse in the pregnant woman if she is detoxified from methadone at this time. As with any drug therapy, the benefits versus the risk must be considered.

Because some studies have shown that the degree of neonatal withdrawal may be correlated with the maternal methadone dose during the last trimester of pregnancy, detoxification on a maintenance dose of <20 mg has sometimes been recommended. However, the relationship between maternal methadone dose and the presence of withdrawal symptoms has been difficult to establish. Ostrea, Chavez, and Strauss (1976) and Madden et al. (1977) both reported a significant relationship between severity of withdrawal and methadone dose during pregnancy. However, other investigators (Blinick et al. 1973; Stimmel et al. 1982) found no relationship between severity of withdrawal and maternal methadone dose. Kaltenbach et al. (1990) examined maternal methadone dose during pregnancy and infant outcome for 147 women maintained on a low dose (5–40 mg), a moderate dose (41–60 mg), or a high dose (>60 mg) during pregnancy. They found no differences among groups in the number of days that the infant required medication for abstinence, birth weight, or gestational age. Multiple regression was used to determine factors predicting gestational age, birth weight, or days on medication for abstinence. There was no significant association for polydrug abuse, opiate use, use of drugs other than opiates, average methadone dose, total months on methadone, or sex of the infant.

Neonatal Abstinence

Infants born to heroin- or methadone-dependent mothers have a high incidence of neonatal abstinence. Neonatal abstinence is described as a generalized disorder characterized by signs and symptoms of central nervous system hyperirritability, gastrointestinal dysfunction, respiratory distress, and vague autonomic symptoms that include yawning, sneezing, mottling, and fever. Neonates often suck frantically on their fists or thumbs, yet they may have extreme difficulty feeding because they have an uncoordinated and ineffectual sucking reflex. Infants who undergo abstinence generally develop tremors, which are initially mild and occur only when the infant is disturbed but which progress to the point where they occur spontaneously without any stimulation. High-pitched crying, increased muscle tone, and irritability develop.

The onset of withdrawal symptoms varies from minutes or hours after birth to two weeks of age, but the majority of symptoms appear within 72 hours. Many factors influence the onset of abstinence in individual infants, including the type of drugs used by the mother, both the timing and the dose before delivery, the character of labor, the type and amount of analgesia and anesthetic given during labor, maturity, nutrition, and the presence of intrinsic disease in the infant. The withdrawal syndrome may be mild and transient, may be delayed in onset, may have a stepwise increase in severity, may be intermittently present, or may have a biphasic course that includes acute neonatal withdrawal signs followed by improvement and then the onset of a subacute withdrawal reaction (Desmond and Wilson 1975).

With appropriate pharmacotherapy, neonatal abstinence can be satisfactorily treated without any untoward neonatal effects. It is recommended that an abstinence scoring system be used to monitor the passively addicted neonate comprehensively and objectively to assess the onset, progression, and diminution of symptoms of abstinence (Finnegan 1990). The score is used to monitor the infant's clinical response to pharmacotherapeutic intervention necessary for the control of withdrawal symptoms and for detoxification (fig 10.1).

Neurobehavioral Characteristics

The neurobehavioral characteristics of newborns undergoing abstinence uniformly have been investigated using the Brazelton Neonatal Behavioral Assessment Scale (Brazelton 1973). A number of researchers consistently found that infants born to narcotic-dependent women differ from infants born to non-drug-dependent women on several behaviors (Chasnoff et al. 1984; Jeremy and Hans 1985; Kaplan et al. 1976; Strauss et al. 1976; Strauss et al. 1975). Narcotic-exposed infants are more irritable, are less cuddly, exhibit more tremors, and have increased tone. Several studies also reported that narcotic-exposed infants are less responsive to visual stimulation. However, infants undergoing abstinence are less likely to maintain an alert state; thus, the orientation items of the Brazelton assessment often cannot be completed. Strauss et al. (1975) reported that, when elicited, the orientation behavior of infants exposed to narcotics was comparable to that of non-drug-exposed infants.

An important aspect of these neonatal behavioral characteristics is their implications for mother/infant interaction. A study investigating the effect of neonatal abstinence on the infant's ability to interact with the environment found that infants born to women maintained on methadone were deficient in their capacity for attention and social responsiveness during the first few days of life (Kaltenbach and Finnegan 1988). These deficiencies were present regardless of whether the neonatal abstinence was severe enough to require treatment. The interac-

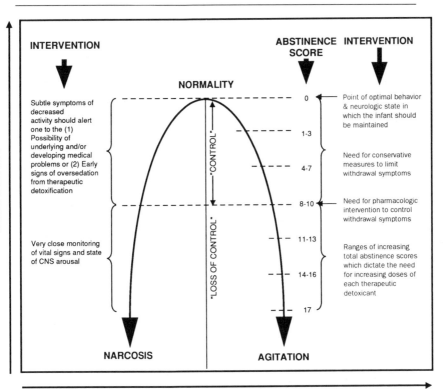

Figure 10.1. The management of the neonatal abstinence syndrome.
Source: Finnegan, L. P. 1990. Neonatal abstinence syndrome. In *Current Therapy in Neonatal-Perinatal Medicine—2*, ed. N. Nelson, 315. Ontario, Canada: B.C. Decker.

tive behavior seemed to be affected until the infant was free of abstinence symptoms and detoxification was complete. Fitzgerald, Kaltenbach, and Finnegan (1990) studied patterns of interaction between drug-dependent women and their infants and non-drug-exposed dyads. Mothers and infants were videotaped at birth and at four months of age. Interaction behavior was evaluated by the Greenspan-Lieberman Observational System (GLOS), the Newborn GLOS, and the Clinical Global Rating System. At four months of age, infants were assessed by the Bayley Scales of Infant Development, including the Infant Behavior Record. Mother's life stress and social support were evaluated by the Social Readjustment Rating Scale and by structured interviews, respectively. Drug-dependent mothers and their newborn infants had significantly lower global ratings of dyadic interaction quality than had comparison dyads. Both drug-dependent mothers and their newborns performed more poorly on a measure of social engagement. Drug-dependent mothers demonstrated significantly less positive affect and greater detachment, and drug-exposed newborns presented fewer behaviors promoting social involvment. At four months of age, dyadic interaction quality, social engagement, detachment, and negative affect among drug-exposed infants and their mothers no longer differed from comparisons. However, drug-dependent mothers reported significantly higher levels of stressful events during the previous year which were strongly correlated with their negative affect and detachment scores during interaction. Drug-exposed four-month-old infants showed significantly greater body tension and poorer coordination on the Infant Behavior Record.

These findings suggest that drug-exposed infants and their mothers experience a difficult early period during which both are less available, less likely to initiate, and less responsive to social involvement than comparison dyads. Although the infants are better adjusted at four months of age, the life stress and infant behavior findings indicate that maternal addiction treatment programs should provide appropriate intervention to facilitate positive mother/infant interaction.

PERINATAL AND DEVELOPMENTAL OUTCOME

Perinatal outcome in relation to intrauterine growth has been an area of concern. A number of prospective studies have yielded somewhat inconsistent findings. Studies that have compared infants born to heroin-dependent women not maintained on methadone versus infants born to heroin-dependent mothers receiving methadone have found differential effects, with greater birth weights for infants born to methadone-maintained women (Kandall et al. 1977; Connaughton et al. 1977). Some studies that have compared methadone-exposed infants with non-drug-exposed infants found that methadone-exposed infants had lower birth weights than had comparison infants (Chasnoff, Hatcher, and Burns 1982; Lifshitz et al. 1983). Other studies, however, found no differences in birth weights (Rosen and Johnson 1987; Strauss et al. 1976). Smaller head circumferences among methadone-exposed infants were also reported. A more recent study by Kaltenbach and Finnegan

(1987) with a large sample of infants (N = 268) found that methadone-exposed infants had smaller birth weights and head circumferences than had comparison infants. Although differences were found between the two groups, the methadone-exposed infants were not small for gestational age and there was a positive correlation between head circumference and birth weight for both the methadone-exposed infants and the comparison infants (r = .72 and r = .69, respectively). The data from this study suggest that infants born to narcotic-dependent women maintained on methadone during pregnancy may have smaller birth weights and head circumferences than non-drug-exposed comparison infants, but that they are not growth retarded.

A longitudinal study by Pasto et al. (1989) evaluated the cerebral sonographic characteristics of methadone-exposed infants and comparison infants at birth, one month, and six months of age. Sonographic characteristics of the cerebral ventricles (slitlike, i.e., no visible fluid, versus normal) were recorded, as were transverse measurements of the intracranial hemidiameter, the right and left lateral ventricles, the temporal lobe, and the thalamic area (traced in a transaxial view). There were significantly more slit ventricles in methadone-exposed infants at all three examinations, although the number of infants with slit ventricles decreased with age. At birth and one month of age, the intracranial hemidiameters were smaller in the narcotic-exposed infants, but thalamic areas and temporal lobe measurements did not differ at any time. Methadone exposure in utero was highly associated with slit ventricles, which were slower to resolve in lower-birth-weight infants. The smaller intracranial hemidiameters and lateral ventricle measurements suggest possible slower cortical growth.

The incidence of strabismus is greater in infants exposed to narcotics in utero than in the general population. A study by Nelson et al. (1987) of 29 narcotic-exposed infants found a 24% incidence of strabismus in contrast to 5–8% incidence in the general population. Birth weights were lower for the infants with strabismus (p = .05), but average maternal methadone dose during pregnancy was higher, so whether strabismus was related to lower birth weight, narcotic exposure, or a combination of factors is unclear.

Diverse findings among studies reflect the myriad of confounding variables present within human populations. The women differ in daily methadone dose, length of methadone maintenance during pregnancy, and amount of prenatal care. A large percentage of pregnant women maintained on methadone continue to use a number of other drugs, such as heroin, diazepam, cocaine, and barbiturates. In addition, 90% are moderate to heavy smokers, and alcohol consumption is quite prevalent (Rosen and Johnson 1987; Wilson, Desmond, and Wait 1981).

Developmental sequelae associated with methadone exposure in utero has been investigated in a number of longitudinal studies. The assessment procedures used in these follow-up studies are quite similar. Children are evaluated throughout infancy, typically at six-month intervals, with the Bayley Scales of Infant Development. Children born to non-drug-dependent women from comparable socioeconomic and ra cial backgrounds are used as controls.

A study by Strauss et al. (1976) found that both methadone-exposed infants and comparison infants scored well within the normal range of development on the Bayley Mental Development Index (MDI) and the Motor Development Index (PDI) at 3, 6, and 12 months of age. However, PDI scores for the methadone-exposed infants declined with age and differed from comparison infants at 12 months of age. Wilson, Desmond, and Wait (1981) also found no difference in MDI scores among infants at 9 months of age but found lower PDI scores for methadone-exposed infants. Although Rosen and Johnson (1987) found no difference between groups on MDI and PDI scores at 6 months of age, they found that methadone-exposed infants had both lower MDI and lower PDI scores at 12 and 18 months of age. In comparison, Lodge (1977) found no differences between groups on either the MDI or the PDI at 6 and 12 months of age; Hans and Jeremy (1984) reported no difference at 4, 8, and 12 months of age; Kaltenbach and Finnegan (1986) found no difference at 6, 12, and 24 months of age; and Chasnoff et al. (1984) reported no difference at 3, 6, 12, and 24 months of age.

Unfortunately, few studies have been able to follow these children longitudinally past infancy. Wilson et al. (1979) reported differences between narcotic-exposed children and three different comparison groups comprising a drug environment group, a high-risk group, and a socioeconomic comparison group. Narcotic-exposed children performed more poorly than comparison groups on the General Cognitive Index of the McCarthy Scales of Children's Abilities and on the perceptual, quantitative, and memory subscales. In this study, heroin was the predominant drug used; only a few of the mothers were maintained on methadone, so there is some difficulty in comparing the data. Strauss et al. (1979) evaluated children from their 1976 sample when the children were five years of age. They found no differences between groups on the McCarthy Scales of Children's Abilities or on any of the McCarthy subscales. Kaltenbach and Finnegan (1989) also found no differences between groups on the McCarthy Scales or on any of the subscales in their sample of children at $4\frac{1}{2}$ years of age. Although both studies found no difference between groups, there were marked differences in the scores between the two studies. The mean General Cognitive Index in the Strauss data was 86.8 for the methadone-exposed children and 86.2 for the comparison children, whereas the mean General Cognitive Indexes in the Kaltenbach and Finnegan study were 106.5 and 106, respectively. The McCarthy scores in the Kaltenbach and Finnegan study are higher than one would expect. It may well have been that this was a self-selected sample of mothers especially interested in their children's development and thus willing to be involved in a five-year longitudinal study. This argument may be supported by the fact that, while the Strauss sample of five-year-old children were from the Strauss infancy study, they did not participate in an ongoing project (i.e., the first investigation concluded when the children were one year of age and then as many subjects as possible were recruited for assessment at five years of age).

Although neonatal abstinence and the concomitant neurobehavioral characteristics can be directly attributed to methadone exposure in utero, further delineation of the effects of prenatal methadone exposure is a complex task. Perinatal and developmental outcomes associated with prenatal methadone exposure must be viewed within a multifactorial perspective (i.e., the primary pharmacological/toxicological effects produced by the drugs(s), postnatal environmental interactive effects, and possible genetic effects) (Hutchings 1985). Furthermore, it is essential that the use of methadone be viewed within the appropriate context. Methadone is a licit drug used to treat a chronic relapsing disease and, as with any treatment drug, the risk/benefit ratio must be considered. When methadone maintenance is provided for pregnant drug-dependent women within a comprehensive treatment program that addresses the medical, obstetrical, addictive, and pyschosocial issues, maternal and infant morbidity and mortality are reduced, and the developmental and cognitive functioning of the progeny is not impaired.

REFERENCES

Blinick, G., Jerez, E., and Wallach, R. C. 1973. Methadone maintenance, pregnancy, and progeny. *JAMA* 225:447.

Blinick, G., Wallach, R. C., and Jerez, E. 1969. Pregnancy in narcotic addicts treated by medical withdrawal. *Am J Obstet Gynecol* 105:997.

Brazelton, T. B. 1973. *Neonatal Behavior Assessment Scale.* Philadelphia: J. B. Lippincott.

Chasnoff, I. J., Hatcher, R., and Burns, W. 1982. Polydrug- and methadone-addicted newborns: A continuum of impairment? *Pediatrics* 70:210.

Chasnoff, I. J., Schnoll, S. H., Burns, W. J., and Burns, K. 1984. Maternal non-narcotic substance abuse during pregnancy: Effects on infant development. *Neurobehav Toxicol Teratol* 6:277–80.

Cherubin, C. E. 1971. Infectious disease problems of narcotic addicts. *Arch Intern Med* 128:309.

Cherubin, C. E., Kane, S., Weinberger, D. R., Wolfe, E., and McGinn, T. G. 1972. Persistence of transaminase abnormalities in former drug addicts. *Ann Intern Med* 76:385.

Cherubin, C. E., and Millian, S. J. 1968. Serological investigations in narcotic addicts: I. Syphilis, lymphogranuloma venereum, herpes simplex and Q fever. *Ann Intern Med* 69:739.

Cherubin, C. E., Rosenthal, W. S., Stenger, R. E., Prince, A. M., Baden, M., Strauss, R., and McGinn, T. G. 1972. Chronic liver disease in asymptomatic narcotic addicts. *Ann Intern Med* 76:391.

Cherubin, C. E., Schaefer, R. A., Rosenthal, W. S., McGinn, T. G., Forte, F., Purcell, R., and Walmsley, P. 1976. The natural history of liver disease in former drug users. *Am J Med Sci* 272:244.

Connaughton, J. F., Finnegan, L. P., Schut, J., and Emich, J. P. 1975. Current concepts in the management of the pregnant opiate addict. *Addict Dis* 2:21–35.

Connaughton, J. F., Reeser, D., and Finnegan, L. P. 1977. Pregnancy complicated by drug addiction. In *Perinatal Medicine*, ed. R. Bolognese and R. Schwartz, 265–76. Baltimore: Williams & Wilkins.

Connaughton, J. F., Reeser, D., Schut, J., and Finnegan, L. P. 1977. Perinatal addiction: Outcome and management. *Am J Obstet Gynecol* 729:679–86.

Cushman, P., and Grieco, M. H. 1973. Hyperimmunoglobulinemia associated with narcotic addiction: Effects of methadone maintenance treatment. *Am J Med* 54:320.

Desmond, M. M., and Wilson, G. S. 1975. Neonatal abstinence syndrome: Recognition and diagnosis. *Addict Dis* 2:113–21.

Dole, V. P., and Kreek, M. J. 1973. Methadone plasma level: Sustained by a reservoir of drug in tissue. *Proc Natl Acad Sci USA* 70:10.

Finnegan, L. P. 1990. Neonatal abstinence syndrome. In *Current Therapy in Neonatal-Perinatal Medicine—2*, ed. N. Nelson, 314–20. Ontario, B.C.: Decker.

Finnegan, L. P., and Wapner, R. 1987. Narcotic addiction in pregnancy. In *Drug Use in Pregnancy*, ed. J. R. Neibyl, 203–22.

Fitzgerald, E., Kaltenbach, K., and Finnegan, L. P. 1990. Patterns of interaction among drug-dependent women and their infants. *Pediatr Res Abstr* 27(4):10A (abstr).

Hans, S. L., and Jeremy, R. J. 1984. Post-neonatal motoric signs in infants exposed in utero to methadone. Paper presented at the Fourth International Conference on Infant Studies, New York.

Hutchings, D. E. 1985. Prenatal opioid exposure and the problem of causal inference. In *Current Research on the Consequences of Maternal Drug Use*, ed. T. M. Prinkert, 6–19. National Institute on Drug Abuse Research Series (DHHS Publication No. ADM 85-1400). Washington, D.C.: U.S. Government Printing Office.

Inturrisi, C. E., and Verebely, K. 1972. A gas-liquid chromatographic method for the quantitative determination of methadone in human plasma and urine. *J Chromatogr* 65:361.

Jeremy, R. J., and Hans, S. L. 1985. Behavior of neonates exposed in utero to methadone as assessed on the Brazelton Scale. *Infant Behav Dev* 8:323–36.

Kaltenbach, K., and Finnegan, L. P. 1986. Developmental outcome of infants exposed to methadone in utero: A longitudinal study. *Pediatr Res* 20:57.

———. 1987. Perinatal and developmental outcome of infants exposed to methadone in utero. *Neurotoxicol Teratol* 9:311–13.

———. 1988. The influence of the neonatal abstinence syndrome on mother-infant interaction. In *The Child in His Family: Perilous Development. Child Raising and Identity Formation under Stress*, ed. E. J. Anthony and C. Chiland, 223–30. New York: John Wiley.

———. 1989. Children exposed to methadone in utero: Assessment of developmental and cognitive ability. *Ann Acad Sci* 562:360–62.

Kaltenbach, K., Thakur, N., Weiner, S., and Finnegan, L. P. 1990. The relationship between maternal methadone dose during pregnancy and infant outcome. *Pediatr Res Abstr* 27:227A (abstr).

Kandall, S. R., Albin, R. S., Gartner, L. M., Lee, K. S., Eidelman, A., and Lowinson, J. 1977. The narcotic dependent mother: Fetal and neonatal consequences. *Early Hum Dev* 1:159–69.

Kandall, S. R., Albin, S., Lowinson, J., Berle, B., Eidelman, A. J., and Gartner, L. M. 1976. Differential effects of maternal heroin and methadone use on birth weight. *Pediatrics* 58: 681–85.

Kaplan, S. L., Kron, R. E., Phoenix, M. D., and Finnegan, L. P. 1976. Brazelton neonatal assessment at three and twenty-eight days of age: A study of passively addicted infants, high risk infants, and normal infants. In *Critical Concerns in the Field of Drug Abuse*, ed. H. Alksne and E. Kaufman, 726–30. New York: Marcel Dekker.

Kreek, M. J. 1973. Plasma and urine levels of methadone. *NY State J Med* 23:2773.

Kreek, M. J., Schecter, A., Gutjahr, C. L., Bowen, D., Field, F., Queenan, J., and Merkatz, I. 1974. Analyses of methadone and other drugs in maternal and neonatal body fluids: Use in evaluation of symptoms in a neonate of mother maintained on methadone. *Am J Drug Alcohol Abuse* 1:409.

Lifshitz, M. H., Wilson, G. S., Smith, E., and Desmond, M. 1983. Fetal and postnatal growth of children born to narcotic-dependent women. *J Pediatr* 102:686–91.

Lodge, A. 1977. Developmental findings with infants born to mothers on methadone maintenance: A preliminary report. In *Symposium on Comprehensive Health Care for Addicted Families and Their Children*, ed. G. Beschner and R. B. Rotman, 79–85. Washington, D.C.: U.S. Government Printing Office.

Madden, J. D., Chappel, J. N., Zuspan, F., Gumpel, J., Meija, A., and Davis, R. 1977. Observation and treatment of neonatal narcotic withdrawal. *Am J Obstet Gynecol* 127:199–201.

Naeye, R. L., Blanc, W., Leblanc, W., and Khatamec. 1973. Fetal complications of maternal heroin addiction: Abnormal growth, infections, and episodes of stress. *J Pediatr* 6:1055–61.

Nelson, L. B., Ehrlich, S., Calhoun, J. H., Matteucci, T., and Finnegan, L. P. 1987. Occurrence of strabismus in infants born to drug-dependent women. *Am J Dis Child* 141:175–78.

Ostrea, E. M., Chavez, C. J., and Strauss, M. E. 1976. A study of factors that influence the severity of neonatal narcotic withdrawal. *J Pediatr* 88:642–45.

Pasto, M. E., Ehrlich, S., Kaltenbach, K., Graziani, L., Kurtz, A., Goldberg, B., and Finnegan, L. P. 1989. Cerebral sonographic characteristics and maternal and neonatal risk factors in infants of opiate-dependent mothers. In *Ann NY Acad Sci* 562:355–57.

Rosen, T. S., and Johnson, H. L. 1987. Children of methadone-maintained mothers: Follow-up to 18 months of age. *J Pediatr* 101:192–96.

Stimmel, B., Goldberg, J., Reisman, A., Murphy, R., and Teets, K. 1982. Fetal outcome in narcotic-dependent women: The importance of the type of maternal narcotic used. *Am J Drug Alcohol Abuse* 9:383–95.

Strauss, M. E., Lessen-Firestone, J. K., Chavez, C. J., and Stryker, J. C. 1979. Children of methadone-treated women at five years of age. *Pharmacol Biochem Behav (Suppl)* 11:3–6.

Strauss, M. E., Lessen-Firestone, J. K., Starr, R. H., and Ostrea, E. M. 1975. Behavior of narcotic-addicted newborns. *Child Dev* 46:887–93.

Strauss, M. E., Starr, R. H., Ostrea, E. M., Chavez, C. J., and Stryker, J. C. 1976. Behavioral concomitants of prenatal addiction to narcotics. *J Pediatr* 89:842–46.

Sullivan, H. R., and Blake, D. A. 1972. Quantitative determination of methadone concentration in human blood, plasma, and urine by gas chromatography. *Res Commun Chem Pathol Pharmacol* 3:467.

Wilson, G. S., Desmond, M. M., and Wait, R. B. 1981. Follow-up of methadone-treated women and their infants: Health, developmental, and social implications. *J Pediatr* 98:716–22.

Wilson, G. S., McCreary, R., Kean, J., and Baxter, C. 1979. The development of preschool children of heroin-addicted mothers: A controlled study. *Pediatrics* 63:135–41.

Zelson, C. 1973. Infant of the addicted mother. *N Engl J Med* 288:1391–95.

11

Phencyclidine: Experimental Studies in Animals and Long-term Developmental Effects on Humans

Gaylia Jean Harry, Ph.D., and Judy Howard, M.D.

T HE USE OF phencyclidine (PCP, "angel dust") and its derivates had an auspicious beginning in 1956 at the Product Development Department of Parke-Davis and Company. Medicinal chemists were looking for safe agents for general anesthesia and, initially, PCP seemed to be a promising candidate because it offered a level of safety—as measured by its therapeutic index—well above those of anesthetic agents in use at that time. Unfavorable hallucinatory side effects, however, led to the discontinuation of its use.

After the preliminary use of PCP to anesthetize animals, the drug was first administered to humans in 1957. Soon after, it was noted that approximately 30% of patients complained of peculiar sensations upon awakening from anesthesia. Their most common distressing symptoms included loss of sensation in the extremities and a feeling of floating in outer space (Domino 1980).

Subsequent to reports of these problems, researchers contacted a psychiatrist, Elliot Luby, who was interested in the phenomenon of sensory isolation in schizophrenic patients. He proposed that the post-anesthetic complications of PCP were similar to those behaviors observed during acute schizophrenic episodes (Luby et al. 1959). Thus, PCP emerged as a research model for schizophrenia.

Over a period of several years, it became apparent that PCP and its derivatives stimulated unique dose-related responses in both animals and humans (Domino 1980). Based on research involving adults from various animal species, it was determined that the higher the cortical functioning of the species, the smaller the amount of PCP required to elicit the anesthetic dose. For instance, the dose needed to anesthetize a mouse is large in comparison with that required for a rat; the required dose is smaller as one ascends up the species scale, with the smallest dose required for humans. Thus, the potency of a very small amount of PCP upon the adult human brain cannot be overestimated. In light of this information, we must begin to raise suspicions about the potential effects of such a drug upon the developing brain of the human fetus.

Although the mechanism of action of PCP is unclear, we know that it alters several neurotransmitter systems and produces a psychoticlike state resembling schizophrenia (Domino 1981). This drug lends itself to abuse, and, in 1973, evidence of PCP abuse surfaced in emergency rooms across the nation (Crider 1986). Acute intoxications and deaths continued to escalate in number until 1978, when the epidemic reached its first peak. Over the following three years, an actual decline occurred in the number of reported cases of acute PCP intoxication.

There seem to be several reasons for this decline: officials from health and law enforcement had warned the population of the complications caused by PCP use, penalties for possession of PCP with intent to sell were stiffened (Crider 1986), some individuals exhibiting psychoticlike symptoms due to PCP intoxication were diverted directly from emergency rooms to psychiatric services (Gorelick, Wilkins, and Wong 1986; Yago et al. 1981), and others under the influence of PCP asked friends to care for them rather than seeking treatment in emergency rooms. A study conducted in Los Angeles County, for example, revealed through street-level interviews with PCP abusers that 56% (22 of 39) sought help from friends in recovering from drug-related emergency complications (Green 1983).

Beginning in 1982, PCP surfaced once again as a primary drug of abuse. More than eight million persons were reported as having used PCP during that year (Miller et al. 1983). Geographic areas where PCP use was extremely high included New York City, Washington, D.C., and Los Angeles County (Crider 1986). In Los Angeles County, the quantity of PCP-laced cigarettes confiscated by police in 1982 was 294,817, rising to 2,551,299 in 1983—an increase of 765%. PCP liquid was also seized, at rates of 69,558 ml in 1982 and 112,454 ml in 1983—up 62% (Husson 1984).

The number of identified cases of PCP intoxication seen in emergency rooms in Los Angeles County rose from 1,567 in 1980 to 3,001 in 1983—an increase of 92%. Approximately 30% of these individuals were women of childbearing age (Husson 1984). In 1986, the Los Angeles County Child Abuse Prevention Program received notification that

Table 11.1 Routes of PCP Use in a
Clinic Population ($N = 1000$)

Route	%
Smoked	72.6
Sniffed/snorted	13.3
Ingested	12.3
Injected intravenously	1.8
Used by two or more routes	1.0

Source: McCarron et al. 1986.

12.5% of 915 newborns had positive urine toxicology screens for PCP (Durfee 1986).

PCP and its six or more analogs can be made inexpensively in home laboratories and commonly are sold on the street in liquid form or, occasionally, in pill form (Jasinski 1981). PCP is used most often in combination with marijuana, cocaine, heroin, and/or alcohol (Crider 1986; McCarron 1986; McCarron et al. 1986; Silber et al. 1988), and the routes of use include inhalation, ingestion, and, less frequently, parenteral administration. When smoked, PCP liquid commonly is dripped onto the brown wrappers of Sherman or More cigarettes. When ingested, it usually is mixed with another liquid, such as alcohol. Less frequently, it may be injected intravenously. Table 11.1 provides an overview of routes of PCP use.

Street names for PCP differ according to geographic regions. In Southern California, it may be referred to as "Kools," "Sherms," "Dust," "Koolly High," "Wet Daddies," and "Juice," whereas East Coast street names for PCP include "Angel Dust," "Dust," "Zoot," "He-Man," "Omen," and "White Devil" (Street Talk 1988).

THE KINETICS OF PCP

In humans, PCP transfers across the placental barrier (Kaufman et al. 1983) and also is present in the urine of seven-day-old human infants (Marble et al. 1980). The presence of PCP in the urine of infants one to seven days after birth was seen when the mothers had discontinued

PCP use at least three months before childbirth (Ahmad 1987). In an experimental animal model using the pig, Cummings (1979) examined the placental transfer of PCP and found that the concentration of PCP in piglet plasma was tenfold higher than in maternal plasma. When PCP was administered to sows just before delivery, it not only crossed the placental barrier, but also remained in the plasma of the piglet at significant levels for at least 48 hours after delivery (Cooper, Cummings, and Jones 1977). The transfer of PCP across the placental barrier also occurs in both the rabbit and the mouse (Nicholas, Lipshitz, and Schreiber 1982). In the mouse, the concentration of PCP in the fetal plasma was seven times higher than that in the plasma of the dams. Of interest is the observation that there was no apparent metabolism of the administered PCP in the fetuses. PCP also is transferred from the dam to the suckling offspring via the breast milk (Nicholas, Lipshitz, and Schreiber 1982). This transfer offers an additional and continued route of exposure during development.

Fico and VanderWende (1988) determined the half-life of PCP in the fetal central nervous system. During two overlapping developmental periods, phencyclidine was administered subcutaneously to the dam at a dose of 20 mg/kg body weight. The first dosing regimen (gestational days 6–15) occurred during organogenesis and produced a decrease in maternal weight gain. The second dosing regimen (gestational days 12–18) was specifically designed to occur during the period of development of the PCP receptor in the central nervous system (Sircar and Zukin 1983). No alterations in maternal weight were evident during this second dosing period. On the final day (either day 15 or day 18), the dams received a known quantity of [^{3}H]PCP, and the level of labeled phencyclidine was quantitatively determined in fetal brain tissue at various times after the subcutaneous injection (at 15, 30, 60, 120, 240, or 480 minutes). Within 15 minutes, [^{3}H]PCP was detectable in the brain. For both dosing periods, the peak concentration of [^{3}H]PCP in the brain was reached by 30 minutes. The peak concentrations were 0.473 and 1.108 μg/g wet weight of tissue for days 15 and 18, respectively. For each of the two dosing periods examined, the time course of [^{3}H]PCP accumulation was virtually identical through 120 minutes. At 120 minutes after injection, the concentration of labeled PCP at gestational day 15 was approximately half that of day 18 (0.3 μg and 0.5 μg/g wet weight of tissue, respectively). The calculated half-life of PCP in brain tissue was 126 minutes at gestational day 15 and 27 minutes at day 18. The two major metabolites of PCP, 4-phenyl-4-piperidinocyclohexanol (PPC) and 1-(1-phencyclohexyl)-4-hydroxypiperidine (PCHP), followed a similar time course. By 24 hours, no detectable levels of labeled PCP or metabolites were evident.

A further examination, based on these findings, was conducted by Ahmad, Halsall, and Bondy in 1987. In this study, maternal dosing (5 mg PCP per kg) was initiated at one of four different times and continued for three consecutive days. PCP was administered to dams on gestational days 9, 10, and 11 in Group I; on days 12, 13, and 14 in Group II; on days 15, 16, and 17 in Group III; and on days 18, 19, and 20 in Group IV. On gestational day 22, all dams and offspring were killed, and serum and brains were collected and analyzed for PCP content. Under these dosing regimens, no differences were noted in fetal viability, physical characteristics, or brain and body weights. The only rats showing circulating blood levels of PCP were in Group IV (dams: 0.34 ± 0.17 ng/ml serum; pups: 1.08 ± 0.39 ng/ml serum). Of interest is the observation that the cerebral concentration of PCP in the offspring (17.22 ± 2.40 ng/g brain tissue) was approximately 16 times the corresponding serum level (1.08 ± 0.39 ng/ml serum) and 11 times the level in maternal brains (1.51 ± 0.84 ng/g brain tissue). There were detectable amounts of PCP in the brains of the progeny of Groups II (2.13 ± 0.75 ng/g brain tissue), III (2.39 ± 0.35 ng/g), and IV (2.39 ± 0.35 ng/g). When injections of PCP (5 mg/kg) were given on gestation day 20, within 30 minutes the fetal serum level of PCP (646–2,079 ng/ml) was elevated relative to the maternal serum level (127–816 ng/ml). The possible absence of a barrier to the free diffusion of PCP from the fetal serum to the fetal brain was indicated by the similarity of PCP levels in the brain (200–2,734 ng/g brain tissue) and in the serum. In contrast, the PCP concentration in the maternal brain was only 2% of the level in the serum. There is evidence to indicate a prolonged persistence of PCP in the adult brain and adipose tissue after a single intraperitoneal injection and an accumulation after multiple doses (Mistra, Pontani, and Bartolomeo 1979). The persistence of drug tissue levels suggests that the exposure risk to the developing organism continues even after the cessation of maternal exposure. Ahmad, Halsall, and Bondy (1987) examined the persistence of PCP in the fetal brain after multiple dosing and reported a level of 17.2 ng PCP per g wet brain weight 24 hours after cessation of dosing. This collection of data indicates that perinatal exposure to PCP results in a substantial exposure of the developing central nervous system and suggests the possibility of an effect on the maturation of that system.

THE TERATOGENIC PROPERTIES OF PCP

Gestational exposure to phencyclidine produces a variety of gross morphological defects. Most of these effects, however, occur only at dose levels producing maternal toxicity. In 1979, Jordan et al. conducted a series of experiments to evaluate the teratogenic properties of phencyclidine. During a midgestational period (days 6–15), dams were exposed daily to intraperitoneal injections of 10, 15, 20, 25, 30, or 40 mg PCP per kg body weight. Alternatively, dams were given an injection of 60 mg PCP per kg body weight on gestational days 10–14. A late-gestational exposure group (days 15–20) was exposed only to a dose level of 40 mg PCP per kg on gestational day 10, 11, 12, 13, or 14. The overall decrease in weight gain for the PCP-treated maternal animals was dose related in that it varied from an average of 20 g less in the 10-mg/kg dose group to approximately 60 g less in the highest dose group. The greatest suppression of weight gain was seen in the animals receiving 40 mg/kg during the late stage of gestation, with an average weight gain of only 20 g during gestation. Even with decreased maternal weight gain, no significant decrease was found in birth weight. In contrast, Nabeshima et al. (1987) reported that prenatal exposure to 10 mg PCP per kg body weight per day resulted in a mild decrease in maternal weight gain and a modest reduction in birth weights.

In the higher-dose groups, PCP treatment induced a threefold increase in the number of resorbed fetuses and a subsequent reduction in the viable litter size (Jordan et al. 1979). A total malformation rate of 45–65% was observed in the offspring of dams that had received the higher dose levels of PCP (25–40 mg/kg) over days 6–15 of gestation or had received PCP during days 15–20. An acute injection of 60 mg PCP per kg during midgestation was effective in producing malformations in 43–56% of the fetuses surviving to day 20 of gestation. These total malformation rates comprise gross, visceral, and skeletal malformations. Exposure during the late gestational period to 40 mg PCP per kg resulted in approximately 10% of the fetuses displaying gross malformations.

The most common malformations were cleft lip/palate, foreshortened snout, micrognathia, and limb dysplasia. When dams were dosed during the midgestational period by either an acute or a repeated dosing regimen, the pups displayed a prominent incidence of visceral defects such as malformations of the urinary system. Hydrocephalus also was commonly noted. The largest percentage of malformations, however, involved the skeletal system. Various skeletal defects were seen, with the most frequently occurring malformations being dysplasias of the interparietal, supraoccipital, and premaxillary bones of the skull. These malformations were seen regardless of dose level or duration of treatment.

Similar teratogenic results were found in mice exposed to phencyclidine during gestational days 6–15. External, visceral, and skeletal alterations were examined in the offspring of dams dosed by gavage with 60, 80, 100, or 120 mg PCP per kg body weight per day from gestational day 6 to day 15 (Marks, Worthy, and Staples 1980). All four doses produced maternal toxicity characterized by initial hyperactivity followed by ataxia, a transient hind-limb paralysis, and decreased body weight gain. A significant increase in the percentage of malformed fetuses was seen only at 120 mg/kg/day, which also produced maternal toxicity. A variety of malformations was found, with a prominence of exencephaly and cleft palate. In contrast to the rat study of Jordan et al. (1979), Marks, Worthy, and Staples (1980) reported a significantly lower average birth weight for all dosed mice offspring. Marks et al. concluded that all four doses produced maternal and embryofetal toxicity. With the administration of 20 mg PCP per kg during a midgestational period, Fico and VanderWende (1988) also reported lower birth weights in both male and female mouse offspring, with no effect on the average litter size.

THE EFFECTS OF PRENATAL PCP EXPOSURE ON ANIMAL OFFSPRING

Postnatal Maturation and Behavioral Development

Examinations of the behavioral alterations following prenatal exposure to phencyclidine have utilized nonteratogenic doses. After a dose-ranging study and subsequent evaluation of the teratogenic properties of phencyclidine, Jordan et al. (1979) chose a nonteratogenic intraperitoneal dose of 10 mg PCP per kg with which to conduct a postnatal evaluation of the effects on the offspring. A dosing regimen of daily injections from gestational day 6 to day 15 produced a transient depression in maternal weight gain; however, by parturition these differences were no longer present. The experimental design utilized both nonfostered and cross-fostered experimental groups of rat pups. The results yielded mild yet measurable differences in several maturational and behavioral parameters. Emphasizing the importance of maternal health and behavior, all pups reared by dams treated with PCP during the gestational period tended to weigh less and to gain weight less rapidly than did control pups. Within one week after weaning, detectable differences in body weight were no longer seen. The fostering environment and possibly a prolonged exposure to PCP via the nursing dam seem to influence the appearance of standard developmental landmarks. The nonfostered drug-treated group showed a fairly consistent retardation of specific landmarks (eye opening, pina detachment, incisor eruption, and piliation). Overall, PCP produced only minimal effects on physical development, with no evidence of a uniform developmental retardation. Periodic examination of pup brains revealed no alterations in brain weight or volume, brain weight/body weight ratios, or gross brain morphology due to PCP exposure, regardless of the fostering environment.

No alterations were seen in the righting reflex of the pups or in the acquisition of locomotor skills (i.e., from no movement to pivoting, crawling, and walking) and climbing abilities. Subsequent experiments found that PCP delayed the initial appearance of these skills and delayed the transition between skill levels within each task. The group of nonfostered pups gestationally exposed to PCP seems to be considerably slower to develop locomotor skills and climbing ability.

The developmental effects of PCP in mice are similar to those in rats. Goodwin et al. (1980) exposed adult female Cox Swiss albino mice to phencyclidine at a dose of 5 mg/kg. Dosing began five days before mating and continued during both gestation and lactation. At the time of mating, no apparent effect was seen in the females. During gestation, from day 1 to day 17, each dam was given a daily subcutaneous injection of 5 mg PCP per kg body weight. The prenatal weight gain of the dams, the length of gestation or parturition, and the size and birth weight of the litters were not altered by drug exposure. All pups were cross-fostered within two hours of birth, and further investigation revealed no gross phencyclidine-induced alterations in maternal behavior. Physical development was unaltered, as measured by neonatal weight gain, the appearance of developmental landmarks, or the ontogeny of sensorimotor reflexes including the righting reflex, cliff-drop aversion, the visual placing response, or bar-holding ability. Observations of open-field behavior gave no indication of an increase in general ambulatory behavior; however, when mice were challenged with a single dose of PCP, an increase in rearing behavior was observed.

In 1983, Nicholas and Schreiber extended the examination of the developmental effects of PCP exposure by utilizing a dosing regimen including gestational and/or lactational exposure to PCP. ICR Swiss mice were given daily injections of 5, 10, or 20 mg PCP per kg body weight during gestation and/or lactation. From birth until weaning, the offspring were observed for the appearance of specific reflex behaviors using a modified version of the Fox battery (Fox 1965). The results indicated that there was a PCP-induced delay in the appearance of walking, crawling, and vibrissal placement and stroking. The righting reflex was decreased, and the disappearance of the cross-extensor reflex was delayed. The overall rate of growth was decreased in PCP-exposed animals until 15 days of age.

Nabeshima et al. reported the effects of phencyclidine on the behavioral development of rat offspring (1987, 1988). After the administration of a nonteratogenic dose of phencyclidine (10 mg/kg/day) on gestational days 7–21, there was a decrease in maternal weight gain, as well as a modest reduction in birth weights and body lengths, a decreased male/female ratio, and a moderate decrease in the viability of offspring. Gross morphological abnormalities were not observed after PCP exposure. Physical development of the offspring was not altered by phencyclidine exposure. Although there were alterations in a number of behavioral functional measurements (i.e., delay in the development of ambulation, negative geotaxis, bar-holding and rope-descending behaviors), these effects were transient and were no longer apparent within 1 week after birth.

Motor Activity

Further examination of the ontogeny of locomotor behavior of the rat and the influence of gestational exposure to PCP was conducted by Hutchings, Bodnarenko, and Diaz-DeLeon in 1984. Two dose levels below the teratogenic threshold were administered by gastric intubation to gravid rats during the last two weeks of gestation. At birth, treated and control litters were both fostered to normal lactating dams. Locomotor activity was measured as total litter activity until the pups were past the age of 30 days. There was a distinct ontogenic pattern of motor activity with increasing age. Offspring exposed to phencyclidine during gestation displayed identical patterns of motor development when compared with control offspring. When the rats reached 60 days of age, locomotor activity was measured in individual animals as the level of maze activity recorded during a ten-minute period. Both treated and control offspring displayed a sex difference in activity level, with females exhibiting a higher level of activity. A pattern of acclimation to the test situation was seen over the three-day test period. No difference was seen in the level or pattern of maze activity as a result of PCP exposure.

Fico and VanderWende (1988) also reported that neither PCP administration nor the treatment period had an effect on the total locomotor activity score as monitored by an activity meter for one hour. Alterations in motor activity were seen when prenatally exposed male mouse offspring were pharmacologically challenged with PCP. Following the same gestational dosing regimen as previously used, male offspring on postnatal days 34–36 received a subcutaneous injection of 0, 2.5, 5, or 7.5 mg phencyclidine hydrochloride per kg. Immediately after the injection, activity counts were recorded for one hour. Ataxia was simultaneously scored by observation for a total of 50 minutes. Prenatal exposure to phencyclidine had no effect on the postnatal drug-induced increases in activity following challenge with PCP on days 34–36. However, PCP challenge-induced ataxia was significantly increased in the offspring exposed to PCP during the late gestational period.

Aggressive Behavior

As mentioned earlier, Fico and VanderWende (1989a, 1989b) examined the half-life of gestationally administered phencyclidine in the CF-one mouse fetal central nervous system for two distinct treatment periods. Pregnant dams received a daily injection of 5, 10, or 20 mg PCP per kg body weight during a period in either midgestation (days 6–15) or late gestation (days 12–18). Within 14 hours of parturition, all pups were fostered to surrogate dams. Because the behavioral parameter to be examined, isolation-induced aggression, is a male-specific behavior, only male pups were maintained past postnatal day 21. On postnatal days 34–36, the male offspring were individually housed, and testing began on the following day. Testing continued until either the test male initiated a fight or 15 test days elapsed without a fighting episode. The percentage of animals that exhibited aggressive behavior was not influenced by gestational exposure to phencyclidine. No alterations were seen in the ontogeny of aggressive behavior or the intensity of fighting. It is of interest, however, that the stress of handling associated with treatment (by either drug or vehicle alone) exerted a profound influence on the aggressive behavior of all offspring.

Learning and Memory

In 1988, Nabeshima and co-workers published their findings on the effects of gestational phencyclidine exposure on learning and memory. Until this time, no published articles had addressed the issue of the possible long-term effects of gestational phencyclidine exposure on the cognitive functioning of adolescent or adult offspring. Phencyclidine in doses of either 10 or 20 mg/kg was intraperitoneally injected on days 7–17 of gestation. A second group of animals was given a dose of 10 mg/kg during gestational days 7–21. At four weeks of age, animals exposed to PCP showed an impaired retention in both a one-trial step-down passive avoidance task and a step-through active avoidance task. At seven weeks of age, the acquisition of an active avoidance behavior (pole climbing) was significantly disrupted in PCP-treated rats. These alterations cannot be attributed to a general alteration in pain threshold, since no treatment effect on pain response was seen as measured by tail-flick response. In a previous study, Nabeshima et al. (1987) had reported that an identical dosing regimen produced decreased brain and body weights. The subsequent study reported that these decreases were still evident even at four weeks of age (Nabeshima et al. 1988). The absolute weight of individual brain regions was decreased, with the exception of the striatum. Therefore, it seems as if the weights of specific brain regions are less influenced by PCP exposure than is overall body weight. Nabeshima and co-workers (1988) suggested the possibility that prenatal PCP exposure may impair the functioning of the cholinergic neuronal system via an activation of the serotonergic neuronal system. It must be noted, however, that the data collected from experiments utilizing challenges with pharmacological agents were collected from control adult mice, not gestationally exposed offspring. Therefore, conclusions about neurotransmitter involvement drawn from the reported 1988 data are speculations based upon adult PCP exposure.

Neurochemical Alterations

PCP exposure has been used to generate a rat model of affective disorders in which to examine alterations in neurotransmitter concentration. In this model both the male and the female of a mating pair were exposed to PCP. When the exposure was continued during the periods of gestation and lactation, alterations were seen in noradrenaline and dopamine concentrations in discrete brain regions (Tonge 1973a; Tonge and Leonard 1973). By three months of age, concentrations of noradrenaline were increased in the cortex and pons/medulla but decreased in the striatum and hypothalamus. Dopamine concentrations were also increased in the cortex and the pons/medulla. These alterations seemed to be permanent, as determinations made at either six or nine months of age were at similar concentrations. Examination of 5-hydroxytryptamine showed an increased concentration in various brain regions: striatum, thalamus, midbrain, pons/medulla, and amygdaloid bodies (Tonge 1973b). The concentration of its metabolite, 5-hydroxyindoleacetic acid, however, was increased only in the pons/medulla and was decreased in the hypothalamus (a region that showed no alteration in 5-hydroxytryptamine concentration). Although no gross behavioral changes were observed in these offspring, a systematic assessment of the behavior was not conducted, leaving the functional significance of these alterations unclear. When exposure to PCP continued throughout the 21-day gestational period of rats, an increase in the concentrations of acetylcholine and choline in the frontal cortex and striatum was observed (Howard 1988). When the exposure regimen was limited to a three-consecutive-day period during gestational days 9–20, Ali and co-workers (1988, 1989) reported no PCP-induced alterations in the muscarinic, cholinergic, or dopamine receptor binding sites of maternal or fetal brains. The concentrations of these neurotransmitters also were unaltered (Ali et al. 1988).

Phencyclidine-induced modifications in the ontogeny of the PCP receptor in gestationally exposed male offspring were examined by Ali et al. in 1988. PCP exposure (5 mg/kg, subcutaneous) during any of the later periods of three consecutive days between gestational days 9 and 20 significantly decreased the number of PCP binding sites in the fetal brain on gestational day 21; maternal values were unchanged. The down-regulation of PCP binding after gestational exposure to PCP may be associated with the receptor ontogeny. No effect on receptor binding was seen after early PCP exposure during gestational days 9–11 (Ali et al. 1989). When specific brain regions were examined on postnatal day 21, Fico and VanderWende (1989a, 1989b) demonstrated an increase on postnatal day 21 in the number of [³H]PCP binding sites in the cortex and striatum, but not in the hippocampus. This was apparently a transient increase; by postnatal day 35, the increase was no longer evident. It also could reflect prolonged PCP exposure via the maternal dam. No alteration was seen in dopaminergic, muscarinic, or cholinergic receptor binding or in the concentrations of these neurotransmitters.

Summary of the Results of Experimental Studies in Animals

Experimental studies have documented the structural teratogenic properties of phencyclidine and the behavioral alterations it induces during the preweaning and early postweaning stages of rodent development. Few studies have examined gestational PCP-induced neurochemical alterations. Studies of alterations induced by gestational exposure to phencyclidine have been limited in number, breadth of factors examined, and the length of time over which the animals were examined. According to the literature, there is little, if any, evidence to suggest that, in experimental models, gestational exposure to phencyclidine produces long-term alterations in the functioning of the exposed offspring. Although minimal effects have been reported, the limited depth of the literature does not allow solid conclusions to be drawn. Still yet to be examined are the possible subtle effects of gestational phencyclidine exposure on the cognitive functioning of the adult. A consensus seems to be that gestational exposure to subteratogenic doses of PCP produces mild, if any, long-term alterations in the functioning of the offspring. The most promising lead stems from the observations made by Ali and co-workers (1988, 1989) of a selective down-regulation of the PCP receptor in offspring in the absence of maternal alterations. However, experiments have yet to be reported that are specifically designed to examine the subtle changes that could be present as a result of gestational exposure to phencyclidine.

CLINICAL STUDIES OF PCP ABUSE DURING THE PRENATAL PERIOD

There is a dearth of published information discussing the effects of PCP upon the developing fetus and the long-term developmental consequences of prenatal PCP exposure. However, PCP has been detected in human amniotic fluid (Kaufman et al. 1983; Petrucha, Kaufman, and Pitts 1982; Strauss, Modanlu, and Bosu 1981). It also has been found to accumulate in the placenta of treated mice and to cross into the fetus (Chari-Bitron et al. 1979). Fetal blood levels are ten times greater than maternal levels after acute administration in the mouse (Nicholas, Lipshitz, and Schreiber 1982) and pig (Cooper, Cummings, and Jones 1977). Based on these findings, one would expect that PCP affects the developing central nervous system; in fact, Jordan et al. (1979) found that pups from dams treated during pregnancy with nonteratogenic doses showed delayed development. More specifically, the pups showed delayed development even in simple behavioral skills such as locomotion and climbing. Furthermore, some prenatally PCP-exposed offspring observed for 60 days were unable to accomplish specific motor tasks, suggesting permanent deficits. Goodwin et al. (1980) showed that prenatal PCP exposure caused significantly increased behavioral activity in mice at 60 days of age. These findings support the notion that prenatal exposure to PCP does have harmful effects that can be observed in laboratory animals.

In 1980, Golden, Sokol, and Rubin were the first to document placental transfer of PCP in humans through a clinical description of a neonate's neurobehavioral symptoms. This infant's mother had smoked an average of six joints of marijuana dusted with PCP per day. The baby's behaviors emerging shortly after birth included extreme jitteriness, coarse flapping movements in response to slight auditory or tactile stimuli, nystagmus, poor visual tracking, and hypertonicity. At two months of age, the infant continued to exhibit coarse tremors, roving eye movements, and hypertonicity. Furthermore, the child had dysmorphic features. Subsequent to this report, Strauss, Modanlou, and Bosu (1981) described two other infants who had been exposed prenatally to PCP. These newborns also displayed signs of irritability, tremulousness, and increased muscle tone; however, no congenital anomalies were noted.

Chasnoff et al. (1983) described the behavior of seven infants whose mothers used PCP daily throughout pregnancy, in addition to using various other drugs intermittently. As compared with a control group of 27 infants, the PCP-exposed newborns had rapid changes in level of consciousness, exhibiting lethargy alternating with irritability. Further-

Table 11.2. Characteristics of 49 Newborns Exposed Prenatally to PCP

| | Number of Newborns | | | |
Study	Total	Preterm	SGA[a]	Full-term
Howard et al. 1986	12	7	0	5
Tabor et al. 1989	37	2	12	23

[a] Infants born small for gestational age (SGA) are from the full-term sample.

more, these infants were very sensitive to auditory stimuli and also evidenced tremors and facial grimacing.

In 1986, Howard, Kropenske, and Tyler described the clinical characteristics of 12 newborns and their mothers, whose primary drug of abuse during pregnancy was PCP. More recently, Tabor, Smith-Wallace, and Yonekura (1989) compared the characteristics of offspring of 37 women who abused PCP during pregnancy with behaviors of children whose mothers preferred cocaine.

These 49 mothers were similar with regard to the following areas: all had low incomes, the majority were single, and most were members of ethnic minority groups. Over 65% received inadequate prenatal care. Table 11.2 summarizes the newborns' status in terms of preterm delivery (<37 weeks gestation), small size for gestational age (<10% in weight at full-term birth), and full-term delivery.

The complexity of unraveling the causes for the prematurity and/or growth retardation in utero of these newborns is obvious, since poor prenatal care, polysubstance abuse, alcohol use, and nicotine use all interfere with gestation and growth in utero (Brar and Rutherford 1988; Carlson 1988; Finnegan 1985; Keirse 1984; Streissguth et al. 1981). In 1989, Tabor, Smith-Wallace, and Yonekura found that prenatally PCP-exposed infants were likely to be born less prematurely than were cocaine-exposed infants. However, they also noted that 32.4% of their PCP-exposed infants were born small for gestational age, as compared with 18.9% of their cocaine-exposed infants.

Almost 100% of the 49 newborns reported in the programs described above exhibited tremors within 48 hours after delivery. Hypertonicity and irritability occurred in approximately 50%. Autonomic nervous system symptoms, including diarrhea, vomiting, and/or temperature instability, were seen in less than 20%.

Treatment of the newborns' symptoms ranged from 58% in the first 12 cases reported (Howard, Kropenske, and Tyler 1986) to 5% in the 41 cases comprising our ongoing longitudinal research project. This treatment pattern reflects a shift in focus from our initial response, which was to calm the infants medically through the use of diazepam, phenobarbital, or paregoric, to a less dramatic response utilizing environmental manipulation (i.e., swaddling, use of pacifiers, and decreased noise).

The interpretation of the observed neonatal behaviors as they relate to future functioning is unclear. Are these temporary behaviors, reflecting withdrawal symptoms similar to those seen in adults? Or will they eventually tie in with future developmental problems?

Growth Parameters

In another study, Howard and colleagues (currently in progress) are evaluating the long-term growth and developmental outcomes in 41 children whose mothers' primary drug of abuse throughout pregnancy was PCP. All 41 mothers abused PCP; however, 67% also reported cocaine use during pregnancy. These women and children were compared with a non-drug-using group of women and their offspring. The 41 infants who are enrolled in the longitudinal study at UCLA have been compared on the basis of height, weight, and head circumference with infants of mothers in the non-drug-using control group. The physical growth scales employed are those published by the National Center for Health Statistics, using percentiles based on the work of Hamill and colleagues (1979).

At 15 months, the drug-exposed infant group had a mean head circumference and weight that were less than those for the control group with a statistical significance at $p < .01$. This finding is worrisome, because a head circumference that is disproportionately less than a child's height is cause for concern regarding interference with brain growth.

The Developmental Outcomes of Infants

For determination of developmental outcomes in children younger than three years of age, standardized tests have been administered in a

Table 11.3. Gesell Developmental Evaluation of 11 Infants at 16.6 Months (± 2)

Developmental Area	Developmental Quotient
Gross motor	108
Fine motor	78
Adaptive	84
Language	90
Personal-social	97
Aggregate score	94

Table 11.4. Gesell Developmental Evaluation of Eight Children at 35 Months (± 4)

Developmental Area	Developmental Quotient
Gross motor	103
Fine motor	97
Adaptive	90
Language	88
Personal-social	111
Aggregate score	100

structured fashion. These measures include the Bayley Scales of Infant Development and the Gesell Developmental Evaluation (Gesell and Amatruda 1954), whereby the infants' and young children's gross motor, fine motor, adaptive, language, and personal-social behaviors are assessed and scored. This provides a developmental age (DA) and a developmental quotient (DQ) for each behavioral area (ascertained by dividing the chronological age into the developmental age for each of the five areas of behavior), as well as an aggregate DA and DQ. For those infants who were born preterm, correction for gestational age is made at least until 24 months. The average DQ is 100.

In a clinical follow-up of 11 children exposed prenatally to PCP, the Gesell Developmental Evaluation was administered repeatedly. The findings at a mean age of 16.6 months are described in table 11.3, and the DQs of 8 of those children at a mean age of 35 months are listed in table 11.4.

The results of these developmental evaluations appear deceptively benign. Unfortunately, the quality of a child's individual performance is not within the purview of the assessment measure. Almost all of the children in the previous follow-up clinically demonstrated problem behaviors in fine motor, language, and personal-social areas of development. Almost all displayed fine motor incoordination, including fine tremors, splayed and extended fingers, and/or overshooting of the hand in tasks requiring eye-hand coordination. Speech was generally indistinct and difficult to understand, and attention spans were short. Distractibility and poor social interaction skills, as seen in PCP-exposed adults (Lewis and Hordan 1986), were major problems that could later interfere with the children's ability to attend in educational and social situations.

In studies of the developmental course of infants and young children who have been exposed prenatally to PCP, these children demonstrate behaviors that are difficult to categorize. During early infancy, they have increased muscle tone and a strong tendency to maintain an asymmetrical posture, which at times gives the appearance that these infants are avoiding direct gaze with the examiner. By nine months of age, fine motor movements are jerky, with fingers extended and splayed (Howard, Kropenske, and Tyler 1986). As more complex cognitive, social, and language behaviors emerge during the second year of life, these infants appear dull, with flat affect. In addition, they continue to demonstrate minimal meaningful vocalizations and poor gestural communication (H. Chipman, personal communication, 1989). However, the more traditional developmental milestones observed by practitioners (e.g., sitting, crawling, and walking) are reached at normal times.

The developmental sequence observed in children exposed prenatally to PCP corresponds to some behaviors noted in adults who have abused this drug. Adult PCP users show affective distrubances, poor reflective thinking, and poor problem-solving skills, even while IQ scores may remain within the normal range (Lewis and Hordan 1986). Since PCP has been observed to interfere with higher cortical functioning in more advanced species, including humans, one would anticipate that children exposed prenatally to PCP will demonstrate difficulties in abstract thinking, affective behaviors, and organized play activities, rather than gross congenital malformations of the organ systems, including the brain. This view is corroborated by the children's normal scores on standardized structured developmental tests.

Howard and colleagues were convinced that the structured developmental tests they used were not identifying the children's disabilities. Their clinical observations of the children while placed in nonstructured situations with toys indicated disorganized attempts at play and poorly executed social interactions. In addition, the children frequently made purposeless movements about the room and only limited vocalizations.

Normal development is characterized by the organization and integration of social, emotional, and cognitive abilities; therefore, a standardized measure assessing such skills in young children during play was used (Ungerer and Sigman 1983). In addition, to distinguish the effect of environment upon the child's developmental performance, investigators assessed security and insecurity in the attachment relationship between child and caregiver using a standardized paradigm, the Strange Situation (Ainsworth et al. 1978). A sample of 18 toddlers (18 months old) who had been prenatally exposed to a variety of drugs, including PCP, cocaine, heroin, and methadone, was selected. The results of their developmental scores, play events, and attachment behaviors were compared with those of a group of 57 preterm infants who had not experienced prenatal exposure to drugs. All of these preterm children had ventilatory assistance after birth, and the two groups were matched according to socioeconomic status.

The drug-exposed toddlers differed from the preterm group in the following ways: (1) in structured tasks the drug-exposed group performed at the low end of the average range; (2) in self-initiated play the drug-exposed toddlers showed more serious delays with regard to goal-directedness, organization, and self-regulation; (3) the majority of the drug-exposed toddlers had insecure relationships with their caregivers; and (4) insecurity of attachment exacerbated the drug-exposed toddlers' difficulties with organization and purposefulness (Rodning, Beckwith, and Howard 1989).

In Howard and colleagues' current research project involving the 41 PCP-exposed infants and the non-drug-exposed control group, the drug-exposed children are scoring in a similar consistent fashion—that is, they have lower overall developmental scores, and show evidence of neurological dysfunction including poor fine motor coordination and an inability to communicate appropriately, either through vocalization or gestures.

The researchers do not think that the developmental problems observed in the children are entirely due to their environments. All children have received, from birth, ongoing health care and home-based intervention services from social workers, public health nurses, and/or early childhood educators.

No doubt there is a continuum of problems in children who have been exposed prenatally to PCP. These problems may range from aborted fetuses, to obvious disabilities, to subtle behavioral dysfunction, to a few children who seem resilient and demonstrate normal development. Based on this research, Howard and colleagues conclude that the majority of children do not escape the deleterious effects of prenatal substance exposure, despite comprehensive and consistent intervention. Even though the children are scoring in the low normal range on the structured developmental evaluation, they once again are demonstrating disorganized and inappropriate behaviors in the independent, nonstructured play situation. Through an open-field or nonstructured test, the toddlers' higher cortical function, which controls organized and meaningful play, is revealed. The structured setting, which provides strict guidelines about use of specific test items and allows the examiner to model appropriate behaviors for the child, may be tapping developmental function on a less complex level.

CONCLUSIONS

As Domino stated (1980), PCP is a "bastard" drug that, despite its auspicious beginnings, now is extracting a heavy cost from society. It is only as we are able to compare infants and young children exposed to PCP with non-drug-exposed groups that the reality of its deleterious effects upon the children's development can become fully understood.

This represents a new frontier for study. Is it possible that some children will improve once higher centers of learning have matured? Or will we continue to see dysfunction in the growing child, similar to that observed in some adults who have abused PCP?

This information will be forthcoming as researchers in the field collaborate regarding their findings. Ultimately, by identifying these children's specific behavioral difficulties, clinical practitioners from the fields of medicine, social work, public health, education, drug treatment, and psychology will be able to develop coordinated efforts to serve these children and families appropriately and help them attain their full developmental potential.

REFERENCES

Ahmad, G. 1987. Abuse of phencyclidine (PCP): A laboratory experience. *Clin Toxicol* 25:341–46.

Ahmad, G., Halsall, L. C., and Bondy, S. C. 1987. Persistence of phencyclidine in fetal brain. *Brain Res* 415:194–96.

Ainsworth, M., Blehar, M., Waters, E., and Wall, F. 1978. *Patterns of Attachment*. Hillsdale, N. J.: Lawrence Erlbaum Associates.

Ali, S. F., Ahmad, G., Slikker, W., and Bondy, S. C. 1988. Gestational exposure to phencyclidine (PCP) in rats decreases PCP binding sites in term fetal brain. *Int J Dev Neurosci* 6:547–52.

————. 1989. Effects of gestational exposure to phencyclidine: Distribution and neurochemical alterations in maternal and fetal brain. *Neuro toxicology* 10:383–92.

Brar, H. S., and Rutherford, S. W. 1988. Classification of intrauterine growth retardation. *Semin Perinatol* 12:2–10.

Carlson, D. E. 1988. Maternal diseases associated with intrauterine growth retardation. *Semin Perinatol* 12:17–22.

Chari-Bitron, A., Simon, G. A., Kadar, T., and Motola, L. 1979. Whole body autoradiography of ^{3}H-phencyclidine in mice. *Arch Toxicol* 43:85–92.

Chasnoff, I. J., Burns, W. J., Hatcher, R. P., and Burns, K. A. 1983. Phencyclidine: Effects on the fetus and neonate. *Dev Pharmacol Ther* 6:404–8.

Cooper, J. E., Cummings, A. J., and Jones, H. 1977. The placental transfer of phencyclidine in the pig: Plasma levels in the sow and its piglets. *J Physiol* 267:17–20.

Crider, R. 1986. Phencyclidine: Changing abuse patterns. In *Phencyclidine: An Update*, ed. D. H. Clouet. *NIDA Res Monogr* 64:163–73.

Cummings, A. J. 1979. Transplacental disposition of phencyclidine in the pig. *Xenobiotica* 9:447–52.

Domino, E. F. 1980. History and pharmacology of PCP and PCP-related analogs. *J Psychedelic Drugs* 12(3–4):223–27.

————. 1981a. Abnormal mental states induced by phencyclidine as a model of schizophrenia. In *PCP (Phencyclidine): Historical and Current Perspectives*, ed. E. F. Domino, 401–18. Ann Arbor, Mich.: NPP Books.

————. 1981b. *Phencyclidine: Historical and Current Perspectives*, 537–69. Ann Arbor, Mich.: NPP Books.

Durfee, M. 1986. Los Angeles County neonatal withdrawal reports, Child Abuse Prevention Program. January–December.

Fico, T. A., and VanderWende, C. 1988. Phencyclidine during pregnancy: Fetal brain levels and neurobehavioral effects. *Neurotoxicol Teratol* 10:349–54.

———. 1989a. Effects of prenatal phencyclidine on ³H-PCP binding and PCP-induced motor activity and ataxia. *Neurotoxicol Teratol* 11:373–76.

———. 1989b. Phencyclidine during pregnancy: Behavioral and neurochemical effects in the offspring. *Ann NY Acad Sci* 562:319–26.

Finnegan, L. 1985. Smoking and its effect on pregnancy and the newborn. In *The At-Risk Infant: Psycho/Social/Medical Aspects*, ed. S. Harel and N. J. Anastasiow, 127–36. Baltimore: Paul H. Brookes Publishing.

Fox, M. W. 1965. Reflex-ontogeny and behavioral development in the mouse. *Animal Behav* 13:234–41.

Gesell, A., and Amatruda, C. S. 1954. *Developmental Diagnosis*. New York: Hoeber.

Golden, N. L., Sokol, R. J., and Rubin, L. L. 1980. Angel dust: Possible effects on the fetus. *Pediatrics* 65:18–20.

Goodwin, P. J., Perez, V. J., Eatwell, J. C., Palet, J. L., and Jaworski, M. T. 1980. Phencyclidine: Effects of chronic administration in the female mouse on gestation, maternal behavior, and the neonate. *Psychopharmacology* 69:63–67.

Gorelick, D. A., Wilkins, J. N., and Wong, C. 1986. Diagnosis and treatment of chronic phencyclidine (PCP) abuse. In *Phencyclidine: An Update*, ed. D. H. Clouet. *NIDA Res Monogr* 64:218–28.

Green, J. O. 1983. Los Angeles County street ethnography study: Final report. Public Health Foundation of Los Angeles County, California.

Hamill, P. V., Drizd, R. A., Johnson, C. L., Reed, R. B., Roche, A. F., and Moore, W. M. 1979. Physical growth: National Center for Health and Statistics percentiles. *Am J Clin Nutr* 32:607–29.

Howard, J., Kropenske, V., and Tyler, R. 1986. The long-term effects on neurodevelopment in infants exposed prenatally to PCP. In *Phencyclidine: An Update*, ed. D. H. Clouet. *NIDA Res Monogr* 64:237–51.

Howard, S. G. 1988. The effect of prenatal exposure to phencyclidine on the postnatal development of the cholinergic system in rat brain. *Abstr Neurotoxicol* 18.

Husson, B. S. 1984. Trends and epidemiology of drug abuse in Los Angeles County, California, 1980–1983. In *Epidemiology and Drug Abuse: Trends in Selected Cities*. Vol. 1, 84–107. Rockville, Md.: National Institute for Drug Abuse.

Hutchings, D. E., Bodnarenko, S. R., and Diaz-DeLeon, R. 1984. Phencyclidine during pregnancy in the rat: Effects on locomotor activity in the offspring. *Pharmacol Biochem Behav* 20:251–54.

Jasinski, D. R., Shannon, H. E., Cone, E. J., Vaupel, D. B., Risner, M. E., McQuinn, R. L., Su, T. P., and Pickworth, W. B. 1981. Interdisciplinary studies on phencyclidine. In *PCP (Phencyclidine): Historical and Current Perspectives*, ed. E. F. Domino, 331–400. Ann Arbor, Mich.: NPP Books.

Jordan, R. L., Young, T. R., Dinwiddie, S. H., and Harry, G. J. 1979. Phencyclidine-induced morphological and behavioral alterations in the neonatal rat. *Pharmacol Biochem Behav (Suppl)* 11:39–45.

Kaufman, K. R., Petrucha, R. A., Pitts, F. N., and Weekes, M. E. 1983. Phencyclidine in amniotic fluid and breast milk: A case report. *J Clin Psychiatry* 44:269–70.

Keirse, M. J. 1984. Epidemiology and aetiology of the growth-retarded baby. *Clin Obstet Gynecol* 11:415–36.

Lewis, J. E., and Hordan, R. B. 1986. Neuropsychological assessment of the phencyclidine abuser. In *Phencyclidine: An Update*, ed. D. H. Clouet. *NIDA Res Monogr* 64:190–208.

Luby, E. D., Cohen, B. D., Rosenbaum, G., Gottlieb, J., and Kelly, R. 1959. Study of a new schizophrenomimetic drug—Sernyl. *AMA Arch Neurol Psychiatry* 81:363–69.

McCarron, M. M. 1986. Phencyclidine intoxication. In *Phencyclidine: An Update*, ed. D. H. Clouet. *NIDA Res Monogr* 64:209–17.

McCarron, M. M., Schulze, B. W., Thompson, G. A., Condor, M. C., and Goetz, W. A. 1986. Acute phencyclidine intoxication: Incidence of clinical findings in 1,000 cases. *Ann Emerg Med* 10:237–42.

Marks, T. A., Worthy, W. C., and Staples, R. E., 1980. Teratogenic potential of phencyclidine in the mouse. *Teratology* 21:241–46.

Miller, J. D., Cisin, I. H., Gardner-Keaton, H., Hanell, A. V., and Fishburne, P. M. 1983. *National Survey on Drug Abuse: Main Findings 1982*, 48. Washington, D.C.: U.S. Government Printing Office. Department of Health, Education, and Welfare (DHEW) Publication (ADM) 83-1263.

Mistra, A. L., Pontani, R. B., and Bartolomeo, J. 1979. Persistence of phencyclidine and metabolite in brain and adipose tissue: Implications for long-lasting behavioral effects. *Res Commun Chem Pathol Pharmacol* 24:431–45.

Nabeshima, T., Hiramatsu, M., Yamaguchi, K., Kasugai, M., Ishizaki, K., Kawashima, K., Itoh, K., Ogawa, S., Katoh, A., Furukawa, H., and Kameyama, T. 1988. Effects of prenatal administration of phencyclidine on the learning and memory processes of rat offspring. *J Pharmacobio dyn* 11:816–23.

Nabeshima, T., Yamaguchi, K., Hiramatsu, M., Ishikawa, K., Furukawa, H., and Kameyama, T. 1987. Effects of prenatal and perinatal administration of phencyclidine on the behavioral development of rat offspring. *Pharmacol Biochem Behav* 28:411–18.

Nicholas, J. M., Lipshitz, J., and Schreiber, E. C. 1982. Phencyclidine: Its transfer across the placenta as well as into breast milk. *Am J Obstet Gynecol* 143:143–46.

Nicholas, J. M., and Schreiber, E. C. 1983. Phencyclidine exposure and the developing mouse: Behavioral teratological implications. *Teratology* 28:319–26.

Petrucha, R. A., Kaufman, K. R., and Pitts, F. N. 1982. Phencyclidine in pregnancy: A case report. *J Reprod Med* 27:301–3.

Rodning, C., Beckwith, L., and Howard, J. 1989. Characteristics of attachment and play organization in prenatally drug-exposed toddlers. *Dev Psychopathol* 1:277–89.

Silber, T. J., Iosefsohn, M., Hicks, J. M., Getson, P. R., and O'Donnell, R. 1988. Prevalence of PCP use among adolescent marijuana users. *J Pediatr* 112:827–29.

Sircar, R., and Zukin, S. R. 1983. Ontogeny of sigma opiate/PCP binding sites in rat brain. *Life Sci* 33:255–57.

Strauss, A. A., Modanlou, H. D., and Bosu, S. K. 1981. Neonatal manifestations of maternal phencyclidine (PCP) abuse. *Pediatrics* 68:550–52.

Street talk: A glossary of street names for drugs. 1988. *Adolescent Counselor*, June/July, p. 11.

Streissguth, A. P., Martin, D. C., Martin, J. C., and Barr, H. M. 1981. The Seattle longitudinal prospective study on alcohol and pregnancy. *J Behav Toxicol Teratol* 3:223–33.

Tabor, B. L., Smith-Wallace, T., and Yonekura, M. L. Perinatal outcome associated with PCP versus cocaine use. *Am J Drug Alcohol Abuse*. In press.

Tonge, S. R. 1973a. Neurochemical teratology: 5-Hydroxyindole concentrations in discrete areas of rat brain after the pre- and neonatal administration of phencyclidine and imipramine. *Life Sci* 12 (Part 1):481–86.

―――. 1973b. Catecholamine concentrations in discrete areas of the rat brain after the pre- and neonatal administration of phencyclidine and imipramine. *J Pharm Pharmacol* 25:164–65.

Tonge, S. R., and Leonard, B. E. 1973. Some persistent effects of the pre- and neonatal administration of psychotropic drugs on noradrenaline metabolism in discrete areas of rat brain. *Br J Pharmacol* 48:364–65.

Ungerer, J. A., and Sigman, M. 1983. Developmental lags in preterm infants from one to three years of age. *Child Dev* 54:1217–28.

Yago, K. B., Pitts, F. N., Jr., Burgoyne, R. W., Aniline, O., Yago, L. S., and Pitts, A. F. 1981. The urban epidemic of phencyclidine (PCP) use: Clinical and laboratory evidence from a public psychiatric hospital emergency service. *J Clin Psychiatry* 42:193–96.

12

The Effects of Maternal Use of Tobacco Products or Amphetamines on Offspring

Joan C. Martin, Ph.D

THIS CHAPTER focuses on the amphetamines, central nervous system (CNS) activators par excellence, and tobacco, the most widely abused drug of this class, as models for agents that cause similar behavioral, neurochemical, and morphological effects.

TOBACCO PRODUCTS AND FETAL EFFECTS

The Varieties of Tobacco Products

Nicotine, Tars, and Smoke

Although smoking is on the decline in this country, far fewer woman manage to stop smoking during their pregnancies than stop drinking (Rubin, Craig, and Gavin 1986). Since tobacco and alcohol are both addictive drugs, perhaps the pervasive advertising, with its focus on young, attractive people, plays a role in this failure. Smoking is negatively correlated with level of education, which is not true of alcohol use (Kruse, LeFevre, and Zweig 1986), and advertising is more persuasive with less-educated individuals.

Most studies in animal models of the effects of prenatal exposure to tobacco have used nicotine, as it is the primary toxic agent in tobacco, although carbon monoxide and dioxide, cyanide, and over 450 other compounds in tobacco are toxic to some degree (Jarvik 1973). Compelling evidence for nicotine as the addictive agent was reviewed in a Surgeon General's report in 1988. Nicotine causes a marked reduction in uterine blood flow and in intrauterine oxygen tension (Hammer, Goldman, and Mitchell 1981). Nicotine and tar levels are positively correlated in cigarettes, so it is difficult to separate out the effects of each in human smokers, although this can be accomplished easily in animal models. Smoke inhalation has been used in several studies, although it suffers from the drawback that the animal is rendered somewhat hypoxic through this method. In his annotated bibliography on smoking and reproduction, Abel (1984) cited 30 studies that administered nicotine to the gravid animal, 9 that used smoke inhalation, and 8 that administered other constituents of tobacco such as cotinine, the tobacco stalk and plant, carbon monoxide, cigarette smoke condensate, ethylnitrosourea, and diethylnitrosamine.

Chewing Tobacco and Snuff

The only published studies on the effects of the use of smokeless tobacco in pregnant humans are from third-world countries, where the practice is more popular than it is in more-developed areas. This method of tobacco administration is on the rise in the United States and may pose a threat to fetal health in a few years. The results of the published studies are similar to those of cigarette smoking (e.g., increased rates of stillbirths and spontaneous abortions as compared with control groups of nonusers) (Krishna 1978; Vaisrub 1979).

Passive Smoke or Particle Inhalation

There have been several tantalizing studies on women who worked in poorly ventilated tobacco factories and exhibited increased rates of spontaneous abortion (Gavrilescu 1973; Athayde 1948; Mgalobeli 1931). I can recall discussing our results of increased resorptions in the rat with a chemist in a tobacco company laboratory, and his reply was that he was not surprised. They had performed a study on women who worked in their factories and found increased rates of spontaneous abortions as compared with their peers who did not work in the factories. I never saw this study in print.

The Maternal Effects

Smoking women and nicotine-exposed rodents gain less weight during pregnancy, which is partially due to reduced food consumption. Gravid rats exposed to tobacco smoke deliver offspring whose body and organ weights are significantly reduced compared with those of offspring whose dams were pair-fed to the smoke-exposed dams, indicating that tobacco constituents have an effect in addition to reduced food intake (Haworth and Ford 1972). Such dams and humans have an increased rate of either resorptions or spontaneous abortions dependent upon the species (Kline et al. 1977). The increased risk has been linked to placental insufficiency (Rowell and Clark 1982), retarded placental growth (Garrett 1975), and placental infarctions. The evidence for premature delivery is less certain, and the small and undergrown infants are, in all likelihood, small for gestational age rather than premature (Surgeon General's Report 1980); however, investigators continue to report evidence for prematurity when the length of gestation is controlled (Hoff, Wertelecki, and Blackburn 1986). Rat deliveries, in contrast, are significantly delayed after nicotine exposure (Becker, King, and Little 1968; Becker and Martin 1971; Martin et al. 1976). This may be a species difference, as third-trimester exposure to nicotine in the mouse causes earlier deliveries (Nasrat, Al-Hachim, and Mahmood 1986).

The Effects on Offspring

Structure and Viability

There is an increased risk of stillbirth or neonatal death for the infants of women who smoke. Abruptio placentae is postulated as one of the causal factors (Goujard et al. 1978). This incidence of abruptio placentae is dose related, and primarily low-birth-weight infants are affected, as described by Steele and Langworth (1966), Meyer and Tonascia (1977), and investigators in places as diverse as India, Northern Finland, Paris, New Haven, Boston, California, and Maryland. Smoking also increases the risk of sudden infant death syndrome (SIDS) (Bergman and Wiesner 1976; Naeye 1978; Naeye, Ladis, and Drage 1976).

Until recently, there was little indication that maternal smoking resulted in teratogenic effects, perhaps because most studies were not large enough to show an effect. Now there is evidence from the Collaborative Perinatal Project for a greater incidence of anencephaly, and animal models have shown increases in lung abnormalities (Wang et al. 1984); skeletal abnormalities, primarily of the limbs (Keeler et al. 1981; Aro 1983); and cardiovascular abnormalities (Fazel and Goeringer 1983). DeMarini (1980, 1983) reported that cigarette smoke condensate was mutagenic and induced chromosome aberrations and cell transformation in vitro. However, present evidence, or the lack of it, suggests that smoking is unlikely to be responsible for a large increase in malformations at birth. This means that functional deficits may often be masked because the children of smoking mothers do not look different.

Neurological and Neurochemical Effects

Receptor sites for specific actions of psychoactive drugs appear very early in fetal life, and hence drug interaction with receptor sites can affect the biochemical parameters of the transmitter system involved (Lichtensteiger and Schlumpf 1987). DNA and protein levels in fetal brain are reduced, which may lead to developmental delay postnatally (Hudson, Merrill, and Sands 1974).

Maternal exposure to cigarette smoke resulted in deficits in whole brain and cerebellar weights in neonatal rats, with decreases in hippocampal cells (Barnes et al. 1981); reduction in cell number in the hindbrain (Haworth and Ford 1972); brainstem injury in the form of fewer cells in the medulla, with implications for sudden infant death syndrome (Krous et al. 1981); lower rates of brain protein synthesis in newborn rats exposed to nicotine in utero (Sershen et al. 1982); suppression of DNA synthesis in rat brain postnatally after prenatal nicotine exposure (Slotkin, Greer, and Faust 1986); and increases in adrenergic receptor binding in rat cerebral cortex in male offspring only (Peters 1984).

I located only one human study, which analyzed the data from the U.S. Collaborative Perinatal Project and found clinical implications for subtle brainstem alterations in children born to smoking mothers (Elliott 1979). It is not known which of the described neural and neurochemical alterations cause the concomitant functional deficits that continue past the neonatal period.

Growth and Development

The early postnatal period is the most thoroughly studied in both humans and animal models, perhaps for economic as well as theoretical reasons. Abel (1983a) devoted an entire chapter to this topic. Human studies have been almost entirely confined to birth weight data, and there have been hundreds of these since Simpson's first report of over 7,000 women in 1957. All of these studies reported that birth weights were negatively correlated with increasing numbers of cigarettes smoked. The curve is displaced downward for blacks (Niswander and Gordon 1972; Lubs 1973). Miller and Jekel (1987) found that, although low birth weight occurred more often in blacks, smoking had less of an effect than did adverse maternal practices. A few studies, notably the Queen's Birthday Study (also known as the British Perinatal Study), followed the children to older ages (Butler, Goldstein, and Ross 1972; Butler and Goldstein 1973). The male, but not female, children were still significantly shorter in height at age 16 (Fogelman 1980).

A smaller study on Finnish children found that male children were still significantly shorter at age 14, although differences in height were extremely small (Rantakallio 1983). That this smaller size is due to components in the tobacco and not to self-selection factors has been supported by studies on animal models and by studies of women who smoked during one pregnancy but not another and whose infants were differentially affected (Naeye 1981). Animal investigations, which were usually performed on rodents, showed decreased birth weight and transient growth deficits, which disappeared by 60 days of age (Martin and Becker 1971; Martin et al. 1976; Martin, J. et al. 1979), or growth-retarded fetuses when the offspring were not carried to term (Younoszai, Peloso, and Haworth 1969; Bassi et al. 1984).

Maturation, as measured by developmental batteries in neonatal animals or motor, reflexive, and perceptual tests for infants and young children (e.g., the Brazelton), has been studied extensively. We found maturational differences after the administration of moderately high doses of nicotine to the rat; the doses were empirically selected to yield underweight, immature newborns equivalent to those produced by smoking women. The dose levels typical of human consumption (e.g., 0.5, 1.0, or 1.5 mg/kg) typically do not result in underweight rodent offspring. It is not surprising that differences in outcome measures are often nonsignificant in studies in which these amounts are administered.

Methamphetamine and amphetamine, which have CNS effects similar to those of nicotine, have more detrimental effects on developmental delay, offspring weight reduction, and change in neonatal activity levels. One other difference is length of gestation. Methamphetamine-exposed dams deliver prematurely, whereas nicotine-exposed rat mothers have extended gestational periods. Nicotine-exposed newborn rats exhibited some of the features typical of the human postmaturity syndrome, including meconium staining and a wrinkled, undernourished appearance. Other features, however, were typical of premature deliveries (e.g., delayed ossification, shorter vibrissae, and shorter claws). The nicotine-exposed offspring were described as immature postmature pups (Becker, King, and Little 1968; Becker and

Martin 1971; Martin et al. 1976), whereas amphetamine-exposed animals were true premature pups.

Krsiak (1973) administered a low dose of nicotine (0.25 mg/kg) to Wistar rats during the 21-day gestational period and found significant delays in incisor eruption, righting on day one of life, eye opening on postnatal day 11, and rearing on day 13. We found delays in ear pinnae uncurling on day 3 and righting from a vertical drop on day 13 (Martin 1982; Martin et al. 1982).

Two-day-old human infants of smoking mothers exhibited better learning on two operant tasks as compared to infants of drinking mothers, drinking and smoking mothers, and nonsmoking and nondrinking mothers. This may have been due to the simplicity of these paradigms, which rewarded a more rapid rate of response rather than indicating a real cognitive difference. Activity levels were not measured in these infants, and a higher activity level could explain the results. When initial baseline measurements were taken before conditioning, the effects of maternal smoking were detrimental. The infants of smoking mothers had longer latencies to the initiation of sucking on a nonnutritive nipple, took longer to complete the required schedule, and exerted less pressure than did control infants (Martin, D., et al. 1979). However, with the addition of dextrose water reinforcement, the nicotine-exposed infants overcame these problems and outperformed the infants of nonsmoking mothers on two simple tasks. A weak suck is usually indicative of an infant at some risk. Picone (1980) found that babies of smoking mothers had increased auditory thresholds and poorer performance on neonatal neurobehavioral tasks, particularly those related to autonomic regulation. There is strong evidence, then, that exposure to tobacco products in utero alters the neurochemistry of brain so as to retard development. Studies on older animals could reveal whether these effects are transitory or irreversible.

Voluntary Activity

Assessments of postnatal activity are fewer in number. A retrospective study of clinically diagnosed hyperactive children indicated that significantly more of their mothers had smoked during pregnancy as compared with mothers of dyslexic children and children who were in the clinic for unrelated reasons (Denson, Nanson, and McWatters 1975). These mothers had continued to smoke heavily, so prenatal and postnatal effects were confounded.

Peters, Taub, and Tang (1979) found that cross-fostering the rat did not attenuate the increased activity in the light at puberty (60–80 days of age) that follows nicotine exposure in utero. The rat is a nocturnal animal and is more active in the dark, so group differences might be masked in the dark. Baer, McClearn, and Wilson (1980) found depressed open-field activity in neonatal mice to whose dams tobacco smoke had been administered. The open-field test is a complex measure, and performance cannot readily be separated from factors of "emotionality" or "timidity." We used the Wahmann activity wheel and found increased voluntary activity in offspring at 50–60 days of age after nicotine administration to the dams during pregnancy and the nursing period, but not when the drug exposure was during pregnancy alone. However, these effects were also found in animals exposed to hypoxic episodes during the gestational period alone. Effects in nicotine-exposed offspring were even more marked during the second week of testing, whereas control animals habituated to the activity wheel and decreased their levels of activity (Martin and Becker 1970). A replication of this study in another laboratory found that these effects were not present at 6 months of age, when the animals were tested for the first time (Martin et al. 1982). Assessments were continued until the animals' natural deaths, and nicotine-exposed animals were no more active than were saline-exposed control offspring from 3 to 36 months of age (Martin and Martin 1981). The increased activity in offspring exposed perinatally to nicotine, although present shortly after birth and lasting until 60 days of age, seems to be a transitory phenomenon.

Learning and Performance

The long-term effects of maternal smoking on children's educational performance have been hotly debated since the publications of the British group who followed every child born on one day in England from birth to age 16, when presumably their formal schooling ended. The results in these 17,000 children were consistent and show retardation in reading and mathematics skills from age 7 to age 16, as well as other deficits (Davie, Butler, and Goldstein 1972; Butler and Goldstein 1973; Fogelman 1980). These researchers consistently argued that the causative factor is the smoking itself, rather than the type of mother who smoked, although this cannot ever be proven in human studies. The mothers who stopped smoking before the fourth month of pregnancy delivered children whose scores were indistinguishable from those of controls. Other investigators who did not find these results used much smaller samples (Hardy and Mellits 1972; Lefkowitz 1981; Dunn et al. 1977); the effect may be manifested only with large samples.

Naeye and Peters (1984) examined the data from the Perinatal Collaborative Study on 50,000 U.S. pregnancies and found hyperactivity, short attention span, and lower scores on spelling and reading tests for the children of smoking women. Cognitive scores were only 2–4% lower and related to elevated neonatal hemoglobin levels and low birth weights, suggesting that fetal hypoxemia may have contributed to these results. Broman, Nichols, and Kennedy (1975) studied the same group and found no correlation between test scores and the number of years that the mother had smoked. They found an unexpected reverse correlation in black children; nonsmoking was correlated with slightly higher intelligence scores, although the reported three-point advantage is probably within the test error variance and certainly would not have been clinically significant.

Sexton, Fox, and Hebel (1986) compared three-year-old children whose mothers continued to smoke versus those whose mothers had stopped during pregnancy and found that the first group had higher scores on the McCarthy Scales of Children's Abilities, even after adjustment for sociodemographic and anthropometric measures. Rantakallio (1983) followed 1,800 Finnish children whose mothers had smoked during pregnancy. When tested at age 14, such children were less healthy and had lower school achievement, and their mothers had often left the household. Other sociobiological factors were equally or more important than maternal smoking, and paternal smoking had equally detrimental effects. Garn et al. (1980) gave the Bayley motor test to 34,000 black and white full-term infants. The newborns of heavy smokers scored markedly lower than did the babies of nonsmoking controls.

Johns et al. (1982) reported that guinea pigs prenatally exposed to nicotine were not able to learn maze problems as well as controls and were particularly impaired on reversal problems, where they exhibited perseveration. This deficit pattern paralleled that of animals subjected to lesions of the dorsomedial thalamus or hippocampus or to hypoxic episodes. Bertolini, Bernardi, and Genedani (1982) tested 60-day-old rats that had been exposed to smoke in utero and found that they acquired an avoidance response faster than did controls. This would be consistent with the increased activity levels found by us at this age, as a faster response is more efficient in simple avoidance paradigms. We found similar results after methamphetamine exposure in utero.

Sprague-Dawley-derived rat offspring that had been exposed to nicotine during gestation and nursing received fewer reinforcements on simple continuous reinforcement (CRF) operant appetitive schedules, discriminated contingencies less well when reinforcement alternated between right and left bars (variable interval one-minute schedule), and were less able to relearn when contingencies were reversed (i.e., they perseverated in a no-longer-rewarded response). This perseveration was similar to the results in the Johns study described above. Animals exposed to hypoxia in utero did even more poorly in this regard (Martin and Becker 1970). Since the experimental animals in this study were lighter in weight when the operant testing began at 80 days of age and were maintained at that weight throughout the study, they may have been differentially motivated for a food reinforcer, and the results should be interpreted cautiously. However, it is difficult to see how this would affect performance on the reversal schedule. There were lifelong irreversible changes in taste discrimination for preferred fluids after nicotine exposure in utero (Martin et al. 1983).

Sex Differences

As is true of most drugs of abuse and other prenatally administered agents as well (e.g., x-irradiation), tantalizing indications of shifts in sex ratios have been reported after nicotine exposure in utero. See Martin (1985) for a review and a discussion of possible mechanisms governing such a change. Fewer male births are the usual consequence of human and animal maternal exposure to tobacco products (Ravenholt et al. 1966; Krishna 1978; Ulrich 1982; Fraumeni and Lundin 1964; Herriot, Billewicz, and Hytten 1962; Peters and Tang 1982; Nasrat, Al-Hachim, and Mahmood 1986).

An early human retrospective investigation reported a very low sex ratio of 0.38 in the control group and the reverse effect (i.e., increased numbers of male offspring) in the group of smoking women. Increased numbers of male births were also found by Ordoez (1975) in Mexico. We also found a greater percentage of male rat births in the nicotine- and hypoxia-exposed as compared with two control groups (Becker and Martin 1971). These differences were consistent but did not reach statistical significance ($p = .15$). As the preponderance of evidence, both empirical and theoretical, is in favor of a lower sex ratio (i.e., fewer male births), I tend to favor this hypothesis.

Other sex differences have been found after exposure to tobacco products. These have included greater growth deficits in human males than in females (Wertelecki, Hoff,and Zansky 1987); lower cord blood activity for male human newborns than for females (Bannon, Halliday, and McMaster 1986); alterations of the male gonadal axis and sexually dimorphic behavior in the rat (Lichtensteiger and Schlumpf 1985); poorer avoidance learning in male rats as compared with females similarly exposed to nicotine (Genedani, Bernardi, and Bertolini 1983); and a reduction in the postejaculatory interval in offspring (Bernardi, Genedani, and Bertolini (1982), leading to a higher sex drive for male rats. The male is usually the more affected sex.

Tumor Development

It is a fact that some of the constituents of tobacco products (e.g., polycyclic hydrocarbons and nitrosamines) are cancer-inducing agents. An epidemiological study on 89,000 infants who survived at least seven days after birth found a slightly elevated risk of cancer before age 10 in children whose mothers had smoked during pregnancy. The authors concluded that tobacco smoke did not have a broadly carcinogenic effect but may have a narrower effect confined to one tissue or expressed over a narrow age range (Neutel and Buck 1971). One wonders what may have been found had the investigators extended the age range studied.

The most thorough animal study was performed by Nicolov and Chernozemsky in 1979. They injected cigarette smoke condensate into gravid Syrian hamsters and observed the offspring for two years. They reported that one third of the offspring developed either benign or malignant neoplasms, with females being more affected than males. No tumors appeared in the control groups.

Everson (1980) reviewed the animal and human evidence and concluded that individuals transplacentally exposed to maternal smoking may be at increased risk for developing cancer in adulthood. Further evidence for increased total cancer incidence rates in children of smoking mothers was found by Hinds and Kolonel (1980) in an examination of the Hawaiian Tumor Registry. An increased risk of testicular cancer, especially when the smoking was compounded by low birth weight, was reported by Brown, Pottern, and Hoover (1986). Buckley, Hobbie, and Ruccione (1986) found no such association in a database of 1,800 women and suggested that subtle biases in case selection or faulty memory by parents might be responsible for the positive results found by other investigators. DeMarini (1980, 1983) performed tissue culture studies with tobacco smoke condensate and concluded that elements in the condensate were mutagenic. They found that cigarette smoke can induce somatic cell mutations that may lead to cancer and may induce germ cell mutations that could cause heritable defects. Pour (1986) found increases in ovarian and testicular tumors in rats exposed to nitrosamines during gestation. Finally, Grufferman, Wang, and DeLong (1982) found an increased incidence of rhabdomyosarcoma induction in childhood if the father smoked, even though there was no increased cancer risk if the mother smoked either pre- or postnatally. The balance of the evidence seems to suggest that products from tobacco smoke, which are definitely cancer inducing in the postnatal animal or human being, are capable of cancer induction in the prenatal animal as well. However, additional in vivo studies in different species are necessary before firm conclusions can be drawn.

Irreversible Effects

Life-span studies are both difficult and expensive, and it is little wonder that few of them are performed in either animals or humans. Even cross-sectional studies at different ages are few. We found decreased life-spans in rats exposed to either nicotine or hypoxia in utero (Martin and Becker 1972). We failed to replicate these results when rats were housed under a modified barrier system in which viruses and other illnesses were kept to a minimum, although effects were trending in the hypothesized direction. Riesenfeld and Oliva (1987) studied fertility in two inbred rat strains and found that the life-span was significantly shortened and that fertility was greatly reduced as a consequence of intrauterine nicotine exposure. I know of no life-span studies that have followed humans whose mothers smoked during pregnancy. As with tumor induction, it is possible that prenatal exposure to tobacco lowers the threshold for disease effects and/or hastens the onset of disease, thus effectively shortening life. Additional research with older animals is needed.

Future Research Directions

Some areas that could benefit from additional study are (1) longitudinal research on tumor induction and other disease processes in older animals and their life-shortening effects; (2) effects when tobacco products are paired with concomitant exposure to other drugs with abuse potential, especially alcohol, marijuana, and caffeine, as women who smoke are more likely to use these drugs as well; (3) second generation studies on the offspring of animals exposed to tobacco products and tobacco in combination with other drugs of abuse; (4) life-span studies to determine which effects are transient and which are irreversible; and (5) chemical and neurochemical studies to link the myriad constituents of tobacco with functional deficits.

AMPHETAMINES AND FETAL EFFECTS

The 1971 Congressional Hearings on Amphetamine Legislation, which were held at the height of amphetamine use in the United States, came to this conclusion regarding amphetamine use during pregnancy (Amphetamine Legislation, 1971): "Safe use in pregnancy has not been established. Reproductive studies in mammals at high multiples of the human dose have suggested both an embryotoxic and teratogenic potential. [If] amphetamines [are taken] especially in the first trimester [the] potential benefits must be weighed against possible hazards to mother and infant." Amphetamine use has dropped drastically since that period, primarily because of federal curbs and regulations governing manufacture and sales; however, the use of amphetamine derivatives and designer drugs with similar effects has taken its place.

The biochemical actions of amphetamines and other CNS stimulants were reviewed thoroughly by Kuczenski (1983). He stated that the behavioral effects of CNS stimulants, of which the amphetamines and cocaine are examples, are generally presumed to be mediated through an increase in neurotransmitter activity at CNS catecholamine receptors. He further stated that doses of amphetamines higher than 1–2 mg/kg in nongravid rats produce qualitatively different behavioral effects in rats and qualitatively different biochemical effects on striatal dopamine dynamics than do smaller doses, which seems to indicate a threshold effect. Although there is no mention of the effects on pregnant animals, presumably these would be similar, and dosage should be kept in mind when attempting to reconcile divergent results from different laboratories.

Animal models have primarily utilized *d*- and *l*-amphetamine. Fewer have used methamphetamine, which is more potent.

Drugs Similar to Amphetamines

Methylphenidate has stimulant effects similar to those of amphetamine, but amphetamine is ten times more potent in producing stereotypy and two to four times more potent in increasing locomotor behaviors (Kuczenski 1983). The biochemical effects of methylphenidate are not as well researched as are those of the amphetamines. MDMA (3,4-methylenedioxymethamphetamine), or "Ecstasy," is the *N*-methyl analog of methylenedioxyamphetamine (MDA), which is classified as a hallucinogen. Behavioral effects are similar for the two drugs (Schechter 1987). I found no studies on either drug in pregnant humans or animals.

The Maternal Effects

The only longitudinal study on pregnant, human amphetamine addicts and their children was performed by Eriksson and her colleagues in Sweden when the Swedish drug scene was dominated by amphetamine abuse (Eriksson et al. 1978; Larsson 1980; Eriksson, Larsson, and Zetterstrom 1981; Eriksson et al. 1985; Eriksson, Steneroth, and Zetterstrom 1986). This was a clinical retrospective study of 23–71 women, who were added to the study at different times, hence the variation in numbers in the published reports. There is some difficulty in interpreting these reports because some of these women used other drugs concomitantly, one third of them ceased usage during early pregnancy, they had no standard amount of prenatal care, they used varying amounts of the drug during pregnancy, and the study utilized no controls. The statistics are virtually nonexistent, perhaps because of these limitations. The conclusions were that pregnant addicts made fewer prenatal visits to medical clinics and had higher percentages of premature deliveries and perinatal mortality as compared with the statistically normal Swedish woman.

We found shorter gestations and a dose-related reduction in maternal weight gain as a function of methamphetamine dose in the rat as compared with normal controls (Martin 1975; Martin et al. 1976). Amphetamine is an anorectic drug and, indeed, was often prescribed for weight loss. Although we found significantly lower weight gain in dams receiving 1.0 or 3.0 mg/kg twice daily, others did not report this effect at this dose range (Hitzemann et al. 1976).

The Effects on Offspring

Neural and Neurochemical Effects

The mechanism for one of the most striking behavioral effects of amphetamine exposure in utero—activity change in the offspring—has been linked to a hypothesized irreversible change in the concentration of brain catecholamines. Tonge (1973) found increased noradrenaline and dopamine in hippocampus, hypothalamus, and cortex in nine-month-old rats exposed to methamphetamine during gestation. Middaugh, Blackwell, and Zemp (1971) noted higher levels of norepinephrine in the brains of 30-day-old mice exposed to *d*-amphetamine during the latter part of gestation. These young mice were characterized by bursts of nondirected activity and increased grooming behaviors. Nasello and Ramirez (1978) found increased catecholamine turnover but no increase in catecholamine levels in similarly exposed male offspring. Ramirez, Keller, and Orsingher (1983) and Ramirez and Carrer (1983) reported that adult rats whose dams were given injections of small doses (0.5 mg/kg) of either *d*- or *l*-amphetamine had a significant decrease in binding of brain α-adrenergic receptors, suggesting that amphetamines produce long-lasting alterations in the metabolism of brain catecholamines. In summary, although the direction of biochemical change is not always consistent, the administration of amphetamines during pregnancy alters some facet of brain catecholamines in the offspring, thus accounting for the behavioral changes present in these animals.

Structure and Viability

The evidence for teratogenesis after amphetamine exposure is not compelling. Four of the 69–71 addicts in the Eriksson cohort delivered babies with congenital malformations. Three of the infants had intestinal defects (Eriksson and Zetterstrom 1981). Nelson and Forfar (1971) retrospectively studied 458 abnormal infants and 411 matched controls and found an increase in congenital abnormalities in the infants of women who took *d*-amphetamine during pregnancy. The anomalies included urogenital and cardiac defects, limb deformities, and cleft lip. Milkovich and Van der Berg (1977) found an excess of oral clefts in the five-year-old children of mothers who had been prescribed amphetamines during the first trimester of pregnancy. This was a large-scale prospective study, and no other anomalies were found.

Kasirsky and Tansy (1971) found a dose-dependent increase in anomalies in mice exposed to methamphetamine during the latter stages of gestation and in rabbits administered a smaller dose. Anomalies were exencephaly, cleft palate, and eye abnormalities. Finally, Fein et al. (1987) gave a very high dose of *d*-amphetamine to gravid mice and found extremely high mortality rates in the dams, high resorption rates, and gross malformations in 15% of the surviving embryos, including skeletal and eye malformations and exencephaly.

We found significantly smaller numbers of live-born young at a dose of 1 or 3 mg of methamphetamine per kg (Martin 1975) but failed to replicate this in a second study, although results were in the expected direction (Martin et al. 1976). The Eriksson group cited above noted an increase in perinatal mortality for infants born to amphetamine-abusing women. This has been duplicated in some studies on animal models (Hitzemann et al. 1976), but not in others utilizing the same doses (Martin et al. 1976; Adams et al. 1982).

Growth and Development

We found growth deficits and failure to equal the weight gain of control animals persisting from birth to 16 months of age in methamphetamine-exposed offspring (Martin, J., et al. 1979). Other investigators either did not report growth parameters or, if they did, did not find any differences (Seliger 1973; Hitzemann et al. 1976; Adams et al. 1982; Kutz et al. 1985). Doses and period of exposure differed among the studies, so results are not directly comparable. Hitzemann and we were the only ones to have administered the drug throughout the gestational period, and our dose was higher.

Developmental changes as a consequence of amphetamine exposure in utero include delayed eye opening (Martin 1975; Martin et al. 1976); inability to habituate to stimuli from birth to three months of age (Hitzemann et al. 1976); faster maturation of the electroencephalogram response (Oliverio, Castellano, and Renzi 1975); and delayed development of the electrocardiogram (Fein et al. 1987). The latter is not surprising as another effect of the drug is to increase cardiac anomalies. On the other hand, Kutz et al. (1985) found no evidence for developmental delay.

Activity

Methamphetamine-exposed offspring in our laboratory were significantly more active than either nicotine- or saline-exposed controls from 3 months of age until 36 months, when the experiment was terminated. Differences were particularly evident in late maturity because by that time activity had dropped off markedly in the control group (Martin et al. 1976; Martin and Martin 1981). Several other investigators found increased activity after amphetamine exposure (Seliger 1973; Zemp and Middaugh 1975; Nomura and Segawa 1983). The latter investigators noted that hyperactivity reached a peak on postnatal day 20 and that nerve terminals and receptors in dopamine receptors become functional at later stages of fetal development in these animals. Clark, Gorman, and Vernadakis (1970) and Adams et al. (1982) found no differences in activity levels after amphetamine exposure when activity was tested before puberty.

Perception

We found altered patterns of consumption of sweet solutions and of plain water in both nicotine- and methamphetamine-exposed offspring during middle and late life (15–36 months of age) relative to two control groups. The trauma of maternal injection per se also had an effect on offspring response, as the consumption patterns of saline-exposed offspring fell between those of the drug-exposed offspring and the offspring of noninjected mothers. Holson et al. (1985) found enhanced intake of sweetened solutions up to seven months of age, when their experiment was terminated. Inasmuch as we did not test our rats that early, the results may be age specific. The important finding from both studies is that consumption of preferred solutions was irreversibly altered in mature offspring by maternal exposure to amphetamines. These are the only two studies on perceptual processes that were found in the literature. It is important to investigate the effects of these drugs on other sensory modalities.

Learning and Performance

Few studies have measured learning and performance consequent to prenatal amphetamine exposure. The amphetamine-exposed children in the Swedish study cited above had somewhat lower IQ scores (Terman Merrill) of 104 at age 4 compared with the IQ of the unselected

Swedish population. Their somatic growth and general health did not differ (Billing et al. 1985). Ramirez, Carrer, and Nasello (1979) found that female rats exposed to amphetamine had greater sensitivity to estrogen and estrogen-progesterone for the induction of sexual receptivity than did controls. Significant deficits in escaping from a Y water maze were found in d-amphetamine-exposed rats at prepubertal ages (Adams et al. 1982).

The other published studies on animals used avoidance paradigms. We found that rats prenatally exposed to 5 mg, but not to 3 mg, of methamphetamine per kg made significantly more avoidance responses in a shuttle box, which could be indicative of more efficient learning, as the groups did not differ in numbers of escape responses (Martin 1975). Satinder and Sterling (1983) found a genetic interaction with prenatal amphetamine exposure. A high-avoiding rat strain avoided significantly more often in a shuttle box than did their controls, whereas a low-avoiding strain did not. The authors postulated that prenatal treatment with amphetamine alters baseline levels of physiological arousal in ways that depend upon the nature of the response and the genetic line. Finally, Seliger (1973) found that 5 mg of d-amphetamine per kg during either the first or the second third of gestation was detrimental to the learning of a passive avoidance response at 60 days of age, particularly in animals exposed during the first trimester. An inability to inhibit a response and/or hyperactivity are possible explanations for these results. For a discussion of functional end points, see the review article by Buelke-Sam (1986).

Sex Differences

We found fewer male births among methamphetamine-exposed offspring than among saline-exposed controls (sex ratios, 0.49 versus 0.53). The only other study that mentioned sex differences found that female offspring were more affected by a challenge dose of amphetamine at around 50 days of age than were males, although amphetamine-exposed males were more affected than were control offspring (Adams et al. 1982).

Tumor Development

Methamphetamine-exposed offspring developed significantly more tumors in middle and late maturity than did either nicotine- or saline-exposed or untreated offspring. The group that went to autopsy was small, and this study should be replicated before drawing the definitive conclusion that such exposure in utero may increase the risk of neoplastic development later in life for the offspring (Martin, J., et al. 1979).

Irreversible Effects

Functional effects that are still present in middle and late maturity may be presumed to be irreversible. We found irreversible growth deficits, hyperactivity, and changes in taste perceptions in methamphetamine-exposed offspring. Adams et al. (1982) also noted altered taste responses. Ramirez, Keller, and Orsingher (1983) reported alterations in the metabolism of brain catecholamines in adult rats that had been exposed to either *d*- or *l*-amphetamine in utero, which could account for the observed behavioral differences in older animals. We found no other studies in the literature on older offspring exposed to these drugs in utero.

Directions for Future Research

The effects in humans and animals of exposure to amphetamines have been studied far less than the effects of exposure to tobacco products. Because amphetamine is now prescribed rarely, human populations of amphetamine abusers/users are difficult to obtain. With the sharp rise in the street availability of crystallized, smokable methamphetamine ("ice," "crank"), this picture may change rapidly (Drugs and Drug Abuse 1990; Mack 1990). Prospective human studies on multiple drug use in which amphetamines are used to alter the effects of other drugs (e.g., marijuana or alcohol) have not been done. Subjects for study on animal models which would add to our sparse knowledge might include, (1) the neurochemical mechanisms of action which could explain behavioral changes in offspring, especially irreversible functional changes; (2) comparisons of the effects of amphetamines with those of cocaine, MDMA, or MDA, which have some similar behavioral actions, particularly in the case of cocaine; (3) the correlation of offspring sex differences with neuroendocrine changes; (4) the determination of which functional changes persist to maturity, including new behavioral deficits that begin at maturity; (5) learning and steady-state performance, particularly in response to stress; (6) steady-state performance in response to repeated stress and the effects of such long-term stress on disease onset; (7) tumor formation and disease onset in later life, with possible life shortening; and (8) the effects of such exposure on sensory modalities other than taste.

REFERENCES

Abel, E. 1983a. Effects of smoking on growth and development. In *Marijuana, Tobacco, Alcohol and Reproduction*, ed. E. Abel, 73–95. New York: CRC Press.
———. 1983b. Mechanisms by which smoking may affect fetal development. In *Marijuana, Tobacco, Alcohol and Reproduction*, ed. E. Abel, 97–111. New York: CRC Press.
———. 1984. *Smoking and Reproduction: An Annotated Bibliography*. New York: CRC Press.
Adams, J., Buelke-Sam, J., Kimmel, C., and LaBorde, J. 1982. Behavioral alterations in rats prenatally exposed to low doses of *d*-amphetamine. *Neurobehav Toxicol Teratol* 4:63–70.
Amphetamine Legislation, 1971. 1972. Hearings before the Subcommittee to Investigate Juvenile Delinquency. Legislative Hearings on S.164. Washington, D.C.: U.S. Government Printing Office.
Aro, T. 1983. Maternal diseases, alcohol consumption and smoking during pregnancy associated with reduction limb defects. *Early Hum Dev* 9:49–57.
Athayde, E. 1948. Incidencia de abortos e mortinatal didade nas operarias da industria de fumo. *Brasil Med* 62:237–39.
Baer, D., McClearn, G., and Wilson, J. 1980. Fertility, maternal care, and offspring behavior in mice prenatally treated with tobacco smoke. *Dev Psychobiol* 13:643–52.
Bannon, M., Halliday, H., and McMaster, D. 1986. Glutathione peroxidase activity in cord blood: Effects of fetal sex and maternal smoking. *Bio Neonate* 50:274–77.
Barnes, M., King, M., Goldberg, D., and Harris, J. 1981. Effect of prenatal exposure to cigarette smoke on rat neurogenesis. *Teratology* 23:25A (abstr).
Bassi, J., Rosso, P., Moessinger, A., Blanc, W., and James, L. 1984. Fetal growth retardation due to maternal tobacco smoke exposure in the rat. *Pediatr Res* 18:127–30.
Becker, R., King, J., and Little, C. 1968. Experimental studies on nicotine absorption during pregnancy: IV. The postmature neonate. *Am J Obstet Gynecol* 101:1109–19.
Becker, R., and Martin, J. 1971. Vital effects of chronic nicotine

absorption and chronic hypoxic stress during pregnancy and the nursing period. *Am J Obstet Gynecol* 110:522–33.

Bergman, A., and Wiesner, L. 1976. Relationship of passive cigarette-smoking to sudden infant death syndrome. *Pediatrics* 58:665–68.

Bernardi, M., Genedani, S., and Bertolini, A. 1982. Sexual behavior in the offspring of rats exposed to cigarette smoke or treated with nicotine during pregnancy. *Riv Farmacol Terapia* 12:197–203.

Bertolini, A., Bernardi, M., and Genedani, S. 1982. Effects of prenatal exposure to cigarette smoke and nicotine on pregnancy, offspring development and avoidance behavior in rats. *Neurobehav Toxicol Teratol* 4:545–48.

Billing, L., Eriksson, M., Steneroth, G., and Zetterstrom, R. 1985. Preschool children of amphetamine-addicted mothers: I. Somatic and psychomotor development. *Acta Paediatr Scand* 74:179–84.

Broman, S., Nichols, P., and Kennedy, W. 1975. *Preschool IQ: Prenatal and Early Developmental Correlates*. Hillsdale, N.J.: Lawrence Erlbaum Associates.

Brown, L., Pottern, L., and Hoover, R. 1986. Prenatal and perinatal risk factors for testicular cancer. *Cancer Res* 46:4812–16.

Buckley, J., Hobbie, W., and Ruccione, K. 1986. Maternal smoking during pregnancy and the risk of childhood cancer. *Lancet* 2:519–20.

Buelke,-Sam, J. 1986. Postnatal assessment following central nervous system stimulant exposure: Amphetamines and caffeine. In *Handbook of Behavioral Teratology*, ed. E. Riley and C. Vorhees, 161–70. New York: Plenum Press.

Butler, N., and Goldstein, H. 1973. Smoking in pregnancy and subsequent child development. *Br Med J* 4:573–75.

Butler, N., Goldstein, H., and Ross, E. 1972. Cigarette smoking in pregnancy: Its influence on birth weight and perinatal mortality. *Br Med J* 2:127–30.

Clark, C., Gorman, D., and Vernadakis, A. 1970. Effects of prenatal administration of psychotropic drugs on behavior of developing rats. *Dev Psychobiol* 3:225–35.

Davie, R., Butler, N., and Goldstein, H. 1972. *From Birth to Seven: The Second Report of the National Child Development Study*. National Children's Bureau, Studies in Child Development. London: Longman Group.

DeMarini, D. 1983. Genotoxicity of tobacco smoke and tobacco smoke condensate. *Mutat Res* 114:59–89.

———. 1980. Mutagenicity of cigarette smoke condensate in *Neurospora crassa* and *Salmonella typhimurium*. Ph.D. dissertation Illinois State University. Microfilms International 80-24304.

Denson, R., Nanson, J., and McWatters, M. 1975. Hyperkinesis and maternal smoking. *Can Psychiatr Assoc J* 20:183–87.

Drugs and Drug Abuse Education Newsletter. 1990. Wishing for the good old crack days? Ice holds awesome potential to become worst ever epidemic. 21:44–47.

Dunn, H., McBurney, A., Ingram, S., and Hunter, C. 1977. Maternal smoking during pregnancy and the child's subsequent development: II. Neurological and intellectual maturation to the age of 6½ years. *Can J Public Health* 68:43–50.

Elliot, J. 1979. Maternal smoking and the fetus: One fear buried but others arise. *JAMA* 241:867–68.

Eriksson, M., Billing, G., Steneroth, G., and Zetterstrom, R. 1985. Preschool children of amphetamine-addicted mothers: II. Environment and supportive social welfare. *Acta Paediatr Scand* 74:185–90.

Eriksson, M., Larsson, G., Winbladh, B., and Zetterstrom, R. 1978. The influence of amphetamine addiction on pregnancy and the newborn infant. *Acta Paediatr Scand* 67:95–99.

Eriksson, M., Larsson, G., and Zetterstrom, R. 1981. Amphetamine addiction and pregnancy: II. Pregnancy, delivery and the neonatal period. *Acta Obstet Gynecol Scand* 60:253–59.

Eriksson, M., Steneroth, G., and Zetterstrom, R. 1986. Influence of pregnancy and child-rearing on amphetamine-addicted women: Five-year follow-up after delivery. *Acta Psychiatr Scand* 73:634–41.

Eriksson, M., and Zetterstrom, R. 1981. The effect of amphetamine addiction on the fetus and child. *Teratology* 24:39A (abstr).

Everson, R. 1980. Individuals transplacentally exposed to maternal smoking may be at increased cancer risk in adult life. *Lancet* 2:123–27.

Fazel, A., and Goeringer, G. 1983. Cardioteratogenic effects of nicotine and cigarette smoke in A/J mice. *Teratology* 27:41A (abstr).

Fein, A., Shviro, Y., Manoach, M., and Nebel, L. 1987. Teratogenic effect of *d*-amphetamine sulphate: Histodifferentiation and electrocardiogram pattern of mouse embryonic heart. *Teratology* 35:27–34.

Fogelman, K. 1980. Smoking in pregnancy and subsequent development of the child. *Child Care Health Dev* 6:233–49.

Fraumeni, J., and Lundin, F. 1964. Smoking and pregnancy. *Lancet* 1:173.

Garn, S., Petzold, A., Ridella, S., and Johnston, M. 1980. Effect of smoking during pregnancy on Apgar score and Bayley scores. *Lancet* 2:912–13 (letter).

Garrett, R. 1975. Nicotine and placental iron transport. *Experientia* 31:486–88.

Gavrilescu, G. 1973. Avortul spontan repetat (Spontaneous habitual abortion). *Obstet Ginecol* 21:201–8.

Genedani, S., Bernardi, M., and Bertolini, A. 1983. Sex-linked differences in avoidance learning in the offspring of rats treated with nicotine during pregnancy. *Psychopharmacology* 80:93–95.

Goujard, J., Kaminski, M., Rumeau-Rouquette, C., and Schwartz, D. 1978. Maternal smoking, alcohol consumption, and abruptio placentae. *Am J Obstet Gynecol* 130:738–39 (letter).

Grufferman, S., Wang, H., and DeLong, E. R. 1982. Environmental factors in the etiology of rhabdomyosarcoma in childhood. *J Natl Cancer Inst* 68:107–13.

Hammer, R., Goldman, H., and Mitchell, J. 1981. Effects of nicotine on uterine blood flow and intrauterine oxygen tension in the rat. *J Repro Fertil* 63:163–68.

Hardy, J., and Mellits, E. 1972. Does maternal smoking during pregnancy have a long-term effect on the child? *Lancet* 2:1332–36.

Haworth, J., and Ford, J. 1972. Comparison of the effects of maternal undernutrition and exposure to cigarette smoke on cellular growth of the rat fetus. *Am J Obstet Gynecol* 112:653–56.

Herriot, A., Billewicz, W., and Hytten, F. 1962. Cigarette smoking in pregnancy. *Lancet* 1:771.

Hinds, M., and Kolonel, L. 1980. Maternal smoking and cancer risk to offspring. *Lancet* 2:703.

Hitzemann, B., Hitzemann, R., Brase, D., and Loh, H. 1976. Influence of prenatal *d*-amphetamine administration on development and behavior of rats. *Life Sci* 18:605–12.

Hoff, C., Wertelecki, W., and Blackburn, W. 1986. Trend associations of smoking with maternal, fetal, and neonatal morbidity. *Obstet Gynecol* 68:317–21.

Holson, R., Adams, J., Buelke-Sam, J., Gough, B., and Kimmel, C. 1985. *d*-Amphetamine as a behavioral teratogen: Effects depend on dose, sex, age and task. *Neurobehav Toxicol Teratol* 7:753–58.

Hudson, D., Merrill, B., and Sands, L. 1974. Effects of prenatal and postnatal nicotine administration on biochemical aspects of brain development. *Adv Behav Biol* 8:243–56.

Jarvik, M. E. 1973. Further observations on nicotine as the reinforcing agent in smoking. In *Smoking Behavior: Motives and Incentives*, ed. W. L. Dunn, Jr., 33–51. Washington, D.C.: V. H. Winston & Sons.

Johns, J., Louis, T., Becker, R., and Means, L. 1982. Behavioral effects of prenatal exposure to nicotine in guinea pigs. *Neurobehav Toxicol Teratol* 4:365–69.

Kasirsky, G., and Tansy, M. 1971. Teratogenic effects of methamphetamine in mice and rabbits. *Teratology* 4:131.

Keeler, R., Shupe, J., Crowe, M., Olson, A., and Balls, L. 1981. *Nicotiana glauca*-induced congenital deformities in calves: Clinical and pathologic aspects. *Am J Vet Res* 42:1231–34.

Kline, J., Stein, M., Susser, M., and Walburton, D. 1977. Smoking: A risk factor for spontaneous abortion. *N Engl J Med* 297:793–96.

Krishna, K. 1978. Tobacco chewing in pregnancy. *Br J Obstet Gynaecol* 85:726–28.

Krous, H., Campbell, G., Fowler, M., Catron, A., and Farber, J. 1981. Maternal nicotine administration and fetal brain stem damage: A rat model with implications for sudden infant death syndrome. *Am J Obstet Gynecol* 140:743–46.

Krsiak, J. 1973. The effect of nicotine administration during pregnancy on the postnatal development of the offspring. *Activ Nerv Sup (Praha)* 15:148.

Kruse, J., LeFevre, M., and Zweig, S. 1986. Changes in smoking and alcohol consumption during pregnancy: A population-based study in a rural area. *Obstet Gynecol* 67:627–32.

Kuczenski, R. 1983. Biochemical actions of amphetamine and other stimulants. In *Stimulants: Neurochemical, Behavioral and Clinical Perspectives*, ed. I. Creese, 31–61. New York: Raven Press.

Kutz, S., Fischer, S., Troise, N., and Debaecke, P. 1985. *d*-Amphetamine sulfate: A subcutaneous behavioral teratology study in rats. *Neurobehav Toxicol Teratol* 7:676 (abstr).

Larsson, G. 1980. The amphetamine-addicted mother and her child. *Acta Paediatr Scand Suppl* 278.

Lefkowitz, M. 1981. Smoking during pregnancy: Long-term effects on offspring. *Dev Psychol* 17:192–94.

Lichtensteiger, W., and Schlumpf, M. 1985. Prenatal nicotine affects fetal testosterone and sexual dimorphism of saccharin preference. *Pharmacol Biochem Behav* 23:439–44.

———. 1987. Biochemical correlates for behavioral teratology effects. *Teratology* 36:34–35A (abstr).

Lubs, M. 1973. Racial differences in maternal smoking effects on the newborn infants. *Am J Obstet Gynecol* 115:66–76.

Mack, R. B. 1990. The iceman cometh and killeth: Smoking methamphetamine. *NC Med J* 51:276–78.

Martin, D., Martin, J., Streissguth, A., and Lund, C. 1979. Sucking frequency and amplitude in newborns as a function of maternal drinking and smoking. In *Currents in Alcoholism*, ed. M. Galanter, Vol. V, 359–65. New York: Grune & Stratton.

Martin, J. 1975. Effects on offspring of chronic maternal methamphetamine exposure. *Dev Psychobiol* 8:397–404.

———. 1982. An overview: Maternal nicotine and caffeine consumption and offspring outcome. *Neurobehav Toxicol Teratol* 4:421–27.

———. 1985. Perinatal psychoactive drug use: Effects on gender, development, and function in offspring. In *Psychology and Gender*, ed. T. Sonderegger, 227–66. Lincoln: University of Nebraska Press.

Martin, J., and Becker, R. 1970. The effects of nicotine administration in utero upon activity in the rat. *Psychonom Sci* 19:59–60.

———. 1971. The effects of maternal nicotine absorption or hypoxic episodes upon appetitive behavior of rat offspring. *Dev Psychobiol* 4:133–47.

———. 1972. The effects of chronic maternal absorption of nicotine or hypoxic episodes upon the life-span of the offspring. *Psychonom Sci* 29:145–46.

Martin, J., and Martin, D. 1981. Voluntary activity in the aging rat as a function of maternal drug exposure. *Neurobehav Toxicol Teratol* 3:261–64.

Martin, J., Martin, D., Chao, S., and Shores, P. 1982. Interactive effects of chronic maternal ethanol and nicotine exposure upon offspring development and function. *Neurobehav Toxicol Teratol* 4:293–98.

Martin, J., Martin, D., Radow, B., and Day, H. 1979. Life-span and pathology in offspring following nicotine and methamphetamine exposure. *Exp Aging Res* 5:509–22.

Martin, J., Martin, D., Radow, B., and Sigman, G. 1976. Growth, development and activity in rat offspring following maternal drug exposure. *Exp Aging Res* 2:235–51.

Martin, J., Martin, D., Sigman, G., and Day-Pfeiffer, H. 1983. Saccharin preferences in food-deprived aging rats are altered as a function of perinatal drug exposure. *Physiol Behav* 30:853–58.

Meyer, M., and Tonascia, J. 1977. Maternal smoking, pregnancy complications, and perinatal mortality. *Am J Obstet Gynecol* 128:494–502.

Mgalobeli, M. 1931. Einfluss der Arbeit in der Tabakindustrie auf die Geschlechtssphate der Arbeiterin. *Geburtschilfe Gynakol* 88:237–347.

Middaugh, L., Blackwell, L., and Zemp, J. 1971. The effects of prenatal administration of *d*-amphetamine sulfate (DAMS) on activity and brain catecholamine levels of young mice. Presented at the First

Annual Meeting of the Society for Neuroscience, Los Angeles, Calif.

Milkovich, L., and Van der Berg, B. 1977. Effects of antenatal exposure to anorectic drugs. *Am J Obstet Gynecol* 129:637–42.

Miller, H. C., and Jekel. 1987. The effect of race on the incidence of low birthweight: Persistence of effect after controlling for SES, educational, marital and risk status. *Yale J Biol Med* 60:221–32.

Naeye, R. 1978. Relationship of cigarette smoking to congenital anomalies and perinatal death. *Am J Pathol* 90:289–93.

———. 1981. Influence of maternal cigarette smoking during pregnancy on fetal and childhood growth. *Obstet Gynecol* 57:18–21.

Naeye, R., Ladis, B., and Drage, J. 1976. Sudden infant death syndrome: A prospective study. *Am J Disabled Child* 130:1207–10.

Naeye, R., and Peters, E. 1984. Mental development of children whose mothers smoked during pregnancy. *Obstet Gynecol* 64:601–7.

Nasello, A., and Ramirez, O. 1978. Brain catecholamine metabolism in offspring of amphetamine-treated rats. *Pharmacol Biochem Behav* 9:17–20.

Nasrat, H., Al-Hachim, G., and Mahmood, F. 1986. Perinatal effects of nicotine. *Biol Neonate* 49:8–14.

Nelson, M., and Forfar, J. 1971. Association between drugs administered during pregnancy and congenital abnormalities. *Br Med J* 1:523–27.

Neutel, C., and Buck, C. 1971. Effect of smoking during pregnancy on the risk of cancer in children. *J Nat Cancer Inst* 4:59–63.

Nicolov, I., and Chernozemsky, I. 1979. Tumors and hyperplastic lesions in Syrian hamsters following transplacental and neonatal treatment with cigarette smoke condensate. *J Cancer Res Clin Onocol* 94:249–56.

Niswander, K., and Gordon, M. 1972. The women and their pregnancies. In *The Collaborative Perinatal Study of NINDS DHEW/PHS*. Philadelphia: W. B. Saunders.

Nomura, Y., and Segawa, T. 1983. The ontogenetic development of the striatal dopaminergic system and the influence of neonatal treatment with 6-hydroxydopa. *Teratology* 28:15A (abstr).

Oliverio, A., Castellano, C., and Renzi, P. 1975. Genotype and prenatal drug experience affect brain maturation in the mouse. *Brain Res* 357–60.

Ordoez, B. 1975. Malformaciones congénitas y físico ambiente biológico. *Gac Med Mex* 109:359–68.

Peters, D. 1984. Prenatal nicotine exposure increases adrenergic receptor binding in the rat cerebral cortex. *Res Commun Chem Pathol Pharmacol* 46:307–17.

Peters, D., and Tang, S. 1982. Sex-dependent biological changes following prenatal nicotine exposure in the rat. *Pharmacol Biochem Behav* 17:1077–82.

Peters, D., Taub, H., and Tang, S. 1979. Postnatal effects of maternal nicotine exposure. *Neurobehav Toxicol Teratol* 1:221–25.

Picone, T. 1980. The effects of maternal weight gain and cigarette smoking during pregnancy on pregnancy outcome and neonatal behavior. Ph.D. dissertation, University of Connecticut. University Microfilms International 81-06702.

Pour, P. 1986. Transplacental induction of gonadal tumors in rats by a nitrosamine. *Cancer Res* 46:4135–38.

Ramirez, O., and Carrer, H. 1983. Noradrenergic modulation of neuronal transmission in the offspring of amphetamine-treated rats. *Can J Physiol Pharmacol* 61:766–69.

Ramirez, O., Carrer, H., and Nasello, A. 1979. Prenatal amphetamine exposure: Ovulation, sexual behavior and hypothalamic monoamine content in rats. *Pharmacol Biochem Behav* 11:605–9.

Ramirez, O., Keller, E., and Orsingher, O. 1983. Prenatal amphetamine reduces alpha but not beta adrenergic receptor binding in brain of adult rats. *Life Sci* 32:1835–38.

Rantakallio, P. 1983. A follow-up study up to age of 14 of children whose mothers smoked during pregnancy. *Acta Paediatr Scand* 72:747–53.

Ravenholt, R., Levinski, M., Nellist, D., and Takenaga, M. 1966. Effects of smoking upon reproduction. *Am J Obstet Gynecol* 96:267–81.

Riesenfeld, A., and Oliva, H. 1987. The effect of nicotine and alcohol on the fertility and life span of rats: A cytological analysis. *Acta Anat* 128:45–50.

Rowell, P., and Clark, M. 1982. The effect of chronic oral nicotine administration on fetal weight and placental amino acid accumulation in mice. *Toxicol Appl Pharmacol* 66:30–37.

Rubin, P., Craig, G., and Gavin, K. 1986. Prospective survey of use of therapeutic drugs, alcohol and cigarettes during pregnancy. *Br Med J* 29:81–83.

Satinder, K., and Sterling, J. 1983. Differential effects of pre- and/or postnatal *d*-amphetamine on avoidance response in genetically selected lines of rats. *Neurobehav Toxicol Teratol* 5:315–20.

Schechter, M. 1987. MDMA as a discriminative stimulus: Isomeric comparisons. *Pharmacol Biochem Behav* 27:41–44.

Seliger, D. 1973. Effect of prenatal maternal administration of *d*-amphetamine on rat offspring activity and passive avoidance learning. *Physiol Psychol* 1:273–80.

Sershen, H., Reith, M., Banay-Schwartz, M., and Lajtha, A. 1982. Effects of prenatal administration of nicotine on amino acid pools, protein metabolism, and nicotine binding in the brain. *Neurochem Res* 7:1515–22.

Sexton, M., Fox, N., and Hebel, J. 1986. The effects of maternal smoking on the cognitive development of three-year-old children. *Teratology* 33:31–32C (abstr).

Slotkin, T., Greer, N., and Faust, J. 1986. Effects of maternal nicotine injections on brain development in the rat: Ornithine decarboxylase, nucleic acids and proteins in discrete brain regions. *Brain Res Bull* 17:41–50.

Steele, T., and Langworth, J. T. 1966. The relationship of antenatal and postnatal factors to sudden unexpected death in infancy. *Can Med Assoc J* 94:1165–71.

Surgeon General. 1980. Pregnancy and infant health. In *The Health Consequences of Smoking for Women*. DHHS/PHS report, 191–249.

Surgeon General. 1988. *Nicotine Addiction*. DHHS/PHS.

Tonge, S. 1973. Permanent alterations in catecholamine concentrations in discrete areas of brain in the offspring of rats treated with methylamphetamine and chlorpromazine. *Br J Pharmacol* 47:425–27.

Ulrich, M. 1982. Fetal growth patterns in premature and low-weight newborn infants in relation to maternal smoking, placental abnormalities and other complications of pregnancy. *Acta Paediatr Scand Suppl* 292:27–45.

Vaisrub, S. 1979. There is more (or less) to tobacco than smoking. *JAMA* 242:178.

Wang, N., Chen, M., Schraufnagel, D., and Yao, Y. 1984. The cumulative scanning electron microscopic changes in baby mouse lungs following prenatal and postnatal exposures to nicotine. *J Pathol* 144:89–100.

Wertelecki, W., Hoff, C., and Zansky, S. 1987. Maternal smoking: Greater effect on males, fetal tobacco syndrome? *Teratology* 35:317–20.

Younoszai, M., Peloso, J., and Haworth, J. 1969. Fetal growth retardation in rats exposed to cigarette smoke during pregnancy. *Am J Obstet Gynecol* 104:1207–13.

Zemp, J., and Middaugh, L. 1975. Some effects of prenatal exposure to *d*-amphetamine sulfate and phenobarbital on developmental neurochemistry and on behavior. *Addict Res* 2:307–31.

13

Policy Responses When Women Use Drugs during Pregnancy: Using Child Abuse Laws to Combat Substance Abuse

Alan J. Tomkins, J.D., Ph.D., and Sam S. Kepfield, J.D.

TWO OF THE most visible and pressing social issues involving families are child abuse and drug abuse. Efforts aimed at curbing these social afflictions are varied. In the drug abuse context, intervention strategies have ranged from the primarily educational (such as the "Just Say No" campaign) to comprehensive sociopolitical and legal efforts (such as President George Bush's major "war on drugs" initiated in the fall of 1989). Child abuse intervention strategies are similarly wide ranging and complex (see, e.g., U.S. Advisory Board on Child Abuse and Neglect 1990).

Recently, another contentious topic—the rights and interests of the unborn—has merged with the child abuse and drug abuse issues to provide a controversial approach to dealing with pregnant women who are using substances harmful to their fetuses. Although such matters related to the unborn typically have split people into prochoice and antiabortion camps, there is a potential convergence of interests when the focus is upon the fetus whose mother is using drugs. Fueled in part by laboratory and clinical research (much of which is summarized in this volume), there has been a movement to use child abuse and neglect laws to intervene on behalf of the fetus to prevent or minimize the effects of perinatal exposure to harmful substances. Although the legal policy has been primarily applied in instances of *illegal* substance use (e.g., cocaine), there may be little reason to distinguish *legal* substances such as tobacco and coffee, once the research evidence of the perinatal effects of these substances is made clearer to policy and legal decision makers. Indeed, one need look no further than to the movement to limit alcohol consumption by pregnant women to understand that interventions to prevent substance use may become more widespread if a fetus orientation takes hold in law and society.

In this chapter, we focus primarily upon the use of child abuse and neglect laws as legal justification to intervene in the mother's life on behalf of the fetus. We recognize, however, that the use of child welfare laws as a means to confront the problem of perinatal substance abuse is not readily accepted by all. One problem is that, if one takes a fetal perspective, there is little rationale to restrict prohibitions to only illegal substances. Alcohol and tobacco are presently the top candidates for legal substances to be banned during pregnancy. What activities will future research suggest as harmful? Living in radon houses? Eating beef? Having sexual intercourse during pregnancy? It should not be too difficult to find scientists who would be willing to argue that exposure to radon, eating certain foods, and engaging in sexual relations during certain times in the pregnancy can have an adverse effect on the health of a developing organism. How far will we as a society be willing to pursue regulatory actions in hopes of providing the child-to-be with maximal developmental opportunities?

A major policy and legal problem that challenges those who advocate child welfare, legal interventions to combat maternal substance use is that fetal harm may occur whether or not a woman engages in behavior that is legal or socially sanctioned, as fetal alcohol syndrome so sadly attests.[1] Some courts (e.g., *Matter of Fletcher*[2]) have refused to uphold the use of child welfare laws precisely because we have not yet developed a logical boundary or "bright line" to indicate which maternal behaviors are appropriately regulated by the state and which behaviors are properly beyond state regulation.

Perhaps even more controversially, policies designed to protect fetuses overlap another fundamental issue, the reproductive privacy interests of the mother. Is there a principled rationale to justify restricting the liberty of a cocaine user who is six weeks pregnant under child welfare laws to prevent her from harming her unborn child while at the same time providing her with the right to terminate her pregnancy? This problem is thorny, and, as noted by Janet L. Dinsmore of the American Prosecutors Research Institute of the National District Attorneys Association, it has created "horrendous factions . . . [among] people who were allied on feminist, health and child welfare issues" (Diesenhouse 1989, 5).

It is our opinion that, regardless of one's view about abortion (and, interestingly, the authors' views are quite polar about abortion rights: one of us supports them and the other objects strenuously to them), there is a strong argument to be made that, once abortion is no longer an issue, either because it is prohibited under a state's law or because the pregnant woman has chosen not to abort the fetus, there ought to be a shift in focus from the mother to the fetus. If a fetus is going to be born, it deserves the opportunity to be born with as sound a mind and body as possible. This fetus-focus turns attention to what will promote the health and well-being of the to-be-born. Under a fetal focus, there is a compelling reason to favor short-term interventions against the mother's liberty that will serve to protect the long-term welfare interests of the fetus to allow it to be born as healthy as possible. Put simply, maternal deprivations are only short-term liberty intrusions; the injuries that can be inflicted on the child, however, are for its life. The logic of this argument has been supported, in different fact contexts, by the courts. Although we acknowledge that there are important limitations to adopting a "fetal focus" and to using child welfare jurisdiction to intervene in a parent's life to promote the health and welfare of the unborn, we think that the benefits outweigh the disadvantages. Moreover, the fetal-focus approach provides us with, if not a bright line for distinguishing those adult behaviors properly regulated by the state from those not properly regulated, then at least a somewhat clearer signal as to the direction in which we should be going.

Throughout this chapter the reader will observe that the questions related to the use of child welfare laws to prevent harm to a fetus have been presented to only a handful of appellate courts. Such issues have been the subject of extensive policy debates for only a decade or so. Perinatal policy issues, however, promise to become some of the most hotly debated legal and social issues of the 1990s, and these are issues that have benefitted—and will continue to benefit—from the information provided by biomedical and social scientists who study issues related to the effects of fetal exposure to substances.

BALANCING COMPETING INTERESTS WHEN PARENTAL AND CHILDREN'S RIGHTS CONFLICT

Two extremely important concerns collide when society—and ultimately the courts—addresses the delicate balance between the conflicting rights of women to choose freely what to do with their bodies and of the state to regulate the behavior of pregnant women to protect fetuses from exposure to harmful substances in the womb. The issue of the appropriate balance will, in all probability, eventually be decided by the United States Supreme Court, although it has not done so yet.

Social issues that pit basic (and emotional) concerns against one another and that implicate fundamental liberty interests are among the most difficult for courts to handle. Later in this chapter, we review the case law that has addressed competing maternal and perinatal interests in the substance use context. In this section, we look at several other contexts in which the interests of an adult woman conflicted with the interest of an actual or potential child.

We begin with abortion. In the seminal case of *Roe v. Wade*,[3] the United States Supreme Court directly addressed the conflict of interest between a woman who wants to terminate her pregnancy and "*another* important and legitimate interest [asserted by the state] in protecting the potentiality of human life."[4] The Court identified a major barrier to easy resolution of the problem: when a woman wants to terminate her pregnancy, the woman's interests and the fetus' interests "are separate and distinct."[5] In its decision, the court held that a pregnant woman's interests dominated during the first trimester of pregnancy. After *Roe* and subsequent opinions on abortion, it seems fair to conclude that, as a constitutional matter, a fetus has no protectable rights (until the time when it might be viable outside the womb) that can be asserted against the fundamental, privacy right of a woman to choose to abort. In other words, the dominant interest is that of the pregnant woman: she has the right to choose what she will do with her own body. After the first trimester, the state can continue to regulate abortions in furtherance of protecting maternal health but, after the fetus becomes viable, the balance of interests shifts considerably: the state can structure the balance to favor the fetus completely unless the mother's life or health is in jeopardy. In instances of such maternal risk, protection of the mother's health can dominate over protection of the fetus.

Over the years since *Roe*, several different avenues have been taken by those who wished to argue for the dominance of fetal protections. For example, in 1982 Pennsylvania passed a law that required physicians to perform postviability abortions in a manner that preserved the life and health of the fetus (unless doing so would harm the life or health of the pregnant woman).[6] The constitutionality of such a statute was challenged in the case of *Thornburgh v. American College of Obstetricians and Gynecologists*,[7] in which the Supreme Court held that the requirement was unconstitutional because it exposed pregnant women to increased health risks in an effort to save the viable fetus. The holding again underscored the fact that the balance between competing interests tipped toward the woman and away from the fetus.

One of the major battles to empower a fetus against its mother was waged by Missouri legislators in 1986. They passed several laws aimed at restructuring the balance between pregnant women and their fetuses.

The Missouri statute began with a preamble in which a series of "findings" were made by the legislature. The legislature found that: "(1) The life of each human being begins at conception," and "(2) Unborn children have protectable interests in life, health, and well-being."[8] The statute went on to provide the unborn fetus, from the moment of conception, all state and federal constitutional rights afforded persons except those prohibited by other state statutes and by U.S. Supreme Court decisions.[9] The language contained in the legislation was an explicit attempt by Missouri's lawmakers to change to the "moment of conception" the point in time at which the state could tip the balance of competing interests to the fetus and away from its mother. The U.S. Supreme Court was presented with an opportunity to consider the constitutionality of these efforts to protect the unborn and restrict abortions in *Webster v. Reproductive Health Services*.[10] The Court's 1989 decision in *Webster* did not resolve the debate. Although rightly publicized as an antiabortion decision, particularly in comparison to the *Roe* decision, the *Webster* decision nonetheless avoided overturning *Roe*. The majority of the *Webster* Court did uphold the right of a state to restrict the use of public facilities for nontherapeutic abortions: however, the Court's majority refused to issue a judgment on the preamble of the statute because the language could be interpreted as a state preference for women to choose childbirth over abortion (see *Maher v. Roe*,[11] quoted in *Webster*, in which the Court noted that *Roe v. Wade* does not prohibit states from stating that they value childbirth rather than abortion).[12] Nonetheless, in future years, the *Webster* case may be identified as the case in which the Court solidified its inclination to shift away from a focus on women and toward a focus on the fetus in its abortion analysis.[13]

The Supreme Court had another opportunity to address indirectly the balance of competing interests between a woman and her fetus in the case of *Baltimore City Department of Social Services v. Bouknight*.[14]

In *Bouknight*, the conflict was not between a woman and an unborn child; instead, it pitted a mother's rights versus her infant's rights. More specifically, *Bouknight* involved a mother's constitutional right not to incriminate herself against the state's interest in protecting the health and safety of her child. The fundamental dilemma, however, was quite similar to that which confronts the courts in the perinatal abuse situation: What should the courts do when an offspring's interests can be furthered only by interfering with a basic right of its mother?

The litigation in *Bouknight* arose after a series of unfortunate events. Approximately four months after giving birth to a son, Maurice M., Jacqueline Bouknight lost custody of him after the Baltimore City Department of Social Services showed the court that Mrs. Bouknight had abused her infant. Documented injuries to Maurice included fractures and other traumas to various parts of the body: leg, humerus, scapula, glenoid, and brachial plexus. Staff at the hospital where Maurice was being treated for a broken leg observed Bouknight treating Maurice roughly, including throwing him back into his crib after holding him. Evidence indicated that Bouknight had a background of being abused, that she was emotionally unstable, and that she was a drug user.

After a separation of several months, physical custody of Maurice was returned to his mother. As part of the return agreement, Bouknight agreed to work with Social Services so that she could learn proper parenting techniques, including appropriate punishment behaviors. However, after a period of months, Social Service workers reported that Bouknight was not cooperating with the agency. Moreover, the whereabouts of Maurice were unclear. Bouknight claimed that Maurice was with relatives, but a police investigation indicated otherwise. Fearing that Maurice was in serious danger—if not already dead—Social Services brought Bouknight before the Juvenile Court. The Judge insisted that Bouknight reveal the whereabouts of Maurice or bring him to court. Bouknight refused to do either and was held in contempt of court.

On appeal to the Maryland Court of Appeals, it was held that the contempt finding violated Bouknight's constitutional privilege against compelled self-incrimination.[15] The majority of the Maryland Court indicated that, even if the Fifth Amendment privilege could be balanced against other important interests, Maurice's interests did not outweigh Bouknight's constitutional interests.[16] In opposition, the dissent noted that even such fundamental constitutional interests as the Fifth Amendment privilege against self-incrimination are permissibly balanced against other societal interests. Judge McAuliffe in dissent argued that the "significant societal interest in the welfare of the child,"[17] when balanced against Bouknight's Fifth Amendment interest, overcomes the self-incrimination privilege.

The U.S. Supreme Court agreed with the dissenting Maryland judge's judgment but did not adopt her reasoning completely. The Court framed its decision in large part as a technical analysis of Fifth Amendment, constitutional law. Although the Justices had requested that the attorneys involved in the case argue the balancing of interests issue, the Court did not use *Bouknight* as its opportunity to make a major policy statement about the balancing of competing interests between fundamental parental rights and fundamental children's rights.

The Court had another opportunity to address the balance of interests between a woman and her fetus in the recently decided sex-discrimination case of *International Union, UAW v. Johnson Controls*.[18] The case arose because Johnson Controls, a private employer, adopted a "fetal protection policy" that prohibited women (but not men) from working in the company's battery-manufacturing division during their "fertile" years. The justification for its policy was that Johnson Controls wanted to protect against fetal injury resulting from a pregnant woman's working in battery manufacturing. In support of their position, Johnson Controls cited the extensive scientific literature documenting the harmful effects of perinatal lead exposure.

Although the Court unanimously agreed that a sex-specific fetal-protection policy overtly discriminates against women because it treats pregnant women differently from men in violation of title VII of the Civil Rights Act of 1964,[19] there was not unanimity concerning whether it is ever possible for an employer to justify such a policy under the bona fide occupational qualification (BFOQ) provisions of the statute.[20] Title VII's BFOQ provisions allow an employer to act in a manner that otherwise would be classified as "discriminatory." The importance of the Court's difference of opinion over the BFOQ law is that, under Justice White's concurring opinion (joined by Chief Justice Rehnquist and Justice Kennedy), the sex-specific fetal-protection policy might be a "legitimate concern" of an employer and, consequently, a BFOQ exception to title VII's prohibition against sex discrimination.[21] The majority's opinion, authored by Justice Blackmun and joined by Justices Marshall, Stevens, O'Connor, and Souter, displayed an appreciation of the dilemma concerning the interests of a fetus; however, the opinion intimated that under virtually no circumstances would the Court allow a workplace fetal-protection policy to survive scrutiny under a BFOQ analysis if the employer's actions explicitly discriminated against women, as they did in this case.[22] Because of the nature of Justice Scalia's analysis in his concurring opinion (which was not joined by any other Justice),[23] it is difficult to predict how he would rule on the matter. Of the three opinions, Justice Scalia's was least responsive to the issue of how best to balance fetal interests against women's interests.

Despite the fact that the Court did not base its decision in *Bouknight* or *Johnson Controls* on an analysis of competing interests, the fundamental competition was unavoidably before the Court in both cases. Thus, it is worthwhile to read the cases in conjunction with the abortion decisions and other decisions that implicate the right to privacy[24] to obtain some preliminary indication of the extent to which a state may permissibly intervene in the life of a pregnant woman to protect a fetus from injury through exposure to harmful substances. Nonetheless, until the Supreme Court does issue a clear analysis of how to balance the competing interests between parents and their offspring and whether there is a difference between "children" who are born and those whose life is potential, it will also be helpful to examine the analyses of other courts that have addressed some of these same types of dilemmas.

Several cases have looked at whether a pregnant woman must undergo medical care against her will to protect her fetus. One of the first of these cases, and still one of the most influential opinions, is the New Jersey case of *Raleigh-Fitkin Paul Morgan Memorial Hospital v. Anderson*.[25] The litigation involved the refusal of a pregnant mother, who was a Jehovah's Witness, to accept a blood transfusion on the basis of her religion. The hospital, citing imminent danger to the unborn child, applied to the court for an order to perform the transfusion.

The New Jersey Supreme Court granted the order, stating that "the unborn child [was] entitled to the law's protection.[26] The decision went on to observe that "the welfare of the child and mother are so intertwined and inseparable that it would be impracticable to distinguish between them with respect to the sundry factual patterns which may develop."[27]

Almost two decades later, the Georgia Supreme Court went further than *Anderson*. In *Jefferson v. Griffin Spaulding County Hospital*,[28] the

Court ordered the mother to submit to a cesarean section to protect her unborn child. The hospital diagnosed the mother as having a complete placenta previa. The chances of the child dying during a "normal" delivery were rated at 99%; the mother's chances of survival were put at 50%. The trial court granted the hospital's petition for a forced cesarean; the Georgia Supreme Court denied a stay of the order. A concurrence stated that "it appears that there is no less burdensome alternative for preserving the life of a fully developed fetus than requiring its mother to undergo surgery."[29]

Jefferson and *Anderson* are typical of an entire line of cases ordering transfusions. Generally, courts do not view transfusions as being especially "intrusive" of a mother's rights. In contrast, courts at first were reluctant to force a woman to undergo surgery. Thus, *Jefferson*'s forced cesarean, the first case of its kind, has had an important influence on the willingness of other courts to infringe upon maternal rights for the benefit of unborn children. Taken to their logical end, one could expect these types of decisions to support far-reaching intrusions of the state into a woman's life once the fetus reaches viability (see generally Myers 1984; Robertson 1982). As a circuit Judge in Wisconsin recently explained in an order that permitted the forced cesarean delivery of an Hmong immigrant despite her objections, "the equities are in favor of the child" when there are competing interests between a mother and her fetus (*National Law Journal* 1990, 6).

When considered together, the abortion cases, the *Bouknight* and *Johnson Control* cases, and the forced medical care cases seem, at a minimum, to provide convergent (albeit not clear or strong) legal rationales and case precedents for limiting a woman's most fundamental rights and interests in order to protect her viable fetus. As it now stands, the abortion cases provide a woman with the right to terminate her pregnancy early in gestation (and perhaps even later in gestation if her life or health is at risk). After fetal viability, however, the state has a compelling interest in protecting potential life.

THE USE OF CHILD WELFARE LAWS TO PROTECT AGAINST PERINATAL HARM

Compared to other areas of social controversy, publications relevant to policies designed to protect against fetal abuse are relatively scarce and of recent vintage. Moreover, the literature that exists is almost exclusively either scientific writings, in which little attention is paid to legal implications, or legally focused commentaries or case decisions that all but ignore the empirical data that might support the policies under examination. The press tends to reflect this tendency not to integrate the empirical and the policy/legal perspectives (see, e.g., Blakeslee 1989; Greene 1989; Rosenthal 1990; but see Goodman 1989, 1990). Happily a change is taking place, and it is likely that the scientific and legal policy literature will continue to be extensively cross-referenced; nonetheless, it is helpful to remember the previous autonomy of the two literatures.

As is discussed in detail in this book, the research literature reveals that it is not only illegal substances that cause extensive and long-lasting perinatal harm, but also legal substances. However, simply because a substance causes harm does not mean that the state has the obligation to regulate it or otherwise act affirmatively to prevent harm.[30]

We have already argued that we think it is within states' powers to regulate the behavior of a pregnant woman once she has decided not to terminate her pregnancy. Thus, from the law's point of view it seems to be permissible—but not mandatory—for a state to confront perinatal exposure to harmful substances. It also is within a state's permissible discretion to address itself to harms caused by illegal substances but to ignore the same kinds of harm caused by legal substances. Furthermore, a state could decide to regulate some legal substances—such as alcohol, for example, to prevent fetal alcohol syndrome—but not others, such as tobacco. Again, this would be legally permissible, even if the nature of the harms, as viewed from the perspective of the fetus, might be medically or psychologically indistinguishable.

The next question, then, is, Are the harms caused by perinatal substances already within the scope of states' existing child abuse and neglect laws? Child welfare provisions provide a useful structure within which fetal interests could be protected. They are already in place, and they are the typical kinds of laws that states have chosen to use to protect children from their parents' behaviors.

Child Abuse Statutes

We believe that most state statutes define abuse and neglect broadly enough to encompass activities that affect a child even before its birth. In table 13.1, we list the abuse statutes of the 50 states and the District

Table 13.1. Abuse Statutes and Reporting Statutes

State	Abuse Section	Reporting Section
Ala. Code (1975)	26-14-1	26-14-3–4
Alaska Stat. (1989 Supp.)	47.17.070(1)	47.17.020(b)
Ariz. Rev. Stat. Ann. (1989)	8-546	13-3620(A)–(B)
Ark. Code Ann. (1987)	9-30-103	12-12-504(a)
Cal. Penal Code (West 1988)	273a(1)	11161.8
Colo. Rev. Stat. (1987)	19-3-303(1)	19-3-304
Conn. Gen. Stat. Ann. (West 1988)	53-21	17-38a–c
Del. Code Ann. (1974)	16 § 902	16 § 903
D.C. Code Ann. (1981)	22-901–902	
Fla. Stat. (1987)	415.503(8)(a)(2)	415.504
Ga. Code Ann. (1987 Supp.)	19-14-2	19-7-5
Haw. Rev. Stat. (1989)	321; 350-1	350-1.1–1.3
Idaho Code (1989 Supp.)	16-1602	16-1619
Ill. Ann. Stat. (Smith-Hurd 1988)	ch. 23, para. 2053(3)(b)	ch. 23, para. 2054
Ind. Code Ann. (Burns 1988)	31-6-4-3.0–3.1	31-6-11-3
Iowa Code (1989)	232.68(2)(c)–(d)	232.69(1)–(2)
Kan. Stat. Ann. (1986)	38-1502(8)	38-1522–1522a
Ky. Rev. Stat. Ann. (Baldwin 1985)	530.060–.065	199.335(a)–(b)
La. Civ. Code Ann. (1990 Supp.)	14-403	14-403(c)(1)–(2)
Me. Rev. Stat. Ann. (1989 Supp.)	tit.22, § 4002(1)	tit.22, §4011
Md. Fam. Law Code Ann. (1988 Supp.)	5-701(b); (n)	5-704–705
Mass. Gen. Laws Ann. (West 1988)	ch.209A:1	ch.119 § 51A
Mich. Comp. Laws (1989 Supp.)	722.622	722.623
Minn. Stat. (1989)	626.556	626.556
Miss. Code Ann. (1989 Supp.)	43-23-3	43-21-353
Mo. Stat. Ann. (Vernon 1983)	210.110(1)	210.115(1)–(4)
Mont. Code Ann. (1989)	41-3-102(2)	41-3-201(2)–(3)
Neb. Rev. Stat. (1989)	28-707	28-711

Table 13.1. (*Continued*)

State	Abuse Section	Reporting Section
Nev. Rev. Stat. (1987)	432B.140	432B.202(2)–(3)
N.H. Rev. Stat. Ann. (1977)	169:38(I)	169:40
N.J. Rev. Stat. (1976)	9:6–8.9	9:6–8.10
N.M. Stat. Ann. (1978)	32-1-3	32-1-15
N.Y. Jud. Law (Consol. 1983)	1012(e)	Soc.S. 413–414
N.C. Gen. Stat. (1986)	7A-517(1)(b)–(d)	7A-543
N.D. Cent. Code (1981)	50-25.1-02(2)	50-25.1-03(1)–(2)
Ohio Rev. Code Ann. (Anderson 1976)	2151.03(1)(D)	2151.42.1(A)–(B)
Okla. Stat. Ann. (West 1989)	21 § 845	21 § 846(A)
Or. Rev. Stat. (1989)	418.740(1)	418.750
Pa. Cons. Stat. Ann. (Purdon 1989 Supp.)	11 § 2203	11 § 2204
R.I. Gen. Laws (1989 Supp.)	40-11-2(2)	40-11-3
S.C. Code Ann. (1976)	20-7-490(B)–(D)	20-7-510(A)–(B)
S.D. Codified Laws (1984)	26-8-6	26-10-10
Tenn. Code Ann. (1984)	31-1-102	37-1-403
Tex. Fam. Code Ann. (Vernon 1986)	34.012	34.01
Utah Code Ann. (1989)	62A-4-502(3)	62A-4-503–504
Vt. Stat. Ann. (Supp. 1989)	tit.33 § 682	tit.33 § 683(a)
Va. Code Ann. (1987)	63.1-248.2	63.1-248.3–.4
Wash. Rev. Code Ann. (Supp. 1989)	26.44.020(12)	26.44.030(1)–(2)
W. Va. Code (1986)	49-1-3	49-6A-2
Wis. Stat. Ann. (1987–1988)	48.981(1)(a)	48.981(2)
Wyo. Stat. (Supp. 1986)	14-3-202	14-3-205

of Columbia to allow interested readers to access these laws easily. Statutes may change yearly. The information in table 13.1 was current as of October 1, 1989.

Most statutes are specific as to the age-span that is encompassed and the type of harm that the state is attempting to avoid. Alabama's statute is fairly typical:[31]

Definitions.

. . .

(1) ABUSE. Harm or threatened harm to a child's health or welfare. Harm or threatened harm can occur through non-accidental physical or mental injury. . . .

(3) CHILD. A person under the age of 18 years.

The definition of abuse contained in the statute is quite broad. Virtually any negative physical or psychological effect (or *possibility* of negative influence) on a child which is a result of intentional behavior by another would be recognized by the courts as an example of "abuse." Broad, vague language is common to statutory laws.

New Jersey exemplifies a different approach to the definition of harm:[32]

Definitions.

. . .

c. "Abused or neglected child" means a child less than 18 years of age whose parent or guardian . . . (2) creates or allows to be created a substantial or ongoing risk of physical injury to such child by other than accidental means which would be likely to cause death or serious or protracted disfigurement, or protracted loss or impairment of the function of any bodily organ.

New Jersey's definition is both more encompassing (creation of a risk) and more restrictive (the behaviors must be engaged in by the child's parent or guardian) than the definitions contained in Alabama's statute. It is unknown whether the difference in "harm" language would result in a functional distinction between the types of activities that would be classified as "abuse" in the two different jurisdictions.

As exemplified in the above-discussed statutes, most states define a "child" as a person who has not yet reached the legal age of "majority." The age at which most states deem a person to be an adult for legal purposes is 18 years. Most state statutes, however, do not explicitly cover unborn children. Until recently, most of the problems confronted by the law concerned the *upper* end of the age of minority, not the lower end. Within the last few years, several state legislatures (e.g., Florida, Hawaii, Indiana, Minnesota, Oklahoma, and Utah) passed legislation to address the problem of the lower end of minority and explicitly to include problems related to prenatal substance exposure.

Most importantly, these newer statutes include prenatal injury within their definitions of a child who has been harmed or is in need of services. Florida and Indiana are typical of these new statutes. In Florida:[33]

> (8) "Harm" to a child's health or welfare can occur when the parent or other person responsible for the child's welfare:
> (a) Inflicts, or allows to be inflicted, upon the child physical or mental injury. Such injury includes, but is not limited to: . . .
> (2) Physical dependency of a newborn infant upon any drug or controlled substance . . . with the exception of drugs administered in conjunction with a detoxification program . . . or upon drugs administered in conjunction with medically approved treatment procedures; provided that no parent of such a newborn shall be subject to criminal investigation solely on the basis of such infant's drug dependency.

Under Indiana's statutes:[34]

> A child is a child in need of services if:
> (1) The child is born with fetal alcohol syndrome or an addiction to a controlled substance or a[n illegal] drug; or . . .
> (C) Is at a substantial risk of a life threatening condition; that arises or is substantially aggravated because the child's mother was addicted to alcohol, a controlled substance, or a legend drug during pregnancy.

The Florida and Indiana statutes also raise the issue of reporting abuse. Child abuse reporting statutes (see table 13.1) are a recent phenomenon, attributable to the wave of concern over physical and sexual abuse of children that has developed since the 1970s. Abuse report statutes vary widely from state to state, especially in regard to who is required to report cases of suspected abuse. Many states mandate that health care professionals, law enforcement officers, and day-care workers—that is, *professional* groups coming into contact with children—report suspected abuse to the appropriate agency at once or face a possible penalty. In addition, "any other person" is permitted, but not required, to make a report of abuse in most states.

However, some jurisdictions (e.g., Delaware, Idaho, Illinois, Indiana, Kentucky, Maine, Maryland, Mississippi, New Hampshire, New Jersey, North Carolina, Rhode Island, Tennessee, Texas, Utah, and Wyoming) mandate reporting for *any person* who has reason to believe that abuse is occurring or has occurred. Texas' broad language is typical of this type of reporting statute:

§34.01. Persons Required to Report.
Any person having cause to believe that a child's physical or mental health or welfare has been or may be adversely affected by abuse or neglect shall report in accordance with Section 34.02 of this code.[35]
§34.07. Failure to Report; Penalty.
(a) A person commits an offense if the person has cause to believe that a child's physical or mental health or welfare has been or may be further adversely affected by abuse or neglect and knowingly fails to report in accordance with Section 34.02 of this code.
(b) An offense under this section is a Class B misdemeanor.[36]

Other states include some interesting variations in their reporting provisions. For example, Illinois[37] and Maine[38] include "homemakers" among the persons who must report child abuse. Tennessee[39] makes reporting mandatory for all persons, including neighbors, relatives, or friends."

Reporting statutes such as these, although sometimes broad, do not explicitly cover the reporting of maternal drug use during pregnancy. They are not intended to do so. Recently a few states (e.g., Minnesota, Oklahoma, Utah) enacted reporting provisions that explicitly target such behavior, although these statutes focus on the period after birth, not during pregnancy.

Oklahoma's law targets health-care providers:[40]

Every physician or surgeon, including doctors of medicine, licensed osteopathic physicians, residents and interns, or any other health care professional attending the birth of a child who appears to be a child born in a condition of dependence on a controlled dangerous substance shall promptly report the matter to the county office of the Department of Human Services in the county in which such birth occurred.

Utah's statute is much broader, not restricting its reporting requirement to health-care professionals:[41]

> When *any person*, including a licensee under the Medical Practice Act or the Nurse Practice Act, attends the birth of a child or cares for a child, and determines that the child, at the time of birth, has fetal alcohol syndrome or fetal drug dependency, he shall report that determination to the division as soon as possible.

Minnesota amended its statute in 1989 to broaden the time frame to the first year of life during which reports are to be made in cases where there is evidence that the child was exposed to harmful substances by its mother.[42] The Minnesota law covers

> parental exposure to a controlled substance . . . used by the mother for a nonmedical purpose, as evidence by withdrawal symptoms in the child at birth, results of a Toxicology Test performed on the mother at delivery or the child at birth, or medical effects or developmental delays during the child's first year of life that medically indicate prenatal exposure to a controlled substance.

After receiving a report of possible abuse, the appropriate investigative entity is required to investigate and, if it finds cause to support the allegation of the infant's substance dependency, the case is then prosecuted in the court of jurisdiction (usually a juvenile or family court). For example, Oklahoma's statute requires the state Department of Human Services to investigate the report and then forward its findings to the district attorney's office. The district attorney's office then files the court case.

In practice, it is most usual for the court to uphold the abuse allegation. Part of the reason is related to the personal (and perhaps political) proclivities of judges: most judges are reluctant to err on the side of maintaining legal custody with the mother when it is fairly certain that she is a drug user. However, another factor is that the statutes leave little room for judicial discretion. For example, under the laws of Indiana, Minnesota, Oklahoma, and Utah, the presence of fetal alcohol syndrome or neonatal addiction constitutes prima facie evidence of abuse. Florida requires more corroboration but does not define what is needed. Perhaps a positive drug test by the mother would suffice, although something more, such as a showing of actual harm, would seem to be necessary.

Maternal drug use reporting statutes ordinarily mention the presence of fetal alcohol syndrome or drug addiction as a necessary prerequisite for a finding of abuse. However, the statutes themselves seem to omit definitions for the clinical terms, apparently leaving courts to fill in the gap. Consequently, there is a risk that many cases that could be properly classified as abuse will not be reported. Clinical identification, in many instances, is quite difficult.

Fetal alcohol syndrome has a standard clinical definition (see, e.g., Rosett and Weiner 1984), but the definition is not based on a single, distinctive feature. For example, Rosett and Weiner (p. 6) indicated that the criteria for a diagnosis of fetal alcohol syndrome require:

1. Prenatal or postnatal growth retardation (weight, length and/or head circumference below tenth percentile when corrected for gestational age).
2. Central nervous system involvement (signs of neurological abnormality, developmental delay or intellectual impairment).
3. Characteristic facial dismorphology with at least two of these three signs: (a) microcephaly (head circumference below the third percentile) (b) micro-ophthalmia and/or palpebral fissures (c) poorly developed philtrum, thin upper lip, and or flattening of the maxillary area.

Moreover, because "[n]eurological impairment may not be noticed until the child's cognitive skills are tested[, g]rowth retardation may become obvious only when the child fails to thrive despite adequate nutrition in a supportive environment[, and f]acial dismorphology may be difficult to recognize in the neonate" (Rosett and Weiner 1984, 6), it is likely that many cases are missed. Consequently, statutory attempts to facilitate state intervention, such as that found in Minnesota's "developmental delay" clause, are not likely to make much difference given the uncertainty of detection.

Similar problems exist with drug addiction. Withdrawal symptoms are quite obvious and are indicative of maternal use of drugs such as heroin or cocaine. Should the infant not display withdrawal symptoms, however, the problems of growth retardation, intellectual impairment, and physical defects may not become apparent for months or years. Minnesota's law represents one approach to broadening the period during which there should be professional sensitivity to the possibility of perinatal drug abuse, but it is too soon for data to indicate how successful such laws are likely to be. It seems likely, albeit unfortunate, that there will be little difference in the numbers of newborns who receive state assistance and/or protection in jurisdictions with or without explicit requirements to report maternal drug use.

Whatever their practical limitations, all states have laws that directly or indirectly address the type of harm that results from maternal use of substances during pregnancy. Statutes, however, are only the beginning; they represent the legislative effort to deal with general or specific problems. The courts have the last word in determining the scope of a statute's reach and potency. Courts will limit the reach of a statute if the statute violates a federal or state constitutional provision, if it impermissibly regulates behaviors, or if it does not clearly specify the conduct that it restricts.

Case Law

As of the end of 1989, only a handful of appellate courts had issued opinions that dealt with the question of harm through prenatal drug and substance exposure. Within the last few years, the number of courts that have addressed issues relevant to the matter seems to have multiplied substantially in comparison to even the total number of cases that were decided during the last decade; however, most of these recent cases have been trial level litigation (e.g., Associated Press 1989; Bessent 1989; see generally Sherman 1989),[43] with the result being that the relevant case law still comes from few jurisdictions.[44]

New York first addressed the general issue two decades ago. In the case of *Matter of Three "John" Children*,[45] a consolidated appeal was heard on behalf of nine infants from different families who were removed from their homes because their parents were addicted to drugs. The legal issue was whether section 1012 of the New York Family Court Act was unconstitutional because it presumptively mandated removal of a child from its home in instances of parental drug addiction. In its opinion, the court noted the grave dangers to children born with neonatal drug addiction, although neonatal drug addiction was itself never directly at issue. Nevertheless, the court stated that "a parent who has been committed because of narcotics addiction, thereby 'abuses' her child by reason at least of the abandonment caused by the addiction."[46] The act was upheld, except for a procedural provision declared unconstitutional.

Another New York case a few years later, *Matter of Vanessa F.*[47] involved a child abandoned at birth by her parents, who were addicted to heroin. The parents sought to regain custody of the child, who was born addicted to heroin herself. The court denied custody to the parents, and then, declaring the child to be neglected, stated in *dicta*:[48] "A newborn baby having withdrawal symptoms is *prima facie* a neglected baby under Article 10 of the Family Court Act, and custody of such a child can be held from the parents responsible until after court hearings and other safeguards."[49]

In 1979, *Matter of Male R.* squarely addressed the issue of neglect through fetal drug exposure.[50] The mother used cocaine, barbiturates, and alcohol; not surprisingly, the baby showed signs of withdrawal after birth. The court found that a child *could be* in imminent danger of impairment due to a parent's inability to think clearly while under the influence of drugs. The court, however, did not find actual impairment through prenatal conduct of the mother. Although the court believed that the mother's conduct was clearly responsible for the temporary impairment of the child after birth, such a condition did not by itself give rise to a finding of neglect. Nonetheless, the court did let stand a finding of neglect based on possible parental conduct while using drugs.

Another New York case, *Matter of Smith*,[51] went even further in its analysis. The mother in this case "acknowledged having had a problem, since 15 years of age, with the drinking of alcoholic beverages. [S]he admitted to hospital personnel that she consumed approximately 10 alcoholic beverages on an average of 3 or 4 days every week" during her pregnancy.[52] Although the mother had been advised by social service workers to seek alcohol rehabilitation treatment and prenatal care, she did not. The child was born with classical symptoms of fetal alcohol syndrome: premature (35 weeks gestation), weight in the fifth percentile, jitteriness, irritability, small philrum, thin upper lip, and increased facial hirsutism. A medical record carried the notation that there was a "small possibility" of fetal alcohol syndrome, and the court jumped on this as indicative that there was insufficient evidence to establish actual impairment for a neglect findings. However, the court did find that such evidence was enough to find imminent danger of impairment, along with the mother's failure to obtain prenatal care.

The court then went further. It claimed that, for it to consider an unborn child neglected, there must be a finding that an unborn child is a "person." Citing *Roe v. Wade*,[53] the court held that, although a fetus was not a person for purposes of the Fourteenth Amendment, there was a compelling state interest in protection of the fetus at the point of viability. Hence, for the purpose of article 10 of the New York Family Court Act, a fetus was granted the status of a person.

A subsequent New York case shows that courts will not necessarily intervene under child welfare laws in cases of alleged perinatal substance abuse in the absence of direct legislative language that tells them precisely what to do. In *Matter of Fletcher*,[54] the court was faced with a situation where a newborn tested positive for cocaine, and the mother admitted to cocaine use during her pregnancy (although she was not specific as to amounts or frequency). A neglect proceeding was instituted under the New York Family Court Act. The neglect allegation relied solely upon the mother's prenatal drug use plus the positive toxicology report on the infant. The court dismissed the neglect charge. The judge wrote that

> I see no authority for the State to regulate women's bodies merely because they are pregnant. By becoming pregnant, women do not waive the constitutional protections afforded to other citizens. To carry the Law Guardian's argument to its logical extension, the State would be able to supersede a mother's custody right to her child if she smoked cigarettes during her pregnancy, or ate junk food, or did too much physical labor or did not exercise enough. The list of potential intrusions is long and constitute entirely unacceptable violations of the bodily integrity of women."[55]

Thus, the court in *Fletcher* addressed directly the concern that we raised earlier: in view of the evidence linking tobacco and caffeine to possible birth defects, where is the principled distinction between regulating legal versus illegal behavior? If we let the state assert jurisdiction on welfare grounds based upon fetal harm, might not the state have the authority to intrude in an extensive array of activities that, but for the pregnancy, would be permissible? This conundrum apparently was taken to heart by the judge in the *Fletcher* case.

California is another state that early confronted the intersecting problems of fetal and drug abuse. California courts, like the New York court in *Fletcher*, reveal a reluctance to fashion judicial remedies in this complex social area where the legislature has not directly confronted the matter. For example, *Reyes v. Superior Court* was an appeal from a felony child endangerment conviction in violation of the California

Penal Code.[56] The mother, a heroin addict, received warnings from public health nurses that her use of heroin and her unwillingness to seek prenatal care could endanger her unborn child. Nonetheless, the mother continued to use heroin during pregnancy and did not obtain prenatal care; her twin sons were born suffering from addiction to heroin.

The court ordered dismissal of the case. It found that an unborn child was not a "person" under the meaning of the statute. "Had the Legislature meant to include unborn children among the class of victims described in Penal Code Section 273a, subdivision (1), it could easily have so provided."[57] Thus, to protect a fetus under the "persons" provisions of a statute, the legislature must explicitly indicate its intention to do so.

This is not to imply that all courts will necessarily take such a restrictive view of legislative intent. In another California case, *In re Solomon L.*,[58] the court upheld termination of parental rights under the California Civil Code.[59] During her pregnancy, the mother had used drugs. It may be that this case is indicative of the willingness of some courts to read more into the scope of legislation in the context of civil law but not when the criminal law is involved.

The analyses used by Michigan's courts underscore how proactive courts can be in the face of maternal substance abuse where there are civil, not criminal, proceedings. For example, the case of *Matter of Baby X*,[60] decided by the Michigan Court of Appeals, involved a neglect proceeding for an infant born with signs of drug withdrawal. As a preliminary matter, the court held that a fetus, although not a person in every sense of the word, did have certain rights under the law, for example, tort actions for injury or wrongful death while still in the womb. "This limited recognition of a child *en ventre sa mere* as a child *in esse* is appropriate when it is for the child's best interest. . . . [A] child has a legal right to begin life with a sound mind and body."[61]

The court then addressed whether prenatal conduct of the mother can, by itself, be a basis for a finding of neglect. Noting that in Michigan the abuse of one child can be used as presumptive evidence of parental behavior toward another child, the court drew an analogy. Prenatal conduct, it reasoned, "can be considered probative of a child's neglect as well."[62] Thus, the mother could be deprived of custody, albeit only temporarily, pending a permanent custody hearing.

Another Michigan case, *In re Gentry*,[63] used the *Baby X* analysis in upholding the constitutionality of a statute giving the juvenile court jurisdiction over children when their home environment was unfit. The *Gentry* court held that the section of the code describing causes for finding neglect was not unconstitutionally vague. In addition, the court, citing *Baby X*, stated that "the fact that the child suffered from drug withdrawal at birth constituted strong evidence in itself of neglect."[64]

It is our opinion that an Ohio case, *In re Ruiz*,[65] is an extremely useful case to examine because the court's opinion presents a reasoned analysis of the flexibility and constraints in using child welfare laws to intervene in situations where a pregnant mother is using substances harmful to a fetus. The child at the center of the suit was born prematurely at 35 weeks and was small for his gestational age, and his urine tested positive for heroin. The mother admitted being a heroin addict and that she had used the drug during the two weeks before delivery. A child abuse petition was filed.

The threshold question before the court was whether the unborn child exposed to heroin was a "child" within the meaning of the statute. The court cited areas where the fetus was given the status of a person, such as intestate rights, tort actions, and paternity actions. It noted, as have California courts, that the fetus was not included within the state's homicide statutes but did not apply the criminal standard to the civil child abuse case before it.

Applying a *Roe v. Wade* analysis, the *Ruiz* court reasoned that, once the fetus attains viability, "the state has an interest in the 'child's' care, protection, and physical and mental development."[66] The court held that "a child does have a right to begin life with a sound mind and body, [and further held] that a viable fetus is a child under the existing child abuse statute, and harm to it may be considered abuse."[67] Ohio thus steered a course akin to New York and Michigan, holding the fetus to be a person, at least for abuse statutes. It also adopted an approach consistent with Michigan's jurisprudence, providing the fetus the right to be born with a sound mind and body.

SHAPING POLICIES TO REDUCE SUBSTANCE USE BY PREGNANT WOMEN

Having reviewed much of the relevant legislation and case law, we return to the question, What might states do to protect the unborn from harm due to exposure to substances during pregnancy? Our reviews of the relevant statutes and case interpretations of those statutes suggest that there is legislative and judicial support for tipping the balance of competing interests between a woman and her fetus in favor of the fetus once it reaches viability. We support the shift from a woman to the fetus, especially using child abuse jurisdiction and the analysis offered by courts such as the one in *Ruiz*. The various court opinions also reveal that it is important for legislatures to specify their intent to include prenatal injury and exposure to injury within the relevant abuse statutes.

A major limitation, however, to *Ruiz* types of interventions is that they are fundamentally legal interventions. Such interventions are generally too little, too late. Like the proverbial closing of the barn door after the horse has bolted, legal interventions may not do as much good as is needed because they address the problem too late in the fetus/child development process. The research presented in this volume clearly indicates that it would be most advantageous to prevent fetal exposure to substances such as tobacco, alcohol, and drugs; if exposure cannot be prevented, the next best course of action is to limit the amount and duration of exposure. Laws such as abuse laws can only be applicable after the unwanted behaviors have occurred; since it is precisely these behaviors that we want to prevent, law seems especially ill-suited to be on the forefront of intervention efforts aimed at reducing fetal exposure to drugs, alcohol, and the like.

Nonetheless, we need to consider the proper role of law in the battle. We look to law to tell us which strategies are appropriate and which cross too far over into the rights of others in our society. We also look to the law to provide guidance in our intervention efforts.

Social policy concerns, combined with issues of legal permissibility, lead us to support temporary interventions into the lives of pregnant women—and perhaps even their male partners—to combat the long-term effects of maternal substance use on the fetus. In an ideal world, of course, we would prefer prevention to secondary or tertiary intervention options. However, there is little evidence to suggest that primary prevention strategies are effective in preventing harm from occurring during pregnancy. Therefore, we are resigned to the fact that more intrusive, secondary interventions will be required for the foreseeable future. However, it makes sense to require that interventions be subject to and limited by the principle of the "least restrictive alternative" so that we can minimize the amount of intrusion into the lives of the mother and father while at the same time securing the right for a child to be born as healthy as possible.

Prevention

Prevention in its primary forms would consist of educational programs for both the public and health-care professionals. Not only must the public be made aware of the growing health disaster, but also men and women must be convinced that they and their potential offspring are at risk. Given that much of the use of substances occurs in a social milieu (e.g., drinking coffee, smoking cigarettes, shooting crack), men, as well as women, need to be aware of possible harms, and behavioral changes must occur in both men and women for there to be any real hope of reducing perinatal exposure to harmful substances.

In the past, a great deal of emphasis has been placed on the use of the media to inform people of risks associated with engaging in particular behaviors. There are probably very few people in the United States who have not been exposed to public service announcements telling us that drugs are dangerous, that we should not drive after consuming alcoholic beverages, and that we should not smoke. The public education system has also been used to inform youngsters of the many health risks associated with drug, alcohol, and tobacco use.

These efforts, however, have not resulted in drastic behavioral changes throughout society, and there is little reason to expect that these efforts alone will significantly reduce the numbers of fetuses exposed to substances. Social, educational, and biomedical scientists are just beginning to make inroads in understanding the complex cognitive and sociopsychological processes that are associated with risk assessment and risk behaviors (see, generally, Arkes and Hammond 1986; Kahneman, Slovic, and Tversky 1982). From what we do know, we realize that lay people are not generally good at making risk assessments or effectively using factual data about risks (see, e.g., Slovic, Fischoff, and Lichtenstein 1982). Thus, it is not surprising that a survey conducted by the National Center for Health Statistics (1986) suggested that public awareness of the adverse effects that arise from using alcohol and tobacco during pregnancy is already high. Most women surveyed by the National Center for Health Statistics (NCHS) responded that smoking definitely increased or probably increased the odds of miscarriages (74%), stillbirth (66%), premature birth (75%), and low birth weight (85%). Even greater numbers of women felt that alcohol use during pregnancy increased the chances of miscarriage (87%), mental retardation of the newborn (87%), low birth weight (89%), and birth defects (88%) (NCHS 1986, 9–10). Sixty–three percent said that they had heard of fetal alcohol syndrome (NCHS 1986, 11–12).

Responses like those of the NCHS survey suggest that many women may be aware of the dangers of using alcohol or tobacco, and it is likely that they are aware of the dangers of using illegal drugs. Whether such awareness affected their behavior in using those substances was not addressed by the NCHS research. The knowledge may stop lighter users, but not heavier users. The heavier users, especially of illegal drugs, may know but be unable to stop their habits, or the information may not reach them at all. Whether awareness of fetal alcohol syndrome and drug-related defects and complications works to reduce the drug and alcohol intake of pregnant women has not yet been extensively studied. What does seem clear, however, is that the number of babies known to have been exposed to harmful substances does not seem to be decreasing, despite the fact that more adults seem to know about the harms of perinatal exposure to drugs, alcohol, and other substances. Traditional educational efforts are unlikely to overcome the complex psychosocial reasons that people use drugs and alcohol (see, e.g., Besharov 1989).

This view is supported by the findings of a 1988 New York City task force, the Child Fatality Review Panel. Their report concluded that current educational campaigns are neither extensive nor effective enough to have any significant effect on the behavior of young pregnant women who are also drug users. The review panel noted that there is a tendency for these women to deny that the dangers of drug use are real. Incredibly, some women suggested that the talk on the street is that the use of crack during pregnancy will lead to an earlier and easier delivery!

In light of the above data, it also seems that the use of warning labels, another popular avenue of prevention, will be inadequate to address the problem. The use of warning labels has received scrutiny from the legislatures and the courts. The U.S. Congress passed legislation to require that warning labels be placed on cigarettes.[68] Federal legislation requiring that warning labels be placed on alcoholic beverage containers is in effect,[69] and notices warning of the adverse effects of alcohol on fetuses are found in bars and liquor stores in many jurisdictions across the nation. When mandatory warning efforts have been challenged on legal grounds, they have typically been upheld by the courts. For example, a California appellate court sustained an ordinance requiring that a notice be posted in all establishments serving alcoholic beverages.[70] The notice warned pregnant women of the possible dangers of fetal alcohol syndrome and birth defects resulting from alcohol consumption.

Although there seems to be no legal barrier to using warning labels, there is no convincing evidence to suggest that warning labels are anything other than a minor intervention strategy. They can only be placed on legal substances such as alcohol and tobacco; illegal drugs, of course, are not covered. Moreover, warning labels would seem to be of dubious efficacy in altering the habits of a heavy smoker or an alcoholic.

Finally, we briefly mention the possibility of prevention strategies that take advantage of the medical and allied health communities. It may be that educating health-care professionals about the harmful effects of substance use and teaching them to identify possible risk signs will be an effective prevention strategy in many instances. Educational programs can be effectively delivered to many women by health-care providers and can begin before or early in pregnancy. However, educational efforts may be hampered by the type of mandatory reporting requirements discussed previously. If fetal-risk situations must be reported to state social service authorities, might there not be a drastic reduction in the numbers of at-risk women who avail themselves of prenatal services? Certainly, reporting requirements and possibly even educational interventions may cause some women to avoid prenatal care; thus, it is important to develop programs that do not result in less health care for pregnant women.

Education of health-care providers to spot drug use in mothers or addiction in children will be useful only if the providers come into contact with the women. This is problematic, since many women who use illegal drugs do not seek prenatal care (see, e.g., Connaughton 1977; Finnegan 1988) and, even if they do, it is likely that they will not admit to excessive alcohol or drug use (see, e.g., Hingson 1986). It would be especially regrettable if efforts aimed at promoting fetal health resulted in women avoiding prenatal services, thereby removing one of the interventions most effective in avoiding medical and behavioral problems for both children and their mothers.

In conclusion, then, although primary prevention programs are desirable, there is little evidence to indicate that these techniques will be successful in the short run in stemming the tide of prenatal harms inflicted by pregnant women. However, primary prevention techniques are valuable as policy options because they require the least amount of intrusion into the lives of pregnant women. They also have the potential, in theory, of targeting both women and men and of affecting, in the long run, the complex psychosocial processes that correlate with the use of substances. Thus, it is useful to invest in small-scale prevention programs to uncover the types of prevention activities that might successfully reduce the likelihood of perinatal exposure to harmful substances. It is more reasonable to envision prevention strategies as longterm goals, not immediate solutions.

Early Interventions

Ideally, substance use by pregnant women should never begin. Realistically, however, there may be techniques to stop substance use shortly after it begins or once it is identified. For example, it most likely would be less expensive for the government and private insurance carriers to offer some kind of monetary or free-service inducement to substance users that would require them to obtain prenatal care and allow monitoring of maternal behavior during pregnancy (see, e.g., Winnick 1991). It is important to remember, however, that any intervention ought to adopt a systems perspective. As we indicated in the previous section, women who smoke, drink, or use drugs are most likely part of a social milieu that supports or even encourages the use of such substances. Many women, for example, begin their drug use with their boyfriends or husbands.[71] There is a likelihood of diminished success in programs that intervene only with the at-risk woman but do not include her lover.

If drug use is confirmed, prevention or other forms of early intervention having failed, what punitive measures may the state take to stop the mother's drug use and prevent the child from being born addicted? Cases from an analogous context, forced medical care for pregnant women, suggest that the state may have broad powers, even if the conduct and prosecution occur while the woman is still pregnant.

In a criminal context, a state could ask the court to find a mother guilty under one of a myriad of charges: child abuse or neglect, delivery of controlled substances and/or alcohol to a minor, or contributing to the delinquency of a minor. Once criminal jurisdiction has been pursued, the state could request continuous monitoring of the woman as a condition of probation or as part of a plea bargain.

Monitoring could be requested regardless of whether criminal charges are filed. Civil proceedings also can provide grounds for an order that includes monitoring if a court determines that the child is abused, neglected, or otherwise in need of care. The court might then assert jurisdiction over the unborn child and take necessary measures to ensure that it is not being abused or neglected.[72] One advantage of civil jurisdiction over criminal jurisdiction is that the burden of proof imposed upon the state in criminal cases is "beyond a reasonable doubt"; in civil cases, it is ordinarily a "preponderance" of the evidence. Thus, a civil proceeding may allow for jurisdiction in much closer cases than would a criminal proceeding.

Finally, many jurisdictions provide more severe and extensive interventions, such as incarceration or institutionalization in child abuse cases. Although punishments are legally supported, these interventions are less desirable than the prevention activities. Nonetheless, when a fetus is placed in a position where it is in danger of imminent and serious harm, there is legal justification to support a finding of criminal endangerment. Most abuse and neglect statutes, as we have already discussed, give a court power to assert jurisdiction over a child who is abused. Although most cases have opted to remove the child from the home, additional sanctions against the adult offender may also be available. Shaw (1984, p. 89 and n.173) argued that "an alcoholic or an addict could be institutionalized for the specific purpose of protecting her fetus," since "[i]t is legally permissible to restrain or isolate individuals who pose an imminent danger to others." Myers (1984, 76) suggested that the powers accorded states under decisions like *Anderson* and *Jefferson* are, by their very nature,

> necessarily . . . highly invasive of [the woman's] personal right to privacy since the only way to effectively monitor her drinking [and drug use] would be to keep constant watch on her or require her to report regularly to some official. If she refused . . . the only alternative would be to deprive her of her liberty, a deprivation which in this case would last nearly a quarter of a year.

However, there are several objections to removing the pregnant woman from her home, regardless of whether removal takes place under criminal or civil jurisdiction. One objection is practical. If she has other children, who will be responsible for them? What are the legitimate interests of the other children, and how do we find a balance between the interests of children already in the home and those not yet born?

A second objection is that the use of civil institutionalization is an abuse and misuse of our commitment laws. One fear is that, if we advocate the use of the state's commitment powers to cajole behaviors in this context, might we not allow commitments to be used to shape a wide variety of behaviors that are unpleasant or unacceptable but nonetheless not the kinds of behaviors envisioned by mental health statutes?

A third objection is philosophical/political. Is it justifiable to punish women for behaviors when the reasons that many of these women are engaging in them have to do with the men whose company they keep? The fact that women are discriminatorily the recipients of incarceration but that the men who prompted their use of drugs are free from child-welfare jurisdiction justifiably angers many.

On the other hand, the fact of disparate effect is irrelevant under a fetal focus. In jurisdictions, such as Nebraska,[73] in which there are family-law statutes that focus on the entire family as a unit, it may be possible to intervene against the fetus' father in the same manner that the fetus' mother is targeted in instances in which it can be shown that the father is engaging in the same types of behaviors as the mother. In other words, taking a systems point of view, it is logical to hold a father who refuses to avoid alcohol as responsible for perinatal exposure to the harmful substance as is the mother who drinks with him. It also is a fairer policy. Finally, it is reasonable to presume that, when men are also the targets of heretofore "women only" policies, policy makers will have an added incentive to develop and/or identify intervention strategies that will be less likely to interfere with a man's employment opportunities and liberty interests. Unfortunately, the history of policies and practices designed to reduce drunk driving reveals the reluctance of courts and legislatures to impose punishments (e.g., taking away driving privileges, incarcerating offenders) that interfere with male mobility. It has taken concerted efforts by such groups as MADD (Mothers Against Drunk Drivers) to force the legal community to take consistent and effective actions against typically "male" behavior.

All things considered, we advocate the adoption of a systems, fetal-focus point of view. It not only forces policy makers and legal decision makers to address the complex social contexts in which substance use occurs, it also provides a great motivation to ensure that interventions that are levied are the least restrictive available. In other words, court-mandated, outpatient family therapy would be preferable to inpatient therapies. Any treatments are preferable to imprisonment.

Another potential objection, raised for example in the 1988 New York case of *Matter of Fletcher*,[74] asks just how far the state can go in restricting the use of certain substances or preventing a pregnant woman from engaging in certain behaviors, as a matter of both civil law and criminal law? Can it, as the *Fletcher* court feared, outlaw a woman's smoking, restrict her diet, or regulate the amount of physical labor or exercise done while pregnant? Is there a line that can be drawn, or should a line even be drawn at all?

From the case law, it is evident that a court can cite drug use and addiction or excessive alcohol use and alcoholism as grounds for permanent removal of the child from the home. Parents may be so impaired by their dependence that they will be completely incapable of caring for their children. The law has stopped there, thus far. Although chain smoking, absent any other factors (drug use, alcohol abuse), may be difficult to conceive of as a basis for asserting jurisdiction before or (especially) after birth, there is no reason to believe that states cannot intervene in light of these activities, given a fetal focus in the law.

The problem of which behaviors justify state intervention also affects the use of reporting statutes to combat fetal substance exposure. Under current reporting statutes, in particular those that specifically cover the reporting of fetal alcohol syndrome or neonatal addiction, illegal drugs are covered. Often, excessive alcohol use is covered, too. Cases involving illegal drugs and excessive alcohol use, however, are the easy ones.

What of light alcohol use or smoking? A literal reading of some alcohol and tobacco sale statutes seems to give a prosecutor grounds for arrest and prosecution. Some commentators argue that a strict reading of precedents like *Anderson* and *Jefferson* should allow the state to punish conduct involving moderate or social drinking and even smoking (e.g., Robertson 1982). Should these activities be included in mandatory reporting statutes? What would be the advantages, and what would be the costs? Clearly, requiring the reporting of alcohol and tobacco use is not without its problems. Defining such behavior as abuse and requiring reporting by physicians, for example, could serve to undermine the woman's trust in the confidentiality of the physician-patient relationship. A woman might wonder, if my physician is going to report socially permissible activities, what else might the physician reveal? Another problem, as we discussed before, is that these provisions would seem to encourage pregnant patients to lie about alcohol and tobacco use or, in the extreme, to seek no prenatal care at all because of fear of prosecution.

Summarizing the Policy Dilemma

The scientific communities can and do have an important influence on the policy-making and legal communities. There have been calls for scientists to become actively involved in disseminating research findings on the effects of substances on the developing organisms to decision makers in the legal and policy communities (e.g., Morris and Sonderegger 1984, 1986). To arrive at useful legal approaches and policy interventions, decision makers cannot operate in a vacuum; the issues demand the synthesis of scientific evidence and policy and/or legal reasoning.[75]

No clear policy exists, nor has a consensus emerged, that provides an optimal strategy for dealing with the complex individual and social problems involved in perinatal exposure to harmful substances. Education must be part of any policy. However, it is clear that reliance on education alone cannot be the sole cure. While we await the development of effective interventions, we must act to protect fetuses now in utero and the fetuses of the near future.

A few attempts to address problems specifically using the civil abuse and neglect laws have been pursued in several states. Some states are asking the courts to apply older criminal laws to fit a crime that could not have been envisioned by their drafters.

We urge that new laws be passed.[76] States should allow the presence of fetal alcohol syndrome and neonatal addiction to constitute a prima facie finding of abuse and neglect. States could then require remedial treatments and other appropriate interventions for the infant and the mother (and perhaps for the father and other family members) to stem further harm to the child and any other children who might be born later. States truly interested in preventing damage (or lessening harm) to an unborn child should further enact legislation requiring a report of drug use and excessive alcohol use by a woman during pregnancy and then use the state's resources to provide *treatment* and other, nonrestrictive interventions for the woman, her partner, and other family members.

Some may argue that, concurrent with the enactment of civil legislation, states should enact similar provisions into their criminal codes. Criminal laws could, like civil laws, expressly make drug and alcohol abuse during pregnancy grounds for prosecution. The newer laws could supplement existing provisions, such as those that outlaw the delivery of controlled substances or alcohol to a minor. We do not go so far, however.

We are especially supportive of laws and policies that adopt a fetal focus. Although we are sensitive to the allegations that fetal protection laws unfairly burden pregnant women and excuse the father, we think that the ultimate loser is the child. To remedy the social inequity between mothers and fathers in this context, we also support broad jurisdiction so that, when a pregnant mother is found to be involved in perinatal abuse, there is a (rebuttable) presumption that her mate is also involved in the abuse. From the perspective of a fetal focus, such a policy is warranted. Finally, we support using the least restrictive means available to protect the fetus (see also Manson and Marolt 1988).

The bottom line is this: We think that the balance of competing interests must tip toward the fetus during a woman's pregnancy if she has renounced her option to terminate the pregnancy or she no longer has the legal right to abort. As Robertson (1983, 437) observed, once a woman "decides to forego abortion and the state chooses to protect the fetus, the woman loses the liberty to act in ways that would adversely affect the fetus."

APPENDIX:

Keeping Informed About
Developments in Law and Policy

FOR THE SCIENTIST who is interested in keeping abreast of the legal and policy developments in the area, we suggest developing a relationship with the local law librarian. Even in those locations in which there is not a law school, there are law libraries, often located in buildings that house the courts and serve the local legal community.

Law librarians can show scientists how to use the myriad legal materials that scientists might want to use to track legal and policy developments. For example, if one wishes to find out about cases in this area that have been decided, one might want to know about the state and federal case reporters that publish legal decisions. It may come as a surprise to some to learn that trial court determinations do not have the "authority" of appellate court decisions, even though many trials are highly publicized by the press. Thus, if researchers are interested in ascertaining the "law" of a jurisdiction, they should be particularly interested in the determinations of appellate courts. The most authoritative appellate court, of course, is the United States Supreme Court.

Most legal activity related to maternal substance use has taken place in the state courts; therefore, one would want to follow the decisions of state supreme courts and the decisions of lower-level state appellate courts. (Although some federal trial court opinions are published, very few state trial court opinions are available.) However, the importance of state court determinations may lessen as more states pass laws that attempt to protect the fetus at the expense of the pregnant woman's liberties, thus implicating constitutional issues that will ultimately be resolved in the federal courts.

Although policies are sometimes implemented through control or appropriation of monetary expenditures, most often public policies are promulgated through statutes (i.e., legislative laws). State and federal statutes are published in series of volumes. The meaning of statutes, however, is determined by the interpretations of courts. Thus, statutory reviews are best conducted in conjunction with case analyses.

Another source of information is the legal periodical. Law reviews generally publish articles that summarize the state of the law in a given area; in addition, law review authors generally provide more complex analyses of trends and implications of legal areas. Law review publications are indexed by several services, and these indexes are available at the law library.

There are several other legal resources that will be of use, depending upon the particular goal that a scientist has in mind. *The National Law Journal* is a weekly newspaper/magazine that has become the generic "legal trade paper" across the nation. *The National Law Journal* follows the most important and controversial areas of law; during the past year, it has run dozens of articles and case synopses related to maternal drug abuse and the law. Additionally, one may wish to consider case digests, legal encyclopedias, and annotated case services. Again, the law librarian will be able to assist in determining the types of legal materials that will enable obtaining the information needed. One should not be daunted about utilizing this resource. Legal librarians are known for their willingness to assist regardless of whether they are helping a lawyer or someone without any legal training, and most legal librarians pride themselves on their ability to uncover helpful information.

For a detailed overview on legal reference materials, one may wish to turn to Cohen, Berring, and Olson (1989). This is a source that is used in many law schools around the country to train law students about legal materials. Briefer, more general overviews of legal materials are also available (e.g., Cohen 1985; see also Cohen and Berring 1984; Hodes 1983). Professor Bander and his colleagues publish a collection of legal source materials by topic, including sections on "Family Law," "Legislation," and case law reports (Bander, Bae, and Doyle 1987). The work of Bander et al. is updated via the use of supplements (e.g., Bander, Bae, and Doyle 1989). A brief description of the types of legal materials that are likely to be of use to social scientists, prepared by Professor David Faigman, is contained in appendix C of the introductory textbook on social science and law by Monahan and Walker (1990).

ACKNOWLEDGMENTS

The authors acknowledge the following contributions. Professor Theo Sonderegger (University of Nebraska-Lincoln) and Ms. Mary Fran Flood (Executive Director of the Youth Service System of Lincoln, Nebraska) provided helpful comments and suggestions on earlier drafts of this chapter; Professor Nancy Felipe Russo (Arizona State University) and Dr. Thomas Hafemeister (Staff Attorney, National Center for State Courts) identified important issues and perspectives that contributed to the policy analyses contained herein; and Ms. Phyllis Gerstenfeld (J.D./Ph.D. candidate at University of Nebraska-Lincoln) assisted in the research on the statutes. We thank each of these individuals for their contributions, but the authors assume all responsibility for any errors that we might have made.

NOTES

1. For an excellent, poignant, personal account of what it means to parent a child afflicted with fetal alcohol syndrome, see Dorris (1989).

2. 141 Misc. 2d 333, 533 N.Y.S. 2d 241 (Fam. Ct. 1988).

3. 410 U.S. 113 (1973).

4. 410 U.S. at 162 (emphasis in original).

5. Ibid.

6. Pennsylvania Abortion Control Act of 1982, § 3210(b), reprinted in *Thornburgh v. American College of Obstetricians and Gynecologists*, 476 U.S. 747, 768 n.13 (1986).

7. 476 U.S. 747 (1986).

8. Mo. Rev. Stat. § 1.205.1 (1986), reprinted in *Wester v. Reproductive Health Services*, 109 S.Ct. 3040, 3048 n.4 (1989).

9. Mo. Rev. Stat. § 1.205.2 (1986), reprinted in *Webster*, 109 S.Ct. at 3048 n.4.

10. 109 S.Ct. 3040 (1989).

11. 432 U.S. 464, 474 (1977).

12. *Webster*, 109 S.Ct. at 3049–3050.

13. For example, Chief Justice Rehnquist, joined by Justices White and Kennedy, wanted to uphold the constitutionality of a provision in the Missouri statute requiring a physician to test for fetal viability if the physician believes that the fetus is 20 or more weeks of gestational age. Among their reasons, they argued that states have a compelling interest in protecting the fetus throughout the entire pregnancy. According to Chief Justice Rehnquist's assessment, the "viability-testing provision of the Missouri Act is concerned with the State's interest in potential human life rather than in maternal health." *Webster*, 109 S.Ct. at 3055. These tests "permissibly further[ ] the State's interest in protecting potential human life." Ibid. at 3057. See also *Thornburgh*, 476 U.S. at 794–795 (White, J., dissenting).

14. 110 S.Ct. 900 (1990).

15. 314 Md. 391, 550 A.2d 1135 (1988) [decision issued under case name of *In re Maurice M.*], *reversed*, 110 S.Ct. 900 (1990).

16. 314 Md. at 409.

17. 314 Md. at 415 (McAuliffe, J., dissenting).

18. 111 S.Ct. 1196 (1991).

19. See § 703(a) of the Civil Rights Act of 1964, as amended, 42 U.S.C. § § 2000e–2(a) & 2000e(k).

20. 42 U.S.C. § 2000(e)–2(e)(1).

21. 111 S.Ct. at 1210–1216 (White, J., concurring in part and concurring in the judgment).

22. See especially ibid. at 1206–1210.

23. Ibid. at 1216–1217 (Scalia, J., concurring in judgment).

24. For example, the Court addressed the extent to which a person's privacy interests can be interfered with by a state in the case of *Cruzan v. Director, Missouri Department of Health*, 110 S.Ct. 2841 (1990). In *Cruzan*, the majority of the Court once again indicated its willingness to defer to a state's interest in the "protection and preservation of human life." Ibid. at 2852. Justice Brennan, in dissent, argued that "[t]he State's general interest in life must accede to [a person's] particularized and intense interest in self-determination in her choice

of medical treatment [i.e., Nancy Cruzan's interest in dying rather than being maintained by medical intervention]." Ibid. at 2870 (Brennan, J., dissenting). The majority, however, favored the State's "general interest" in life.

25. 42 N.J. 421, 201 A.2d 537, *cert. denied* 377 U.S. 985 (1964).

26. 42 N.J. at 423.

27. Ibid.

28. 247 Ga. 86, 274 S.E.2d 530 (1981).

29. Ibid. at 91.

30. See, for example, *DeShaney v. Winnebago County Dept. of Social Services*, 109 S.Ct. 998 (1989), in which the Supreme Court noted that "our cases have recognized that the Due Process Clauses [of the Constitution] generally confer no affirmative right to governmental aid, even where such aid may be necessary to secure life, liberty, or property interests of which the government itself may not deprive the individual." Ibid. at 1003.

31. Ala. Code § 26-14-1 (1975).

32. N.J. Rev. State. § 9:6–8.21 (1976).

33. Fla. Stat. § 415.5015 (1987).

34. Ind. Code Ann. § 31-6-4-3.1 (Burns 1988).

35. Tex. Fam. Code Ann. § 34.01 (Vernon 1986).

36. Tex. Fam. Code § 34.07 (Vernon 1986).

37. Ill. Ann. Stat. ch. 23, para. 2054 (Smith-Hurd 1988).

38. Me. Rev. Stat. Ann. tit. 22, § 4011 (1989 Supp.).

39. Tenn. Code Ann. § 37-1-403(8) (1984).

40. Okla. Stat. Ann. 21 § 846(A) (West 1989).

41. Utah Code Ann. § 62A-4-504 (1989) (emphasis added).

42. Minn. Stat. § 626.556, subd. 2(c) (1989).

43. In fact, what does not often make its way into the newspapers is what happens in the aftermath of these trials. Thus, although there was considerable publicity about the juvenile court hearing that resulted in the conviction of a Rockford, Illinois, mother on charges of prenatal child abuse and neglect in light of the mother's use of cocaine during pregnancy and further resulted in the temporary removal of custody of her baby to the state department of social services (see Associated Press 1989), there was much less attention paid to the fact that her baby was returned to her within a month of her conviction (*National Law Journal* 1989). The mother regained custody after another hearing in which the mother's attorney told the court that the mother had successfully completed drug rehabilitation.

44. It is important to remember that case law is made by appellate courts, not by trial courts. Thus, even though there recently have been a substantial number of highly publicized cases in this area, the trials in these cases do not have precedential value. Regardless of whether a defendant is acquitted or convicted or whether a child is removed from its mother's custody or not, the particular case result has limited legal meaning. It does have considerable social and political implications, and that is why prosecutors are interested in bringing these cases to trial.

45. 61 Misc. 2d 347, 306 N.Y.S.2d 797 (Fam. Ct. 1969).

46. 61 Misc.2d at 356.

47. 76 Misc.2d 617, 351 N.Y.S.2d 337 (Surrogate's Ct. 1974).

48. Dictum is essentially "advisory" language found in a legal opinion. It is technically not binding in future cases, although a good argument often becomes law in a future case. Technically, anything not squarely before the court (termed "at issue") is considered dictum. Deciding what is dictum and what is binding opinion is the lifeblood of lawyers and law professors.

49. 76 Misc.2d at 619.

50. 102 Misc.2d 1, 422 N.Y.S.2d 819 (Fam. Ct. 1979).

51. 128 Misc.2d 976, 492 N.Y.S.2d 331 (Fam. Ct. 1985).

52. 128 Misc.2d at 977.

53. 410 U.S. 113 (1973).

54. 141 Misc.2d 333, 533 N.Y.S.2d 241 (Fam. Ct. 1988).

55. 141 Misc.2d at 335.

56. 75 Cal.App.3d 314, 141 Cal.Rptr. 912 (1977).

57. 75 Cal.App.3d at 219; see also *In re Steven S.*, 126 Cal.App.3d 23, 178 Cal.Rptr. 525 (1981). The court refused to hold that an unborn child could be a "person" under a statute conferring jurisdiction to juvenile court over persons under 18 and judged dependent and suggested that the legislature amend the statute if it wanted the unborn included.

58. 190 Cal.App.3d 1106, 236 Cal.Rptr. 2 (1987).

59. Cal. Civ. Code §§ 232(a)(2)–232(a)(3).

60. 97 Mich. App. 111, 293 N.W.2d 736 (1980).

61. 97 Mich.App. at 115.

62. 97 Mich.App. at 116.

63. 142 Mich.App. 701, 369 N.W.2d 889 (1985).

64. 142 Mich.App. at 708.

65. 27 Ohio Misc.2d 31, 500 N.E.2d 935 (Ohio Comm.Pl. 1986).

66. 27 Ohio Misc.2d at 35.

67. 27 Ohio Misc.2d at 35.

68. 15 U.S.C. § 1333(a)(1) (1985 Supp.).

69. Alcohol Beverage Labeling Act, 27 U.S.C.A. § 213 (Supp. 1990).

70. *California Restaurant Association v. City of Los Angeles*, 192 Ca.App.3d 405, 237 Ca.Rptr. 415 (1987) (upholding constitutionality of Los Angeles, Cal., Code § 46.80).

71. Even some judges have been moved to comment on this sociological pattern. For example, the Court in *Matter of Three "John" Children*, 61 Misc.2d at 366–367, noted that "[e]ven if only the father is addicted, the probability is substantial that the pregnant mother will be introduced to narcotics use. The husband and wife, appearing in case after case, are both addicted; young married couples seem especially prone to entice one another to become involved with heroin, if one has become a user."

72. See, for example, *Gloria C. v. William C.*, 124 Misc.2d 313, 476 N.Y.S.2d 991 (Fam.Ct. 1984) (Court issues independent protective order to an unborn child, against the father, protecting against injury from the father's abuse of the mother). In issuing the protective order, the Court noted that violation of the order could result in a jail term for the father. 124 Misc.2d at 992 & 998.

73. Family Policy Act, Neb. Rev. Stat. §§ 43-532–43-534 (1989).

74. 141 Misc.2d 333, 533 N.Y.S.2d 241 (Fam.Ct. 1988).

75. For the scientist who wishes to keep informed of the legal and policy developments, we provided some information on how to do so in the Appendix.

76. A positive example, one that would supplement the use of "child abuse and neglect" laws, is proposed Congressional legislation that would provide 50 million dollars in funds for the purpose of developing programs to prevent perinatal exposure to substances: Child Abuse During Pregnancy Prevention Act of 1989, S. 1444, 101st Cong., 1st Sess. (1989). The bill would fund "five pilot projects for the purposes of demonstrating the effectiveness of, and expense associated with, providing outreach, education, and treatment services concerning substance abuse to pregnant females, postpartum females and their infants." The bill, unfortunately, died in the Senate Committee on Labor and Human Resources.

REFERENCES

Arkes, H. R., and Hammond, K. R. (eds.). 1986. *Judgment and Decision Making: An Interdisciplinary Reader.* New York: Cambridge University Press.

Associated Press. 1989. Cocaine use in pregnancy amounts to child abuse, a judge rules. *New York Times*, May 4, p. A22.

Bander, E. J., Bae, F., and Doyle, F. R. 1987. *Searching the Law.* Dobbs Ferry, N.Y.: Transnational Publishers.

———. 1989. *Searching the Law: Supplement I.* Dobbs Ferry, N.Y.: Transnational Publishers.

Besharov, D. J. 1989. Crack babies: The worst threat is mom herself. *Washington Post*, August 6, pp. B1 et seq.

Bessent, A. E. 1989. Mom's drug use is "child neglect." *Newsday*, July 1, p. 6.

Blakeslee, S. 1989. Crack's toll among babies: A joyless view even of toys. *New York Times*, September 17, pp A1 et seq.

Cohen, M. L. 1985. *Legal Research in a Nutshell.* 4th ed. St. Paul, Minn.: West Publishing.

Cohen, M. L., and Berring, R. C. 1984. *Finding the Law: An Abridged Edition of "How to Find the Law, 8th Ed."* St. Paul, Minn.: West Publishing.

Cohen, M. L., Berring, R. C., and Olson, K. C. 1989. *How to Find the Law.* 9th ed. St. Paul, Minn.: West Publishing.

Connaughton, J. 1977. Perinatal addiction: Outcome and management. *Am J Obstet Gynecol* 129:679–86.

Diesenhouse, S. 1989. Punishing pregnant addicts: Debate, dismay, no solution. *New York Times*, September 10, p. E5.

Dorris, M. 1989. *The Broken Cord*. New York: Harper & Row.

Equal Employment Opportunity Commission. 1988. *Policy Statement on Reproductive and Fetal Hazards under Title VII*. October 3. (Reprinted in 401 *Fair Employment Practice Manual* 6013.)

Finnegan, L. 1988. Influence of maternal drug dependence on the newborn. In *Toxicologic and Pharmacologic Principles in Pediatrics*, ed. S. Kacew. New York: Hemisphere.

Goodman, E. 1989. The fallout of pregnant drug abusers. *Boston Globe*, August 17, p. 23.

———. 1990. The latest target in prosecution: Pregnant women. *Newsday*, February 9, p. 80.

Greene, M. S. 1989. The crack legacy: Ad hoc orphanages. *Washington Post*, September 11, pp. A1 et seq.

Hingson, R. 1986. Maternal marijuana use and neonatal outcome: Uncertainty posed by self-reports. *Am J Public Health* 76:667–69.

Hodes, W. W. 1983. *Legal Research: A Self-teaching Guide to the Law Library*. 1st ed. St. Paul, Minn.: National Institute for Trial Advocacy.

Kahneman, D., Slovic, P., and Tversky, A. (eds.). 1982. *Judgment under Uncertainty: Heuristics and Biases*. New York: Cambridge University Press.

Manson, R., and Marolt, J. 1988. A new crime, fetal neglect: State intervention to protect the unborn—at what cost? *Calif West Law Rev* 24:161–82.

Monahan, J., and Walker, L. 1990. *Social Science in Law: Cases and Materials*. 2d ed. Westbury, N.Y.: Foundation Press.

Morris, R. A., and Sonderegger, T. B. 1984. Legal applications and implications of neurotoxin research of the developing organism. *Neurobehav Toxicol Teratol* 6:303–6.

———. 1986. Perinatal toxicology and the law. *Neurobehav Toxicol Teratol* 8:363–67.

Myers, J. 1984. Abuse and neglect of the unborn: Can the state intervene? *Dusquesne Law Rev* 23:1–23.

National Center for Health Statistics. 1986. *Health Promotion and Disease Prevention Provisional Data from the National Health Interview Survey: United States, January–June 1985*. NCHS Advance-Data: May 14.

National Law Journal. 1989. User gets child back. *Nat Law J*, June 12, p. 6.

———. 1990. C-section ordered. *Nat Law J*, December 17, p. 6.

Robertson, J. A. 1982. The right to procreate and in utero fetal therapy. *J Legal Med* 3:333–66.

————. 1983. Procreative liberty and the control of conception, pregnancy and childbirth. *Va Law Rev* 69:405–64.

Rosenthal, E. 1990. When a pregnant woman drinks. *New York Times Magazine*, February 4, pp. 30 et seq.

Rosett, H. L., and Weiner, L. 1984. *Alcohol and the Fetus*. New York: Oxford University Press.

Shaw, M. 1984. Conditional prospective rights of the fetus. *J Legal Med* 5:63–116.

Sherman, R. 1989. Keeping babies free of drugs. *Nat Law J*, October 16, pp. 1, et seq.

Slovic, P., Fischoff, B., and Lichtenstein, S. 1982. Facts versus fears: Understanding perceived risk. In *Judgment under Uncertainty: Heuristics and Biases*, eds. D. Kahneman, P. Slovic, and A. Tversky, 463–89. New York: Cambridge University Press.

U.S. Advisory Board on Child Abuse and Neglect. 1990. *Child Abuse and Neglect: Critical First Steps in Response to a National Emergency*. Washington, D.C.: U.S. Government Printing Office.

Winick, B . J. 1991. Harnessing the power of the bet: Wagering with the government as a mechanism for social and individual change. *Univ Miami Law Rev* 45:737–841.

Index

Page numbers in italics denote information derived from studies of laboratory animals.

A

Aberrant maternal behavior, *29*
Abnormalities, 226, 293
Abortion: legal issues and, 307–8, 309–10, 314; spontaneous, 78, 92, 94, 280, 281
Abruptio placentae, 186, 190, 281
Acetylcholine, *205*, 265
Acetylcholinesterase, *40*
Acetyltransferase, *40*
Active avoidance, *264*
Activity behavior, *32, 68, 70–71, 141, 141, 192, 202, 211, 283–84*, 284, *284–85, 286, 292, 294*
Adaptive functioning, 110–28
Adrenocortical activity, *37, 61–64*
Aggressive behavior, *203*
AIDS (acquired immunodeficiency syndrome) 11, 24, 79, 241
Alcohol (*see also* Fetal alcohol syndrome [FAS]): administration methods, *16–18*; and behavior, *64–70, 136*; and brain, *34, 35, 37, 38, 55–56, 57*; and drinking patterns, 135; feminizing effect of, on males, *59, 64–65*; genetic susceptibility and, 95–97; and hormones, *58–61, 61–64*; interactions of, with nicotine, 75–76; and maternal behavior, *24, 26–27, 29, 35, 64, 75–76*; maternal consumption of, *19–20, 21, 22,* 73–75, 91–92, 93–95; mechanism

of action of, 144–47; and metabolism, 20, 96; nutrition and, *17–30, 33, 35, 36*; paternal use of, effects on offspring, *16, 70–71, 132–50,* 132–50; pharmacological mechanisms of, *19–20, 97*; programs to prevent birth defects from, 98–100, 128–30; and sexual development, *59–60*; and sperm abnormalities, 143–44, 147
Alcohol effects on pregnancy: labor and delivery, *23*; maternal age/ parity, 97; maternal feeding patterns, *24, 26*; maternal weight gain, *21, 23*; neurochemistry, *24*
Alcohol-exposed fetus: physical features of, *22,* 75–76; sex hormones of, *58–61*
Alcohol-exposed neonate/infant: behavior of, 74, *141–42*; body weight of, *53, 70–71,* 74, 75–76, 93; brain of, *34, 35, 37, 55, 56, 57*; growth and development of, *21–22*; lactation and, *19, 26–27*; neonatal mortality of, *23, 36, 70–71*; physical characteristics of, *21, 34, 36,* 75–76, 93, *140*; sex hormones of, *58,* 72–73; and stillbirths, *23*
Alcohol-exposed offspring/child: behavior of, *34, 35, 61–63, 65–66*; brain of, *34, 35, 37*; physical characteristics of, *34,* 105–10; sex hormones of, *59*

Alcohol exposure, long-term effects
of, 104–30; on behavior, *37, 65–66,*
106–28; on brain, *37, 38, 55–56*; on
growth and development, *54, 75,*
105–6, 107–10; on hormone
responses, *60–61*; on physical
characteristics, 105–6, 107–10,
117, 120, 122, 123; on sexual
behavior, *64*
Amphetamine-exposed neonate/
infant: activity of, *68, 70, 294*;
growth and development of, 283,
293; neural and neurochemical
effects on, *292*; perception of, *294*;
physical features of, 292–93, *293*;
sex differences of, *295*
Amphetamine-exposed offspring/
child: activity of, *68, 70, 294*;
learning and performance of,
294–95, *295*
Amphetamine-exposure, long-term
effects of, *296*
Amphetamines, 290–97; directions
for future research with, 296; drugs
similar to, 291; effects of on
pregnancy, 283, *283*; legal issues
and, 290; mechanism of action of,
290, 292; tumor development and,
295–96
Analgesia: and methadone, *69*; and
morphine, *31, 33, 213*
Angel dust. *See* Phencyclidine (PCP)
Animal models, methodological
issues in, *13–40*
Animal studies, importance of,
13–16, 28
Apgar score, 171, 185, 231
Arousal, and cocaine, 188–89
Artificial rearing-intragastric feeding,
33–35
Avoidance learning, *70–71, 142, 165,
264, 288, 295*

B

*Baltimore City Department of Social
Services v. Bouknight,* 310–12, 313
Barbiturates. *See* Phenobarbital

Bayley Scales of Infant
Development, 177, 231, 245, 248,
270
Behavior, *38–39, 64–70,* 110–28, *136,*
226
Behavioral laterality, *66*
Behavioral teratogenesis, 167, 224,
226
Bender-Gestalt Test of Visual Motor
Function, 228
Binge drinking. *See* Alcohol,
maternal consumption of
Birth weights, *21, 33, 53, 54, 71,* 74,
75–76, 93, 136, *140,* 186, *191,* 240,
246, 247, 282, *283*
Blood/brain barrier, *212*
Body weight, *18, 21, 26–27, 33, 34,
36, 37, 38, 53–55, 56, 71,* 280
Bogus pipeline, 95
Bone development, *22, 54, 259, 281,
293*
Brain: growth, *32, 33, 34, 35, 37, 38,
40, 55–56, 164, 196–202*; growth
spurt, *14–15, 33, 34, 37, 38, 55,* 68;
microcephaly/microencephaly, *34,
35, 55,* 105; opioid receptors, *213*;
sexually dimorphic nucleus, *57*;
weight, *21, 34, 37, 38, 55–56, 71,
164, 282*
Brain structures: cerebellum, *34, 37,
38, 56, 282*; cerebrum, *56*; corpus
callosum, *56*; cortex, *34, 212*;
hippocampus, *34, 57, 67, 193, 212*;
hypothalamus, *57*; neocortex, *56*
Brazelton Neonatal Assessment
Scale, 174, 185, 187, 188, 189, 244
Breast milk. *See* Lactation

C

Calcium membrane transport, *167*
Caldwell Home Inventory (HOME),
177, 231
Cancer, and tobacco, 288–89, *288–89*
Cannabinoids/cannabinol (CBN). *See*
Marijuana
Case laws, on harm through prenatal
drug exposure, 323–27

Catecholamines, *57, 196*
Cell culture, 40
Central nervous system. *See* Brain
Central nervous system deficits, and FAS, 105–10
Child, legal definition of, 318–19
Child abuse: laws to combat substance abuse, 306–37; legal definition of, 318–20; statutes, 315–23
Child welfare laws, 314–27
Cigarette smoking (*see also* Nicotine): interactions of with other drug use, 75–76, 169–71; maternal, effects of on children, 235
Circadian rhythms, *24*
Clinical Global Rating System, 245
Clonidine, *63–64*
Cognitive functioning and marijuana, 177–78
Cocaine, 184–203; dose/response curve, *190*; and glucose utilization, *193–96, 197*; mechanism of action of, 187, *191, 192, 193, 196, 197, 201–2*; neurobehavioral effects of, *191–202*
Cocaine-exposed fetus: development of, *196*; physical characteristics of, *190, 196*
Cocaine-exposed neonate/infant: neurobehavior of, 187, 188–90, 191; pharmacology, *32*; physical characteristics of, 186, 188, 268; psychomotor abilities of, 189
Cocaine exposure, effects of on pregnancy: complications, 185–88, *190*; maternal consumption, 184–85; maternal weight gain, *190, 191*
Cocaine exposure, long-term effects of: on hormones, *193*; on neurobehavior, *192, 193, 197*; on sexual behavior, *193*; on sexual differentiation, *193*
Collaborative Behavioral Teratology Study, *70*

Conditioned emotional response (ability to acquire fear), and morphine, *31, 211*
Continuum of reproductive casualty, 94
Coping skills of, children and adults with FAS, 110–30
Corticosterone, *24, 30, 31, 32, 37, 61–64*
Craniofacial dysmorphologies and FAS, 105–6
Cross-fostering, *26, 27–28, 285*

D

Delay of maturation, *33, 176–77, 209, 214, 228–29, 262, 284,* 293
Detoxification, 242
Diazepam, effects of on offspring, *69*
Discrimination learning, and amphetamines, *70*
DNA damage, 143–50, *282*
Dopamine/dopaminergic pathways, *32,* 167, 191, 196, 202, 212, 265
Draw-a-Person Test, 228
Drug abuse laws, 306–37
Drug administration methods, *16–18, 31–38*; artificial rearing-intragastric feeding, *33*; development stage at treatment time, *16–38*; inhalation, *38*; injection, *31*; intragastric intubation, *36*; mini-osmotic pump, *18, 210*
Drug dosage issues, *15, 24, 29, 34, 37*
Drug education programs, 98, 329–32
Drug effects, second generation, *54–55*

E

Early interventions, for maternal substance abuse, 332–36
Ecstasy, 291. *See also* Amphetamines
Embryo culture, 40
Endogenous opioids, 215–16
Enkephalin, 164
Environmental interactions, and prenatal growth, 78

Estrogen, 73
Ethanol. *See* Alcohol

F

Fetal alcohol effects (FAE), 105. *See also* Fetal alcohol syndrome (FAS); Alcohol
Fetal alcohol syndrome (FAS), 73–74, 75, 90–94, 104–30, 132–50, 173; adaptive functioning in, 110–12; case histories, 117–25; defined, 51, 90; defined by statutes, 322; diagnosis of, 105–6; drinking patterns and, 91–92, 135; historical reports of, 132–35; incidence in U.S., 90–91; intervention strategies and prevention, 128–30; and IQ and achievement, 106–10; as legal evidence of child abuse, 319, 321–22, 324; paternal role in, 132–50; psychiatric and social implications of, 125–28; psychosocial functioning and, 112–17; Symptom Checklist for FAS, 112–17; threshold for, 92, 94
Free radicals and alcohol effects, 147–50

G

Gender-specific body composition, 79
Gender-specific effects, *18, 30, 39, 51–52, 53–72, 72–79, 116, 136–37, 192, 199, 263,* 283, *287–89,* 287–98, *295*
Gender-specific growth and development, 76–79
Gender-specific maturation timing, 77
Gender specificity, mechanisms for, 72–73
Gender-specific susceptibility to disease, 78–79, 287–89, *287–89*
Genetic damage, alcohol effects on, 143–50
Genetic susceptibility to alcohol, 95–97

Gesell Developmental Schedules, 226, 270
Gonadotropins, *60*
Greenspan-Lieberman Observational System (GLOS), 245
Growth and maturation. *See under specific drugs*
Growth Hormone, 73

H

Handling, methodological issues, *17, 29–30, 36–37, 63, 264*
Hashish, 161
Health care providers, and child abuse laws, 320–21
Heroin, 224–37 (*see also* Opioids); addicts as parents, 227–28; clinical studies of, on maturation of drug-exposed infants, 227–35; clinical studies of, on methodological issues, 225–26; and cognitive development, 228; and paternal drug use, 228
Heroin-exposed neonate/infant: neurodevelopment of, 226; socioemotional development of, 228
Heroin-exposed offspring/child: behavior of, 226–27, 233–34; clinical studies of children raised by addicts, 227–28; cross-sectional studies of, 226–27; descriptive studies of, 226; intellectual potential of, 234; neurobehavioral findings of, 233; neurodevelopmental characteristics of, 226; neurological findings of, 232–33; recommended treatment for, 235–37; socioenvironmental findings of, 232; somatic growth of, 235
Heroin exposure, effects of on pregnancy: maternal factors, 224–37; obstetrical complications, 240
Heroin exposure, long-term effects of, 228–37; intellectual potential, 234

Home Observation Measure of the
Environment (HOME), 177, 231
Hormones. *See specific hormones*
Hot plate test, *31, 33, 69*
Human immunodeficiency virus
(HIV) (AIDS), 11, 24, 79, 241
Human studies, methodological
issues in, 41–42
Hyperactivity, 214, 226, 286
Hypothalamo-pituitary-adrenal axis.
See Pituitary-adrenal activity
Hypoxia, prenatal, 77, *212*

I

In re Gentry, 326
In re Ruiz, 327
In re Solomon L., 326
Inhalation methods, *38*
Injection methods, *31*
*International Union, UAW v.
Johnson Controls*, 312–13
Intragastric intubation, *36*
In vitro research, 40

J

*Jefferson v. Griffin Spaulding County
Hospital*, 313–14

L

Lactation, *19, 26–27, 257*
Learning, *211*, 285
Legal information, sources of,
337–39
Legal rights of fetus, 309–14
Legal sanctions, against paternal
drug use, 334
Life-span changes, *289*
Life-style, and drug use interactions,
172, 229, 232, 236–37
Litter size, *33, 70, 140, 210*
Locomotor behavior, *261, 263*
Longitudinal studies: of
amphetamines, 291; of fetal alcohol
syndrome, 117–30; of heroin-
exposed children, 228–35, 248,
249; of maternal smoking, 285; of
phencyclidine, 269
Luteinizing hormone, *58–61, 163, 193*

M

McCarthy Scales of Children's
Abilities, 231, 248, 286
Marijuana, 161–78; cannabinol
(CBN), effects of, *163, 165*; and
cognitive functioning, 177–78;
future research on, 178; historical
background of, 161; interactions of
with other drugs, 168–71, 173;
and maternal behavior, 168–74;
mechanisms of action of, *166–67*;
paternal use of, effects on
offspring, *16*; and tetrahydrocannabinol (THC), effects of, *162,
163, 164, 165*; use and life-style
interactions, 171–72
Marijuana-exposed fetus;
implantations, resorptions, *162–63*;
physical characteristics of, *53, 163*
Marijuana-exposed neonate/infant:
behavior of, *165*, 174–76;
endocrine factors and, *166*; growth
and maturation of, *163*; nervous
system maturation of, 176–77
Marijuana-exposed offspring/child:
behavior of, *164*; physical
characteristics of, 172–74; visual
system of, 176–77
Marijuana exposure, effects of, on
pregnancy: maternal consumption,
162, 168–71, *172*; placental
transfer, 162
Marijuana exposure, long-term
effects of: on behavior, *164–65*; on
cognitive functioning, 177–78; on
fertility, *163–64*; on neurological
development, *164, 166–67*; on
reproductive function, *163, 165*
Maternal behavior, *24, 26–30, 35, 64*;
and drug abuse case law, 306–37
Matter of Baby X, 326

Matter of Fletcher, 325, 335

Maturational timing, gender-specific, 77

Maze performance, *32, 66–67, 68, 69–70, 286*; and alcohol, *64–65*; and amphetamine, *68*; and diazepam, *69*; and marijuana, *165*; and monosodium glutamate, *69*; and morphine, *32*; and opioids, *69, 70*

Mechanisms of drug actions, 144–47, *166–67*, 187, *191, 192, 193, 196, 197, 201–2, 212–13, 215–16,* 242, 255–57, *255–59, 264, 265, 290, 292*

Meconium staining, 185, 188, 283

Methadone, 239–49 (*see also* Heroin; Opioids); detoxification, 242; maintenance, 228–30, 232–35, 239–49; mechanism of action of, 242; paternal use, effects of on offspring, *16*

Methadone-exposed neonate/infant, 248–49; brain abnormalities, 247; size, 246–47; strabismus, 247

Methadone-exposed offspring/child, 248–49; behavior of, *69, 211,* 226; psychomotor development of, 226

Methadone exposure, effects of, on pregnancy: maternal nutrition, 229, 241; obstetrical complications, 229–30, 239, 240–41

Methamphetamine. *See* Amphetamines

Methodological issues, *13–39*, 40–43, *136–37*, 209 (*see also* Drug administration methods); aberrant maternal behavior, *29*; artificial rearing, *33–35*; clinical studies, 209, 225–26, 236, 237, 249; cross-fostering, *26, 27–28, 285*; drug dosage; *15, 24, 29, 34, 37*; gender-specific effects, *39, 136–37*; handling, *17, 29–30, 36–37, 63*; importance of animal studies, *13–16, 28, 196, 209*; life-styles, 172, 229, 232, 236–37; longitudinal studies with humans, 225–26; maternal/infant interactions, *27,*
244; nature of effects, *14*; nutritional issues, *17, 19–27, 29, 30, 33, 36*; pair-feeding, *20–21, 23–26, 31*; polydrug use, 41–42; postnatal drug treatment, *28–31*; rearing in isolation, *30, 33–34*; selection of behavioral tests, *38–39*; self-reported consumption information, 91, 95, 171; sensitivity of outcome measures, *22–23*

Methylphenidate, 291. *See also* Amphetamines

Michigan Alcohol Screening Test (MAST), 95

Microcephaly/microencephaly. *See* Brain

Monosodium glutamate, *69*

Morphine, *40. See also* Opioids

Morphine exposure, effects of on pregnancy: maternal body weight, *210*; pregnancy rate, *210*

Morphine exposure, long-term effects of: activity, *32*; learning, *32, 37*; neurobehavior, *31*; neuroendo-crines, *32*; physical effects, *33, 54–55*; reproductive function (capacity), *33*; second generation effects, *54–55*

Morris water maze, *66–67*

Mother/infant interactions, *27,* 244–46

Mother's vs. infant's rights, 306–37

Motor Development Index (PDI), 248

N

Naloxone, *63*

Naltrexone, *53*

Neonatal abstinence, 235, 243–44, 249; scoring system, 244–46; syndrome, *214,* 224, 225, 235

Neonatal drug withdrawal, 175, *210, 211, 214,* 224, 226, 230, 236, 242–44

Neurobehavioral effects, *33, 174–78, 192, 202,* 236, 237, 244–46, 249, *262, 264,* 284

Neuroendocrine system, *166,* 166

Neurotransmitters, *167, 196, 255, 264, 265*. *See also specific kinds of neurotransmitters*
Newborn narcotic withdrawal syndrome, 235
Nicotine, 279–80 (*see also* Cigarette smoking); and behavior, *68*; and future research directions, 289–90; and life-span, *289*; passive smoke or particle inhalation effects, 280; pharmacology of, 279–80; smokeless tobacco, 280; tobacco, 279–90; varieties of tobacco products, 279–80
Nicotine-exposed neonate/infant: growth and development of, 282–84, *283–84*; litter size of, *18*; neurochemical effects, *282*; neurological effects, 282, *282*; physical features of, *18, 54, 281–82*; sex differences of, 287–88; sex ratios of, 287
Nicotine-exposed offspring/child: activity of, 284, *284–85*; growth and development of, *61, 283*, 283; learning and performance of, 285–87, *286*
Nicotine exposure effects during pregnancy, complications of, *281*, 281
Nicotine, long-term exposure effects of, 285; fertility, 289; physical features, *54*; tumor development, 288–89
Noise, effects of, on prenatal growth, 78
Norepinephrine, *57*, 164, 167, 196, 265
Nose-poke response, *70*
Nutrition (*see also under specific drugs*; Methodological issues): effect of on growth, 76–77; issues in, *17, 19–27, 29, 30, 33, 36*

O

Obstetrical complications: with heroin addiction, 240; with methadone maintenance, 240–41

Open-field activity, *31, 32, 34, 37, 68, 69, 165, 262*
Operant tasks, 66, 284, *287*
Opiates, 52. *See also specific drugs*
Opioid receptors, *212–13, 214*
Opioid-exposed fetus, brain and nervous system of, *212, 214*
Opioid-exposed neonate/infant: behavior of, *210–11*; maturational delay in, *210*; stillborns, *210*
Opioid-exposed offspring/children behavior of, *211*
Opioid exposure, effects of during pregnancy: maternal nutrition, *212*; maternal weight gain, *210*
Opioids, 207–16 (*see also* Heroin; Methadone; Morphine); and behavior, *69–70*; and growth and maturation, *211*; history of use of, 207–8; incidence of use of, 208; mechanism of action of, *212–13, 215–16*; and nervous system, *212, 213*; and perinatal opioid syndrome, 207–16; receptors for, *212–13*
Opioids, endogenous, 215–16
Opium, 207–8
Ottawa Prenatal Prospective Study, 169–71

P

Pain sensation. *See* Analgesia
Pair-feeding, *20–21, 23–26, 31*
Parenting and drug abuse, 117–30, 227–28
Paternal drug use, effects of on offspring, *16, 70–71, 136–43, 228*, 289
PCP. *See* Phencyclidine
Peabody Picture Vocabulary Test, 110, 228
Perinatal complications associated with methadone maintenance, 241
Perinatal developmental outcome, 246–49
Perinatal harm, laws to protect against, 314–27

Perinatal opioid syndrome, 207–16
Perinatal substance abuse: concerns
    for future, 9–11; prevalance of,
    1–3
Phencyclidine (PCP), 254–74; and
    aggressive behavior, *263*; and
    blood/brain barrier, *258*; history of
    use of, 254–56; incidence of use in
    U.S., 255–56; kinetics of
    mechanism of action of, 256–59;
    legal problems with, 255–56;
    mechanism of action of, 255; street
    names for, 256; teratogenic
    properties of, *259–60*; use by
    women of childbearing age,
    255–56; ways used, 256
Phencyclidine-exposed adult: adipose
    tissue of, *258*; behavior of, 271;
    brain of, *258*
Phencyclidine-exposed fetus, *257–60*;
    body weight of, *258, 259–60*; brain
    weight of, *258*; central nervous
    system and brain of, *257–59*;
    physical characteristics of, *258,
    259–60*; serum of, *258, 267*;
    viability of, *258, 259*
Phencyclidine-exposed neonate/
    infant, *260–66*; behavior of, *263,
    267*, 267–69; learning and memory
    of, *264*; maturation and develop-
    ment of, *260–62*, 269; motor
    activity of, *262–63, 267*;
    neurochemical alterations in,
    265–66; physical features of, 267,
    269
Phencyclidine-exposed offspring/
    child, development of, 269–73
Phencyclidine exposure, long-term
    effects of, motor skills, *267*
Phenobarbital, *32*
Pituitary-adrenal activity, *24, 33,
    61–64*
Pituitary-gonadal activity, *58–61, 165*
Placental transfer, 162, *210*, 256, *267,
    267*, 281
Policy issues, substance abuse and
    pregnancy, 306–37

Polydrug abuse, 41–42, 75–76,
    168–71, 226, 230, 248, 268, 269,
    291
Postnatal drug treatment, *28–31*
Pregnancy: complications in, *162,
    168–71, 172*, 185–88, *190*, 239–40,
    241; and detoxification, 242; drug
    abuse laws and, 306–37; heroin use
    during, 224–37; legal rights of
    fetus, 309–14; maternal weight
    gain, *257, 261, 262*; methadone
    maintenance during, 239–49
Prune belly syndrome, 186
Psychiatric diagnosis of drug-exposed
    individuals, 128
Psychosocial functioning
    (socioemotional), 112–17, 228

R

Race: differential susceptability to
    drugs, 96, 104; selection bias in
    treatment, 229
*Raleigh-Fitkin Paul Morgan
    Memorial Hospital v. Anderson*,
    313
Rearing animals in isolation, *30,
    33–34*
Rearing response, *262*
Receptor changes, 197, 202, 212, *265,
    266, 292, 294*
Respiratory disease syndrome, 78
Reynell Developmental Language
    Scales, 177
Roe v. Wade, 309
Rough and tumble play, *64–65*

S

Saccharin preference, *64–65*
Schizophrenia and phencyclidine,
    254–55
Second generation drug effects,
    54–55, 126–27
Selection of behavioral tests, *38–39*
Self-reporting in drug use studies, 91,
    95
Sensitivity of outcome measures,
    22–23

Serotonin, 167, 196, 264
Sex-dependent effects. *See* Gender-
specific effects
Sex hormones. *See specific kinds of
hormones*
Sex ratios, *18, 33, 54, 71,* 75, *140,
162, 190, 262, 287,* 287, *295*
Sexual behavior, *30, 64,* 116, 124,
126, *165, 289*
Sexual dimorphic behavior, *59,
64–65, 288*
SIDS. *See* Sudden infant death
syndrome
Skeletal development. *See* Bone
development
Smoking. *See* Cigarette smoking
Social Readjustment Rating Scale,
245
Spatial learning, *66–67*
Sperm abnormalities, 143–44, 147
Stanford-Binet Vocabulary Sub-test,
228
Startle response, *68,* 175, *192*
Steroids. *See under specific
hormones*
Strabismus, 247
Strange Situation Test, 272
Stress response. *See* Corticosterone
Sudden infant death syndrome
(SIDS), 281, 282
Symptom Checklist, FAS, 112–17

T

Tail bias, *66*
Taste: discrimination, 287;
perception, 294, 296

Teratogenesis, 91, 172, 175, 190, 210,
259, 292
Testosterone, *57, 58, 60, 65, 70, 73,
163*
THC. *See* Marijuana,
tetrahydrocannabinol
*Thornburgh v. American College of
Obstetricians and Gynecologists,*
309–10
Tissue culture, 40, 213, 289
Tobacco. *See* Nicotine
Tolerance development, 99, *164–65*
Tremors, 74, 174, 176, *210,* 268
Tumors, 9, 288, 289, 295

V

Vineland Adaptive Behavior Scales,
110
Visual system anomalies, 173, 175,
247, *267*

W

Waddington's theory of canalization,
76
*Webster v. Reproductive Health
Services,* 310
Wechsler Adult Intelligence Scale,
106
*Wechsler Intelligence Test for
Children,* 106
Wet-dog shake, head-shake, *211*
Wide Range Achievement Test-
Revised, 110
Withdrawal. *See* Neonatal drug
withdrawal

Designed by Edward D. King

Composed by Maryland Composition Company, Inc.
in Times Roman text and display

Printed on 60-lb. Glatfelter Spring Forge,
and bound in Holliston Roxite by Thomson-Shore, Inc.